PROSTATIC CARCINOMA

CLINICS IN ANDROLOGY

E.S.E. HAFEZ, *series editor*

VOLUME 6

1. J.C. Emperaire, A. Audebert, E.S.E. Hafez, eds., Homologous artificial insemination. 1980. ISBN 90-247-2269-1.

2. L.I. Lipshultz, J.N. Corriere Jr., E.S.E. Hafez, eds., Surgery of the male reproductive tract. 1980. ISBN 90-247-2315-9.

3. E.S.E. Hafez, ed., Descended and cryptorchid testis. 1980. ISBN 90-247-2299-3.

4. J. Bain, E.S.E. Hafez, eds., Diagnosis in andrology. ISBN 90-247-2365-5.

5. G.R. Cunningham, W.-B. Schill, E.S.E. Hafez, eds., Regulation of male fertility. 1980. ISBN 90-247-2373-6.

7. S.J. Kogan. E.S.E. Hafez. eds.. Pediatric andrology. 1981. ISBN 90-247-2407-4.

series ISBN 90-247-2333-7

PROSTATIC CARCINOMA
BIOLOGY AND DIAGNOSIS

edited by

E.S.E. HAFEZ
*Departments of Gynecology/Obstetrics and Physiology
and C.S. Mott Center for Human Growth and Development
Wayne State University School of Medicine
Detroit, Michigan, USA*

and

E. SPRING-MILLS
*Department of Anatomy and Urology
State University of New York
Upstate Medical Center
Syracuse, New York, USA*

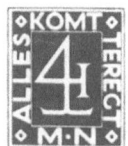

1981

MARTINUS NIJHOFF PUBLISHERS
THE HAGUE / BOSTON / LONDON

Distributors:

for the United States and Canada

Kluwer Boston, Inc.
190 Old Derby Street
Hingham, MA 02043
USA

for all other countries

Kluwer Academic Publishers Group
Distribution Center
P.O. Box 322
3300 AH Dordrecht
The Netherlands

Library of Congress Cataloging in Publication Data   CIP

Main entry under title:

Prostatic carcinoma.

   (Clinics in andrology; v. 6)
   Includes index.
   1. Prostate gland – Cancer. 2. Prostate gland – Cancer – Diagnosis. I. Hafez, E.S.E., 1922-
II. Spring-Mills, Elinor. III. Series.
RC280.P7P77   616.99'463   80-17417

ISBN 13 : 978-94-009-8889-7   e-ISBN-13 : 978-94-009-8887-3
DOI : 10.1007 / 978-94-009-8887-3

TABLE OF CONTENTS

Contributors   VII

Foreword   XI

I. BIOLOGICAL ASPECTS

1. Functional anatomy of the prostate   5
   E. Spring-Mills and A. Krall

2. Quantitative physiopathology of prostatic carcinoma   13
   E.S.E. Hafez

3. Prostatic cytology in the follow-up of prostatic carcinoma   38
   K. Bandhauer, P. Spieler, L. Schmid and H. Toggenburg

4. Histochemistry of prostatic cancer and stromal invasion   44
   D. Kirchheim

5. Endocrine aspects and steroid receptors in prostatic carcinoma   59
   G. Concolino and F. Di Silverio

II. DIAGNOSTIC PROCEDURES

6. Mass screening of prostatic diseases   71
   H. Watanabe, T. Mishina and H. Ohe

7. Clinical markers in prostatic cancer   79
   R.Y. Kirdani, J.P. Karr, G.P. Murphy and A.A. Sandberg

8. Hormonal control of prostatic biochemical markers; acid phosphatase as a marker of
   androgenic control of the ventral prostate   98
   A.F. Clark, M.P. Tenniswood, C.E. Bird, T.G. Flynn, F.A. Jacobs and P.A. Abrahams

9. Prostatic biopsy   109
   N.K. Bissada and A.E. Finkbeiner

10. Serial prostatic biopsies: application in control and management of benign and malignant
    prostatic disease   115
    H. Wolf

11. Bone marrow acid phosphatase in prostate cancer 124
N.A. ROMAS, R.J. VEENEMA and M. TANNENBAUM

12. Radioimmunoassay for human prostatic acid phosphatase 131
B.K. CHOE, N.R. ROSE and E.J. PONTES

III. IN VITRO STUDIES AND ANIMAL MODELS

13. In vitro models 145
M.M. WEBBER

14. Androgen regulation in the prostate of rhesus monkey (Macaca mulatta) 160
R. GHANADIAN

15. Effects of carcinogens and retinoids on prostatic explants 166
D.P. CHOPRA and L.J. WILKOFF

16. Epilogue 175
E.S.E. HAFEZ

Index 191

CONTRIBUTORS

Abrahams, Pamela A., Department of Biochemistry, Pathology and Medicine, Queen's University, Kingston, Ontario K7L 3N6, Canada

Bandhauer, K., Chefarzt urologische Klinik, Kantonsspital, CH-9000 St. Gall, Switzerland

Bird, C.E., Departments of Biochemistry, Pathology and Medicine, Queen's University, Kingston, Ontario K7L 3N6, Canada

Bissada, N.K., Department of Urology, University of Arkansas College of Medicine, 4301 West Markham, Little Rock Arkansas 72201, USA

Choe, B.K., Department of Immunology/Microbiology, Wayne State University School of Medicine, 540E. Canfield, Detroit, Michigan 48201, USA

Chopra, D.P., Southern Research Institute, Cell Biology Division, 2000 Ninth Avenue South, Birmingham, Alabama 35205, USA

Clark, A.F., Department of Biochemistry, Pathology and Medicine, Queen's University, Kingston, Ontario K7L 3N6, Canada

Concolino, G., Clinica Medica V. Università di Roma, via San Marino 30, 00198 Roma, Italy

Di Silverio, F., Clinica Medica V. Università di Roma, via San Marino 30, 00198 Roma, Italy

Finkbeiner, A.E., Department of Urology, University of Arkansas, College of Medicine, 4301 Markham, Little Rock, Arkansas 72201, USA

Flynn, T.G., Department of Biochemistry, Pathology and Medicine, Queen's University, Kingston, Ontario K7L 3N6, Canada

Ghanadian, R., Prostate Research Laboratory, Royal Postgraduate Medical School, du Cane Road, London W12 0HS, United Kingdom

Hafez, E.S.E., Departments of Gynecology/Obstetrics and Physiology, Wayne State University School of Medicine, 550 E. Canfield, Detroit, Michigan 48201, USA

Jacobs, E., Department of Biochemistry, Queen's University, Kingston, Ontario K7L 3N6, Canada

Karr, J.P., Roswell Park, Memorial Institute, 666 Elm Street, Buffalo, New York 14263, USA

Kirchheim, D., 5213 Klahanie Ct. NW, Olympia, Washington 98502, USA

Kirdani, R.Y., Roswell Park Memorial Institute, Buffalo, New York 14263, USA

Krall, Audrey, Department of Anatomy, State University of New York, Upstate Medical Center, 766 Irving Avenue, Syracuse, New York 13210, USA

Mishina, T., Department of Urology, Kyoto Prefectural University of Medicine, Kajii-Cho, Kawaramachi-Hirokoji, Kamigyo-ku, Kyoto 602, Japan

Murphy, G.P., Roswell Park Memorial Institute, Buffalo, New York 14263, USA

Pontes, E.J., Department of Immunology and Microbiology, Wayne State University School of Medicine, 540 East Canfield, Detroit, Michigan 48201, USA

Romas, N.A., Columbia University, College of Physicians and Surgeons, Department of Urology and Pathology, Division of Uropathology, 630 West 168th Street, New York City, New York 10032, USA

Rose, N.R., Department of Immunology/Microbiology, Wayne State University School of Medicine, 540 E. Canfield, Detroit, Michigan 48201, USA

Sandberg, A.A., Roswell Park Memorial Institute, Buffalo, New York 14263, USA

Schmid, L., Departments of Urology and Pathology, Kantonsspital, CH-9000 St. Gall, Switzerland

Spieler, P., Klinik F. Urologie, Kantonsspital, CH-9000, St. Gall, Switzerland

Spring-Mills, Elinor, Departments of Anatomy and Urology, State University of New York, Upstate Medical Center, 766 Irving Avenue, Syracuse, New York 13210, USA

Tannenbaum, M., Department of Urology and Pathology, Columbia University, College of Physicians and Surgeons, 630 West 168th Street, New York City, New York 10032, USA

Tenniswood, M., Department of Biochemistry, Queen's University, Kingston, Ontario K7L 3N6, Canada

Toggenbur, H., Departments of Urology and Pathology, Kantonsspital, CH-9000 St. Gall, Switzerland

Veenema, R.J., Department of Urology and Pathology, Columbia University, College of Physicians and Surgeons, 630 West 168th Street, New York City, New York 10032, USA

Watanabe, H., Department of Urology, Kyoto Prefectural University of Medicine, Kajii-cho, Kawaramachi-Hirokoji, Kamigyo-ku, Kyoto 602, Japan

Webber, M.M., Department of Biochemistry, Biophysics and Genetics. University of Colorado. Medical Center. P.O. Box C319, 4200 E. Ninth Avenue, Denver, Colorado 80262, USA

Wilkoff, L.J., Southern Research Institute, Cell Biology Division, 200 Ninth Avenue, South Birmingham, Alabama 35205, USA

Wolf, H., Department of Urology, 435, Hvidovre University Hospital of the University of Copenhagen, DK-2650 Hvidovre, Denmark

FOREWORD

In the last decade substantial progress has been made in the understanding of prostatic physiopathology by the application of modern techniques and instrumentation in microanatomy, immunology, neurophysiology, pathology, genetics, endocrinology, biochemistry, biophysics and surgery. An attempt is made in this volume to coordinate anatomical, physiological, biochemical, endocrinological, pharmacological and immunological aspects of human prostatic carcinoma. It is hoped that this volume will serve as a stimulus to basic scientists and clinicians to intensify their research for better diagnostic techniques. Thanks are due to the contributors who prepared their chapters meticulously. Thanks also are due to Ms. Lori Rust for her editorial skills, and to Mr. Jeffrey Smith of Martinus Nijhoff for his fine cooperation during the production of this volume.

E.S.E. HAFEZ
Detroit, Michigan

PROSTATIC CARCINOMA: BIOLOGY AND DIAGNOSIS

I. BIOLOGICAL ASPECTS

1. FUNCTIONAL ANATOMY OF THE PROSTATE

E. Spring-Mills and A. Krall

I. EMBRYOLOGY

The prostate gland develops from solid, endodermal outgrowths of urogenital sinus epithelium during the 12th week of gestation. The sinus is formed by the division of the cloaca into ventral (urogenital sinus) and dorsal (rectal) regions by the growth of the urorectal fold from the lateral walls. As the urorectal septum develops, the mesonephric or Wolffian ducts reach the cloaca caudal to the bladder. They aid in delineating the newly formed urogenital sinus and eventually give rise to the ductus deferens, seminal vesicles and ejaculatory ducts. The Müllerian ducts arise independently, lateral to the mesonephric ducts. During the 8th week of development, they grow caudally and rotate medially to contact the urogenital sinus in the midline at the swelling on the posterior urethral wall, the Müllerian tubercle. In the presence of the Müllerian inhibiting factor, these ducts quickly atrophy except for the fused distal remnant known as the prostatic utricle, a small blind-ended tubule (Patten 1968).

The classic study by Lowsley (1912) describes five groups of prostatic epithelial buds according to their relation to the prostatic utricle and ejaculatory ducts (Figure 1). The middle group of cords arises on the posterior wall of the sinus, superior to the utricle and limited by the ejaculatory ducts. Two lateral outgrowths develop from the lateral walls of the sinus. The posterior buds branch caudally to the prostatic utricle while the anterior cords arise from the anterior wall of the sinus. Although this anterior lobe is present in the fetus, it rapidly regresses in the neonate. In the adult, the distinction between the embryological lobes is masked.

As the cords grow, they induce the proliferation and differentiation of the surrounding mesenchyme into smooth muscle cells and collagen secreting fibroblasts. These cells form the stroma which ensheaths the branching glands and ejaculatory ducts as they pass from the junction of the vas deferens and seminal vesicles to the urethra.

The epithelium of a cord varies greatly in appearance. After canalization, it is composed of 2 cell layers with the principal cells cuboidal to low columnar. During the fifth month of gestation, tubules originating from the posterior wall of the urethra near the verumontanum as well as the prostatic utricle sometimes undergo squamous metaplasia. Regression of the metaplasia occurs through the first week postpartum. A PAS-positive lumenal secretion may persist a month or more after birth before subsiding; however, this secretion has not been observed in tubules with squamous metaplasia (Zondek and Zondek 1975, Brody and Goldman 1940).

During childhood, there is little further develop-

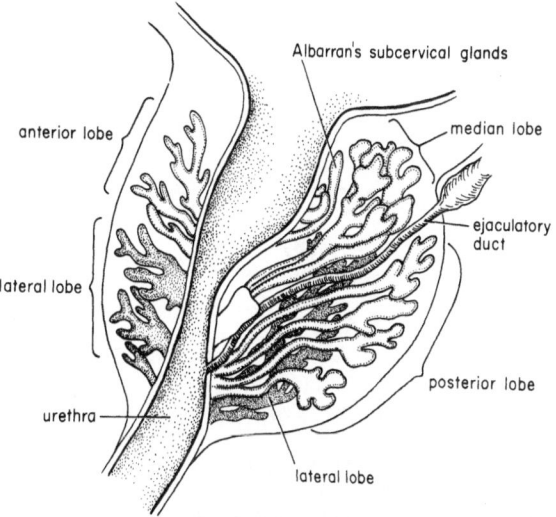

Figure 1. Line drawing illustrating the embryologic origins of the human prostate from the primitive urethra.

6

ment of the prostate. Some acinar proliferation occurs but the epithelium generally is cuboidal and quiescent. Few ducts from the anterior lobe remain; however, the lateral lobes extend anteriorly to encircle the urethra. At puberty, there is a relatively rapid increase in the size of the prostate. There is an expansion of the acini, an increase in lumenal diameter, and the appearance of tall columnar epithlium. Secretion resumes and continues throughout the life of a healthy individual (Swyer 1944).

II. GROSS ANATOMY

The prostate is situated at the neck of the bladder in the inferior portion of the pelvic cavity and surrounds the first segment of the urethra (Figure 2). It is triangular with the apex directed downward, contacting the urogenital diaphragm. The superiorly located base is continuous with the inferior aspect and neck of the bladder, but slightly separated from it by short, lateral and posterior grooves. Two convex lateral surfaces meet the levator ani fascia and join to form a rounded anterior edge. The edge passes posteriorly to the pubic symphysis. The posterior surface of the prostate is flattened and contacts inferiorly the urogenital diaphragm and the inferior rectum. It is this region which is palpated during a rectal examination. Great variation in the size of the prostate has

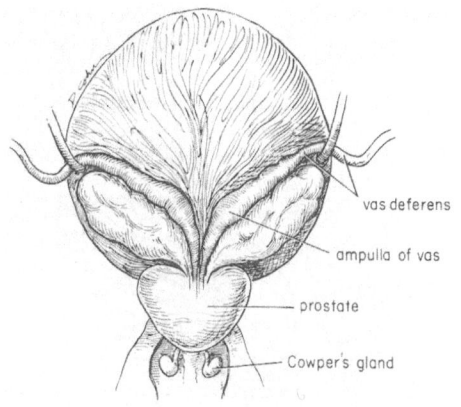

Figure 2. Line drawing illustrating the gross anatomical relationships of the bladder, ampulla of the vas deferens, seminal vesicles (unlabelled), prostate and Cowper's glands. Posterior view. From Spring-Mills E, Hafez ESE: Male accessory organs, In: Human reproduction, Hafez ESE, Evans TN, New York: Harper and Row, 1979.

been observed, but in the adult, it generally has a vertical length of 3 cm, frontal diameter of 4 cm, anteroposterior diameter of 2 cm, and a weight of approximately 20 gms. (Harrison 1972).

The 2 ejaculatory ducts penetrate the posterior surface at the upper border, anteroinferiorly traverse the glandular elements, and open into the urethra laterally to the verumontanum on the posterior wall. These orifices, in conjunction with that of the prostatic utricle, have been used as landmarks in delineating the lobes of the fetal and adult prostates. Although there is a consensus that the prostatic cords arise from 5 distinct regions of the urogenital sinus in the embryo, controversy still surrounds the lobation pattern of the adult gland. This stems from the use of different techniques to examine the gland (histology or step-sections versus gross dissection) and from the dogma established by Lowsley (1912) that benign hypertrophy and carcinoma arise in separate and distinct regions of the prostate. The two most commonly encountered schemas are the three butterfly-shaped pairs of lobes described by Tissell and Salander (1975) and the central and peripheral zones originally described by Huggins and Webster (1948) and later modified by others (Franks 1954, McNeal 1972).

A dense, fascial sheath encircles the entire prostate. The puboprostatic ligaments blend with this sheath anteriorly and laterally to anchor the gland to both the body of the pubis and the fascia of the levator ani muscles. Posteriorly, the prostatic fascia fuses with that of the ampulla of the ductus deferens and seminal vesicles to form the rectovesical septum which separates these structures from the rectum. (Harrison 1972)

Embedded within the fascial sheath are the vessels which form the prostatic venous plexus. The plexus receives blood from the dorsal vein of the penis. It communicates with both the vesical and the vertebral plexuses and drains into the internal iliac vein. The arterial blood supply is usually derived from branches of the internal iliac artery, although it may originate from the umbilical artery as well. Just prior to the terminal division of the internal iliac artery into inferior gluteal and internal pudendal branches, the prostatovesical trunk arises which, in turn, yields the artery to the prostate. The lymph drains to the nodes surrounding the pelvic wall, and terminates mainly in the internal iliac nodes, with the sacral and external iliac nodes receiving some of the flow as well.

Nervous innervation is derived from sympathetic fibers of the inferior hypogastric plexus originating at the lumbar 1 and 2 ventral rami. The prostatic nervous plexus also receives communicating branches from the vesical plexus and some sensory fibers derived from the pudendal nerve.

III. HISTOLOGY AND ULTRASTRUCTURE

The prostate is a compound exocrine gland. Its ducts branch profusely. The secretory portions at the ends of the ducts, however, are especially large and contain very wide lumens. Hence, it is common to refer to the prostate as a compound saccular or compound tubuloacinar gland. The 16-32 excretory ducts within a mature prostate each empty into the urethra on the right and left sides of the colliculus seminalis. Most ducts are lined by simple or pseudostratified columnar epithelium which becomes stratified columnar or cuboidal (transitional) at the level of the urethra.

For convenient description, the 'true' prostate or the prostate proper often is divided into two parts: a central and a peripheral zone. The anatomical relationships are seen to advantage when the prostate is sectioned in a plane parallel to the long axis of the ejaculatory ducts. The central zone is shaped like an inverted pyramid: The base of the prostate rests on the neck of the bladder and its apex surrounds the ejaculatory ducts. In this zone, the epithelium is pseudostratified. It contains cuboidal or columnar principal cells and cuneiform basal cells. Occasionally a third cell of intermediate height is crowded into the highly irregular epithelium. The pseudostratification of the cells is pronounced. The large, pale nuclei lie at different levels in the granular, moderately acidophilic cytoplasm. In addition to the conspicuous crowding of epithelial cells, the central zone also is distinguished by larger and more irregular secretory acini than the acini within the peripheral zone. The stroma is compact and very regularly arranged around the glandular units. Ducts from the central zone open into the prostatic urethra at the level of the verumontanum.

Approximately three quarters of the prostate proper is thought to reside in the peripheral zone.

The stroma is loosely arranged and moderately irregular whereas the glandular units are regularly arranged and quite uniform in appearance. The epithelium is predominantly simple columnar with an incomplete layer of basal cells (Figure 3). In some prostates it is definitely pseudostratified. However, neither epithelial arrangement is associated with the formation of intralumenal ridges or papillae as in the central zone. Ducts from the peripheral zone open into the lower third of the prostatic urethra.

A transitional zone lies anterior to the peripheral zone and above the verumontanum. Although the epithelium resembles the epithelium of the peripheral zone, the stroma is highly irregular and coarse in texture. The connective tissue and smooth muscle fibers often form incomplete rings parallel to the muscle fibers of the sphincter of the urethra. Benign nodular hyperplasia most commonly is seen in the transition zone.

Above the verumontanum lie many small glands and diverticula from the upper part of the prostatic urethra which give rise to the periurethral portion of the prostate. Nodules which form here are neither as large nor as numerous as nodules formed in the transition zone.

Under normal circumstances, the principal or glandular cells exhibit surface and cytoplasmic polarity. Moderate numbers of filamentous mitochondria, free ribosomes and cisternae of the rough endoplasmic reticulum (RER) reside in the infranuclear cytoplasm. A moderately well developed Golgi, some RER, a few lipid droplets, several membrane bound secretory granules, vacuoles, numerous lysosomes and dense bodies reside in the supranuclear cytoplasm. The apical plasmalemma contains many microvilli and intense aminopeptidase activity (Figure 4). Adjacent principal cells are joined by typical junctional complexes and desmosomes.

Basal cells rest on the basal lamina but do not reach the lumen. They appear to be significantly less specialized than the glandular cells. They exhibit little surface or cytoplasmic polarization although they have abundant tonofilaments and pinocytotic vesicles. Basal cells proliferate in response to a number of normal and abnormal stimuli (Kastendieck and Altenähr 1979).

In all parts of normal glands, both the glandular

8

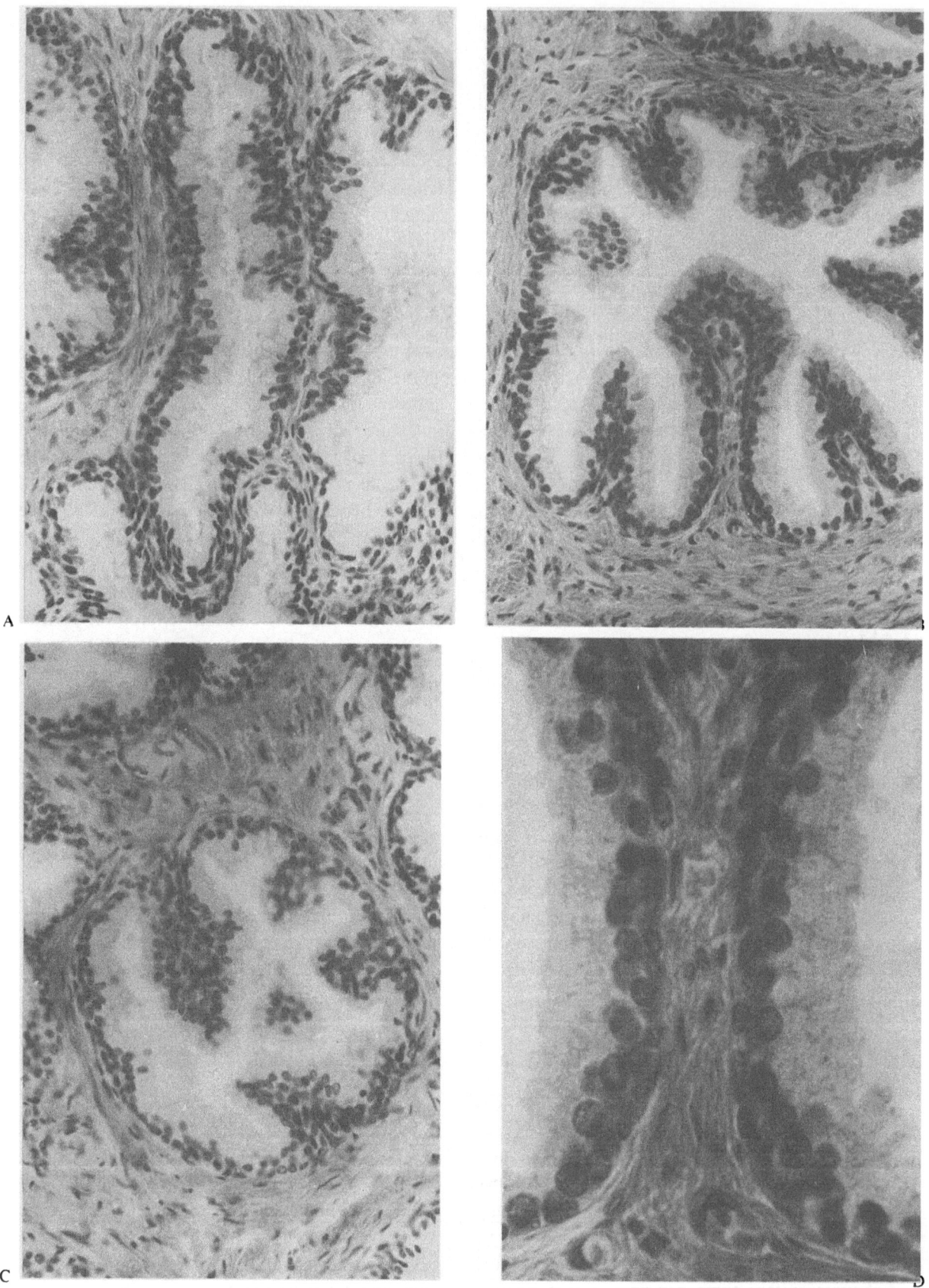

Figure 3. Histologic variations within the human prostate are shown at low (A-C) and high (D) magnification. In certain regions the epithelium is crowded and folds of the mucosa extend into the lumen. In other areas the secretory units are less complicated in structure.

and the basal cells sit on an indistinct basal lamina and an underlying stroma composed of loose to moderately dense connective tissue, smooth muscle cells, elastic fibers and blood capillaries. The connective tissue capsule which covers the exterior of the organ, sends septae into the interior of the gland. The stroma accounts for one-third or more of the prostatic mass. Occasionally, free nerve endings are applied to the epithelia. Nonmyelinated nerve fibers connected to sympathetic ganglia are numerous in the stroma; and the glands of most mammals have a dual sympathetic and parasympathetic efferent innervation (Elbadawi and Goodman 1980). The functional significance of these nerve patterns, however, is a matter of speculation and debate.

Corpora amylacea occur in the lumens of many of the secretory segments (Figures 4, 5, 6). They are lamellated bodies containing proteins and carbohydrates. They increase in size and number with aging, but their significance is not understood.

IV. SECRETIONS

The prostatic fluid constitutes one-tenth to one-third of the total semen volume in an ejaculate (Lundquist 1949). It is clear in appearance and now known to be alkaline, with a pH between 7.4 and 8.0 (Fair and Cordonnier 1978). Prostatic secretions are characterized by an absence of reducing sugars, high levels of acid phosphatase, citric acid, and zinc, and contain factors which stimulate spermatozoal motility. The secretion of products by the principal cells is merocrine and possibly apocrine (Thompson and Heidger 1978).

Gutman and Gutman (1938) report that the amount of acid phosphatase in the prostatic epithelium is an age-related phenomenon. The low levels observed throughout childhood (1.5 King-Armstrong units/g tissue) are followed by higher levels beginning at puberty (73 units) and continue to rise variably throughout adulthood (522-2284 units). Serum levels of acid phosphatase have been utilized in the diagnosis of prostatic carcinoma. Although the prostatic enzyme is normally stored in the tissue epithelium and is found in the seminal fluid, usually it does not diffuse into the general circulation. However, when a metastatic carcinoma from the prostate exists, plasma levels of acid phosphatase show a marked increase, even though the carcinoma cells have less activity than normal cells (Mann 1964, Brandes and Kirchheim 1977).

Citric acid is another standard marker of the functional status of the prostate. Like acid phosphatase, it too is used as an indicator of prostatic carcinoma. The citric acid concentration has a range between 480-2,688 mg/100 ml of prostatic secretion (Huggins and Neal 1942). Citric acid may be involved in the coagulation/liquefaction of the seminal clot, and in establishing seminal osmotic equilibrium. It is also possible that citric acid helps in limiting calculus formation since it binds calcium ions. These ions are suspected of providing a nucleus for the formation of calculi (Mann 1964).

It has been known since the work of Bertrand and Vladesco (1921) that the prostate contains high concentrations of zinc. The functional significance is still uncertain. Zinc is needed as a cofactor in certain enzyme reactions, acts as a seminal bacteriostatic agent, and may be involved in the prevention of DNA degradation in spermatozoa. Differences in concentration have been reported in the various regions of the prostate with values greatest toward the apex (Byar 1974). Although there are reports that the zinc content decreases in prostatic malignancies and increases during benign hypertrophy, the value of zinc measurement as a reliable indicator of disease is still uncertain.

Most proteolytic enzymes originate from the prostate. Two proteinases which are found in relatively high concentrations in prostatic fluid are plasminogen activator and seminin. These proteolytic enzymes are believed to be involved in the liquefaction of the seminal coagulum. This is important clinically as a number of investigators have observed poorly motile spermatozoa in viscous semen and non-liquefaction of the coagulum in sub- and infertile men (Tauber and Zaneveld 1976). Lysozyme and α-amylase, also components of prostatic fluid, may participate in the dissolution process as well.

V. HISTOPHYSIOLOGY

The prostate undergoes many striking morphological and functional changes throughout the life

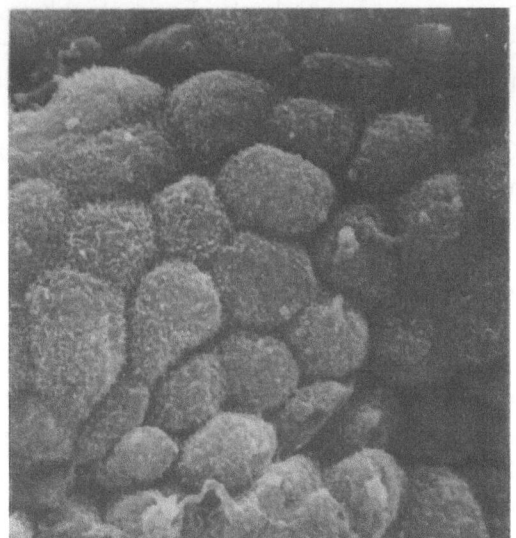

Figure 4. Scanning electron micrograph showing the surfaces of prostatic epithelial cells. From a patient with prostatic carcinoma.

cycle; nevertheless, only very few of the mechanisms initiating or promoting these alterations are known in any species. Unlike the prostates of many rodents, the human gland is more apt to hypertrophy with age than it is to involute. After puberty, cell renewal is dependent upon androgens, especially testosterone (Tuohimaa 1980). In the absence of testosterone, there is a decrease in gland weight followed by a loss in total DNA content. Reduction in secretion generally parallels the loss in gland weight. When a single replacement dose of androgen is given to rodents with post-castration prostatic atrophy, cell proliferation continues for approximately one week and is capable of producing a three-fold increase in cell number (Coffey 1974,

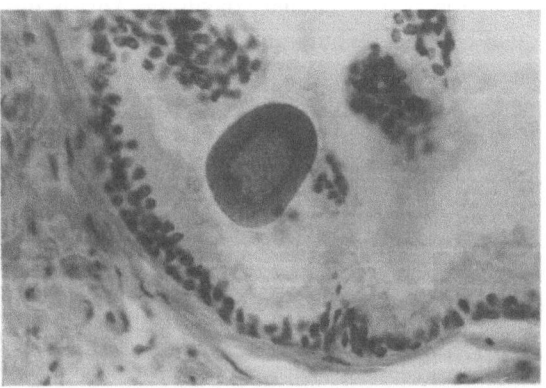

Figure 5. Light micrograph showing a corpora amylacea within the lumen of a prostatic gland.

Bruchovsky and Lesser 1976). It appears, therefore, that either the androgen remains within the prostate for a prolonged period or that in this situation proliferation can continue for some time without additional androgenic stimulation (Österberg and Tuohimaa 1975, Tuohimaa 1980).

The normal prostate has little mitotic activity (Faul and Rabes 1972); and, no significant increase in mitotic divisions has ever been documented in the stroma of large versus small human prostates. Indeed, Alison et al. (1976) postulated that the normal prostate is refractory to cell proliferation and that an increase of mitotic activity may require a real loss in cell number. It is obvious that these mitotic-restraints – if they exist – are less potent in hyperplastic and carcinomatous prostates. Since mitotic inhibition appears to be androgen-dependent, altered steroid metabolism, a change in androgen receptors, decreased plasma androgens or altered stromal influences, alone or in combination, may promote a real or relative decrease in androgens and an increase in mitotic activity of neoplastic prostates (Pietilä et al. 1977, Tuohimaa 1980).

Following castration, the prostatic epithelium atrophies, the RER and mitochondria decrease while lysosomes and lipofusin pigments increase. Appropriate replacement doses of testosterone will restore the histologic and fine structural appearance of the gland. The effects of other hormones are more variable. Estrogens, for example, usually produce epithelial atrophy and stromal hyperplasia in intact animals, but produce little or no change in the prostates of castrated animals given testosterone replacement therapy (Tisell et al. 1976, Thompson and Heidger 1978, Seppelt 1978).

The avidity of the prostatic epithelium for androgens depends upon specific androgen receptors. Anti-androgens, therefore, cause a prompt and profound involution of the prostate (Steinbeck et al. 1971; Neri 1976). In fact antiandrogen atrophy often approximates that caused by surgical castration: the epithelium regresses and the fibromuscular stroma remains abundant. The effects of castration and anti-androgens on prostatic ultrastructure have been studied extensively by Dahl, Tveter and their associates (Tveter and Aakvaag 1969, Dahl and Tveter 1974, Pietilä et al. 1977, Tveter et al. 1978, Tveter et al. 1980).

In appropriate doses antiandrogens reduce cell

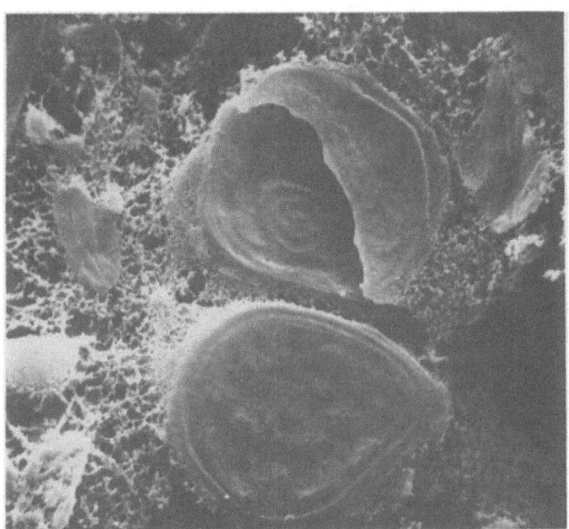

Figure 6. Scanning electron micrograph showing two corpora amylacea. From Spring-Mills E, Jones AL: The prostate gland in SEM of human reproduction, Hafez ESE, ed. Ann Arbor: Ann Arbor Science, 1978.

size, RER, Golgi, secretory material and free ribosomes of the prostatic epithelium. In addition, many of these agents also destroy prostatic cancer cells. Unfortunately, however, even in the most responsive patients, tissue biopsies after anti-androgen therapy all too often reveal abundant, healthy-appearing neoplastic cells.

Synergistic effects of prolactin and testosterone have been observed on the prostates of castrated rodents (Thompson and Heidger 1978). Combined prolactin and testosterone therapy can increase gland weight (Chase et al. 1957, Negro-Vilar et al. 1977), enhance zinc uptake (Moger and Geschwind 1972) and increase ^{3}H-thymidine incorporation into the epithelium (Resnick et al. 1974). The morphological effects of this combination, however, require additional study.

VI. CONCLUDING REMARKS

Since so many questions remain unanswered concerning the normal development, maintenance and function of the prostate, it is not surprising that we understand very little about the pathogenesis and control of its diseases. Hopefully the recent surge of interest in andrology and prostatic carcinoma will foster more basic and clinical research directed at elucidating which factors accelerate or promote growth, whether there are differences in the response of the stroma and epithelium to a given endogenous or exogenous condition and finally what are the best criteria for distinguishing normal from neoplastic prostatic cells.

REFERENCES

Alison MR, Wright NA, Morley AR, Appleton DR: Cell proliferation in the prostate complex of the castrate mouse. J Microsc (Oxf) 106 (2): 221, 1976.

Aumüller G: Lipopigment fine structure in human seminal vesicle and prostate gland epithelia. Virchows Arch B Cell Path 24: 79, 1977.

Bertrand G, Vladesco R: Intervention probable du zinc dans les phénomènes de fécondation chez les animaux vertébrés. Comptes Ren Acad Sci 173: 176, 1921.

Brandes D, Groth DP, Gyorkey F: Occurrence of lysosomes in the prostatic epithelium of castrate rats. Exptl Cell Res 28: 61, 1962.

Brandes D, Kirchheim D: Histochemistry of the prostate. In: Urologic pathology of the prostate. Tannenbaum M, ed. Philadelphia: Lea and Febiger, 1977.

Brody H, Goldman SF: Metaplasia of the epithelium of the prostatic glands, utricle and urethra of the fetus and newborn infant. Arch Pathol 29: 494, 1940.

Bruchovsky N, Lesser B: Control of proliferative growth in androgen responsive organs and neoplasms. Adv Sex Horm Res 2: 1, 1976.

Byar DP: Zinc in male sex accessory organs: distribution and hormonal response. In: Male accessory sex organs: structure and function in mammals, Brandes D, ed. New York: Academic Press, 1974.

Chase MD, Geschwind II, Bern HA: Synergistic role of prolactin response of male rat sex accessories to androgen. Proc Soc Exp Biol Med 94: 680, 1957.

Coffey DS: Effects of androgens on DNA and RNA synthesis in sex accessory tissue. In: Male accessory sex organs: structure and function in mammals, Brandes D, ed. New York: Academic Press, 1974.

Dahl E, Tveter KJ: The ultrastructure of the accessory sex organs of the male rat. V. Effect of the antiandrogen cyproterone acetate. J Endocrinol 62: 251, 1974.

Elbadawi A, Goodman DC: Autonomic innervation of accessory male genital glands. In: Male accessory sex glands, Spring-Mills E, Hafez ESE, eds. Amsterdam: Elsevier – North Holland, 1980.

Fair WF, Cordonnier JJ: The pH of prostatic fluid. A reappraisal and therapeutic implications. J Urol 120: 695, 1978.

Faul P, Rabes H: Thymidine-^{3}H-autoradiographie an cytologischen Prostata-punktaten des Menschen. Urologie A 11: 295, 1972.

Franks LM: Benign nodular hyperplasia of the prostate. A review. Ann Roy Coll Surg Eng 14: 92, 1954.

Franks LM: Atrophy and hyperplasia in the prostate proper. J Path Bact 86: 616, 1954.

12

Gutman AB, Gutman EB: Acid phosphatase and functional activity of the prostate (man) and preputial glands (rat). Proc Soc Exp Biol Med 39: 529, 1938.

Harrison RG: The urogenital system. In: Cunningham's textbook of anatomy, Romanes GJ, ed. London: Oxford Univ Press. 1972.

Huggins C, Neal W: Coagulation and liquefaction of semen: proteolytic enzymes and citrate in prostatic fluid. J Exp Med 76: 527, 1942.

Huggins C, Webster WO: Duality of human prostate in response to estrogen. J Urol 59: 258, 1948.

Kastendieck H, Altenähr E: Role of basal cells in non-malignant lesions of the prostate. Arch Androl 2 (Suppl 1): 64, 1979.

Lowsley OS: The development of the human prostate gland with reference to the development of other structures at the neck of the urinary bladder. Am J Anat 13: 299, 1912.

Lundquist F: Aspects of the biochemistry of human semen. Acta Physiol Scand 19 (Suppl): 66, 1949.

Mann T: The biochemistry of semen and of the male reproductive tract. New York: J Wiley and Sons, 1964.

McNeal JE: The prostate and prostatic urethra: a morphologic synthesis. J Urol 107: 1008, 1972.

Moger WH, Geschwind II: The action of prolactin in the sex accessory glands of the male rat. Proc Soc Exp Biol Med 141: 1017, 1972.

Negro-Vilar A, Saad WA, McCann SM: Evidence for a role of prolactin in prostate and seminal vesicle growth in immature male rats. Endocrinology 100: 729, 1977.

Neri RO: Antiandrogens. Adv Sex Horm Res 2: 233, 1976.

Österberg K, Tuohimaa P: Increased androgen sensitivity with time after castration in the accessory sex glands. 10th Acta Endocr Congr (Kbh). 199 (Suppl): 418, 1975.

Patten BM: Human embryology. New York: McGraw-Hill, 1968.

Pietilä J, Arvola I, Senius KEO, Tuohimaa P: Weight, stroma to gland ratio, and mitotic activity of the human hyperplastic prostate. Invest Urol 15: 90, 1977.

Resnick MI, Walvood DJ, Grayhack JT: Effect of prolactin on testosterone uptake by the perfused canine prostate. Surg Forum 25: 70, 1974.

Seppelt U: Correlation among prostate stroma, plasma estrogen levels, and urinary estrogen excretion in patients with benign prostate hypertrophy. J Clin Endo and Met 47: 1230 1978.

Spring-Mills E, Hafez ESE: Male accessory organs. In: Human reproduction, Hafez ESE, Evans TN, eds. New York: Harper and Row, 1979.

Spring-Mills E, Jones AL: The prostate gland in SEM of human reproduction, Hafez ESE, ed. Ann Arbor: Ann Arbor Science, 1978.

Steinbeck H, Mehring M, Neumann F: Comparison of the effects of cyproterone, cyproterone acetate and oestradiol on testicular function, accessory sexual glands and fertility in a long-term study on rats. J Reprod Fert 26: 65, 1971.

Swyer GIM: Postnatal growth changes in human prostate. J Anat 78: 130, 1944.

Tauber PF, Zaneveld LJD: Coagulation and liquefaction of human semen. In: Human semen and fertility regulation in men, Hafez ESE, ed. Saint Louis: The CV Mosby, 1976.

Thompson SA, Heidger PM: Synergistic effects of prolactin and testosterone in the restoration of rat prostatic epithelium following castration. Anat Rec 191: 31, 1978.

Tisell L-E, Andersson H, Angervall L: A morphological study of the prostatic lobes and the seminal vesicles of castrated rats injected with oestradiol and/or insulin. Urological Res 4: 63, 1976.

Tisell LE, Salander H: The lobes of the human prostate. Scand J Urol Nephrol 9: 185, 1975.

Tuohimaa P: Control of cell proliferation in male accessory sex glands. In: Male accessory sex glands, Spring-Mills E, Hafez ESE eds. Amsterdam: Elsevier – North Holland,

Tveter KJ, Aakvaag A: Uptake and metabolism in vivo of testosterone-1,2-^{3}H by accessory sex organs of male rats: influence of some hormonal compounds. Endocrinology 85: 683, 1969.

Tveter KJ, Dahl E, Aakvaag A: Effect of antiandrogens on the prostate gland. In: Male accessory sex glands, Spring-Mills E, Hafez ESE, eds. (Amsterdam: Elsevier – North Holland, 1980.

Tveter KJ, Otnes B, Hannestand R: Treatment of prostatic carcinoma with cyproterone acetate. Scand J Urol Nephrol 12: 115, 1978.

Zondek T, Zondek LH: The fetal and neonatal prostate. In: Normal and Abnormal Growth of the Prostate, Goland M, ed. Springfield: Charles C Thomas, 1975.

2. QUANTITATIVE PHYSIOPATHOLOGY OF PROSTATIC CARCINOMA

Extensive investigations have been conducted in several countries on the physiopathology of the human prostate with particular reference to prostatic carcinoma. There are remarkable racial and geographical differences in the incidence and mortality rate from prostatic carcinoma which are particularly high in the USA, especially in blacks; and significantly low in Jews and Orientals, especially in native Japanese. Prostatoglandular carcinoma is consistently related to the marital status, with a higher incidence and mortality rate in married than in single men. The following values represent the incidence of prostatic carcinoma in the United States:

number of new cases in 1 year	42.000
number of deaths in 1 year	17.000
% of new cases, potentially curable when first discovered	30%

This chapter deals with quantitative parameters of functional anatomy and functional biochemistry of the normal prostate, structural and ultrastructural differentation of prostatic carcinoma, age related changes, physiopathological and endocrine mechanisms, androgen receptors, diagnostic procedures, experimental approaches to drug therapy and animal models.

I. FUNCTIONAL ANATOMY OF THE PROSTATE

A. Regional physiomorphology

Most of the anterior surface of the prostate is formed by the periurethral gland mass. The dorsal pair of the prostate forms the apex, the lateral surfaces and the dorsal surface of the gland. Between the dorsal and median pairs, the lateral lobes

reach the external surface of the prostate. The median pair of the prostate is centrally located between the firmly attached lateral pair dorsally and the supracollicular segment of the urethra ventrally. The ejaculatory ducts, enclosed by the median pair, are attached dorsally on each side to both lateral and dorsal lobes of the prostate (El-Badawi 1979a).

There are three tissue types: periurethral glands, accessory prostatic glands and the prostate proper (Figure 1). Concepts of lobation of the prostate are based on the clustering pattern of prostatic glands in histologic sections, casts or grossly dissected specimens (Figure 2, 3). Advocates of the zonal arrangement deny the existence of anatomically demarcated separable lobes in the prostate, and instead describe anatomical subdivisions of the 'functional prostate,' based on differential suscepti-

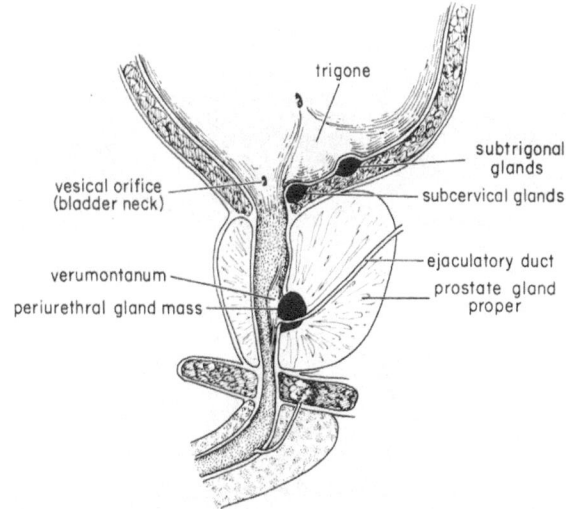

Figure 1. The three masses of prostatic type tissue: prostate gland proper, periurethral gland mass and paraprostate (subcervical and subtrigonal glands); diagram of nearly coronal section with slight obliquity relative to midline to show course of ejaculatory duct (El-Badawi 1979a).

14

bility of parts of the gland to sex hormones and to different disease processes, i.e., nodular hyperplasia vs. carcinoma (El-Badawi 1979a).

The prostate, an aggregate of 30 to 50 tubulo-alveolar glands with 15 to 30 ducts emptying into the prostatic urethra, is not fully developed until puberty. The elongated alveoli and tubules are variable in size and shape. The cuboidal to columnar epithelial cells contain secretory granules

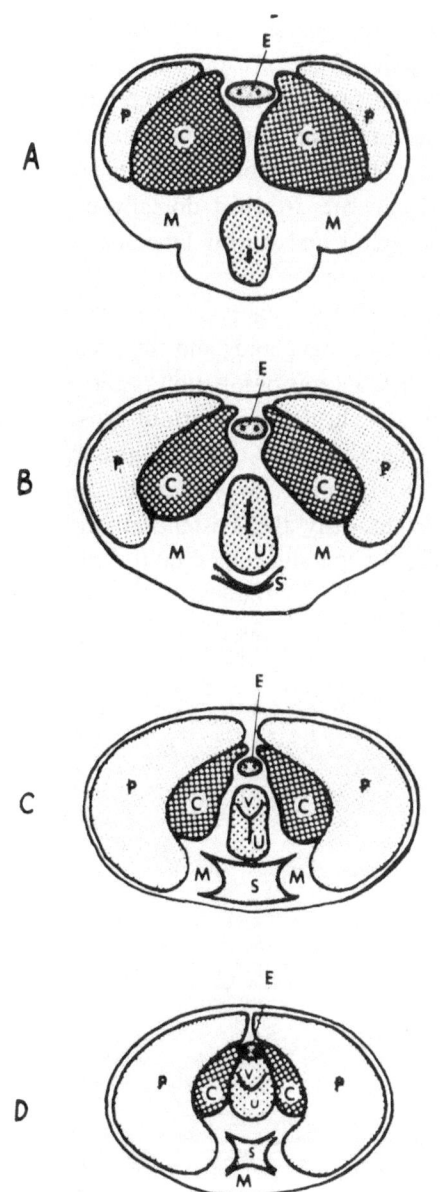

Figure 2. Sections of prostate perpendicular to urethra at equal intervals from cephalic pole to verumontanum. C = central zone, P = peripheral zone, E = ejaculatory ducts, M = smooth muscle, S = striated muscle, U = periurethral stroma, V = verumontanum. (McNeal 1968)

and yellowish, lipoidal droplets. The smaller ducts have irregular lumen, resembling secretory tubules, whereas the terminal excretory ducts near the urethra have pseudostratified epithelium. The differential morphology of the prostate, is of clinical significance in male infertility and particularly in problems associated with sperm motility.

B. Prostatic cysts and prostatic concretions

Congenital cysts and concretions are common characteristics of the prostate. Congenital cysts are caused by blockage of prostate excretion due to maldevelopment of the parenchyma, atresia of the excretory ducts or lack of communication of the ducts with the parenchyma. Endoscopy and radiography are used to identify the direction of expansion and anatomical relationships of prostatic cysts (Figure 4). Sizable cysts are palpable rectally and frequently obstruct the prostatic urethra, producing difficulty of micturition or urinary tract infection (El-Badawi 1979a).

Five types of prostatic concretions are noted: corpora amylacea, corpora calculi, true (endogenous) prostatic calculi, exogenous (false) prostatic calculi and calculi of the prostatic utricle (Figure 5). Corpora amylacea, a product of prostatic secretions, are noted in all parts of the prostate particularly in the larger ducts and acini of the lateral lobes and cephalic part of the posterior lobe. Corpora amylacea, an amorphous mucoprotein matrix, with laminations, are eosinophilic, lipid positive, usually PAS-negative and alcian blue-positive. Corpora calculi differ from prostatic calculi in being the product of natural aging of corpora amylacea, particularly those trapped in prostatic acini.

Deposition of mucopolysaccharides from altered secretions creates a matrix, which becomes highly mineralized by calcium salts. Unlike corpora amylacea and corpora calculi, chronic and/or acute inflammatory changes are constantly present around true prostatic calculi (El-Badawi 1979a).

Exogenous prostatic calculi develop in prostatic diverticula or cavities, or migrate into prostatic ducts from the urinary tract. They are associated with urinary tract infection, urolithiasis or obstructive uropathy, and may cause urethral obstruction or incontinence.

15

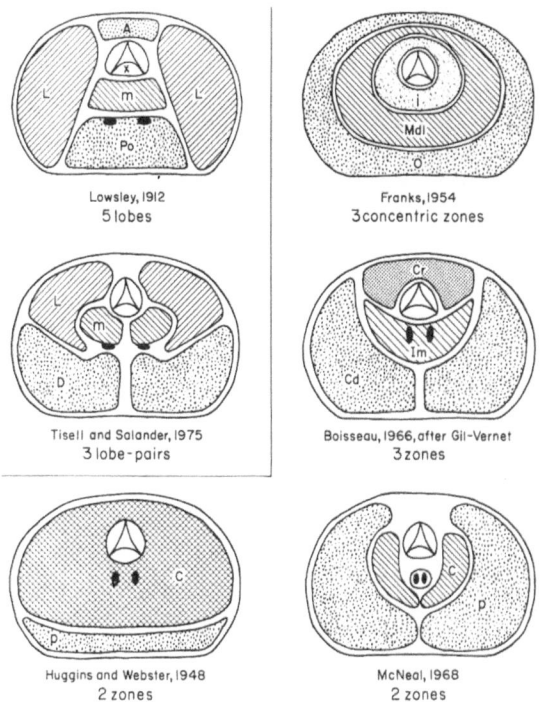

Figure 3. Main concepts of prostatic lobes and zones; diagrams of cross section of prostate gland at level of verumontanum (X). Lobes: A = anterior, L = lateral, M = median, Po = prosterior, D = dorsal. Zones: C = central, p = peripheral, i = inner; Mdl = middle, O = outer, Cr = cranial, In = intermediate, Cd = caudal. (El-Badawi 1979a).

II. ENDOCRINE PARAMETERS

The differentiation, growth, development, regression and physiopathological alterations of the prostate are regulated directly by the action of androgen and prolactin and indirectly by the action of gonadotropins, adrenal and thyroid gland.

A. Androgens

The human testis secretes androstenedione, progesterone and 17α-hydroxyprogesterone (Strott et al. 1969; Vermeulen and Verdonck 1976; Hammond et al. 1977a). The potential biologic significance of the ability of the prostate to convert testosterone into more potent androgens, as well as the apparent synergism between prolactin and androgens, are of special interest. Most of the estrogens in men arise from peripheral conversion of testicular and adrenal precursors, i.e. testosterone and 4-androsterne-3, 17-dione. There is also a certain degree of direct secretion of estradiol-17β by the testis (Marcus and

Korenman 1976).

Androgens play a major 'organizational' or 'morphogenetic' role at specific periods during early development. These effects are essentially irreversible compared with the 'activational' or 'inhibitory' actions of androgens which are often reversible and take place throughout the lifespan of adult animal (Williams-Ashman and Reddi 1972).

The action of androgens in the prostate is mediated by intracellular metabolites of circulating androgens which are primarily testosterone and androstenedione (King and Mainwaring 1974, Offner et al. 1974, Mainwaring 1977).

Androgen deprivation causes remarkable alterations in the metabolic patterns of the prostate. The activity of respiratory enzymes corresponds with these changes with a few exceptions in some target tissues. Respiration-coupled synthesis of fatty acids from acetate by rat ventral prostate slices is depressed by castration to a greater extent than respiration, and is restored to normal levels by testosterone administration (Ahmed et al. 1979). The glycolytic activity and the individual glycolytic enzymes do not seem to respond to androgenic status of the male. In the rat, the ventral prostate exhibits characteristic profiles of glucose-6-phosphate dehydrogenase enzymes which can be altered by exogenous testosterone (Ozols and Hilf 1973).

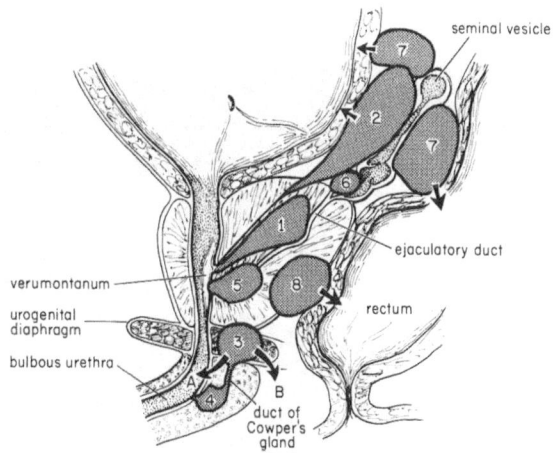

Figure 4. Congenital cysts of the prostate (8), and anatomical relationships and directions of expansion (arrows). 1 =utricular cyst; 2 =Müllerian duct cyst; 3 =Cowper's gland cyst, which on expansion bulges into bulbous urethra (a) or perineum (B); 4 = cyst of duct of Cowper's gland; 5 = ejaculatory duct cyst; 6 = cyst of ampulla of vas deferens, an extremely rare anomaly; 7 =seminal vesicle cyst. (El-Badawi 1979a).

16

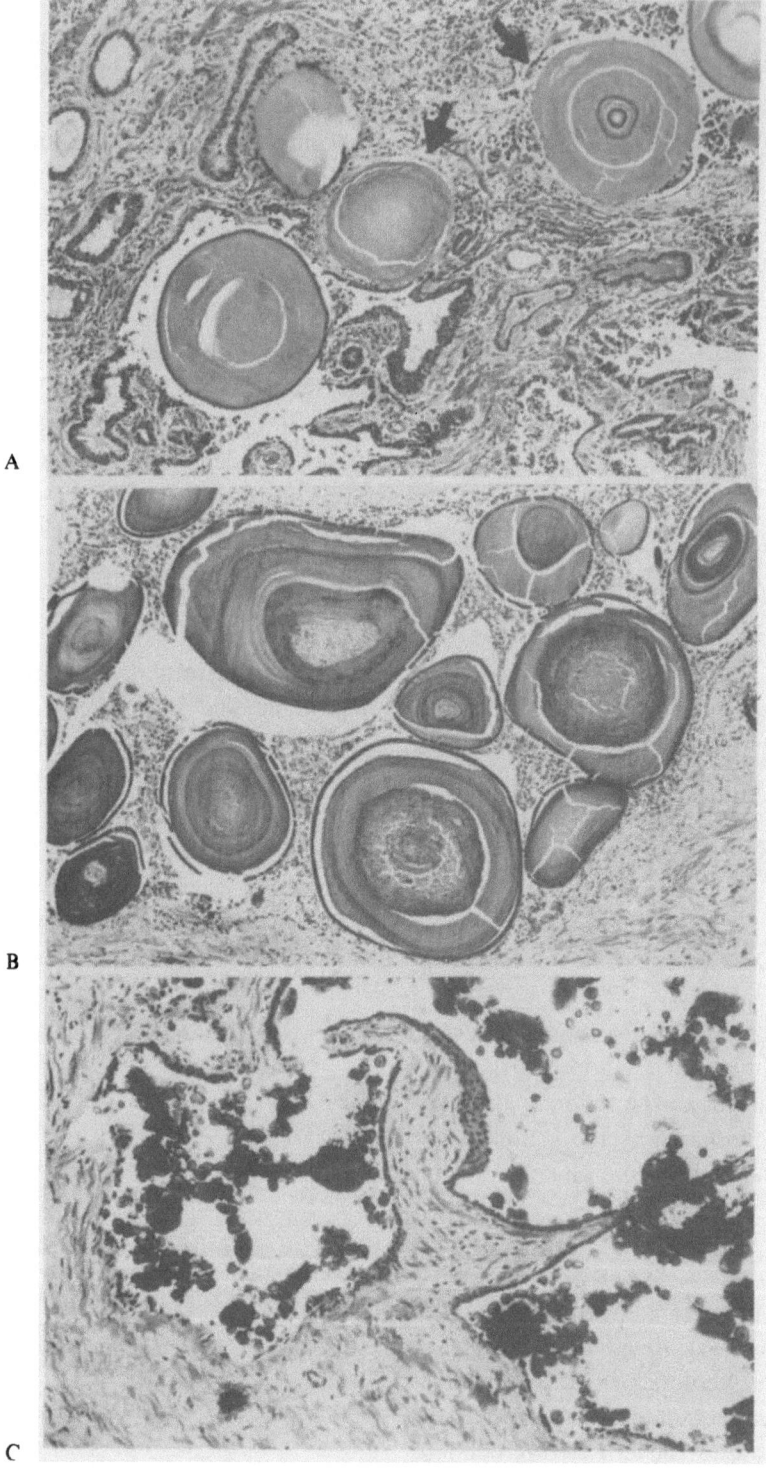

Figure 5. Three types of prostatic concretions. (A) Corpora amylacea in area of parenchymal atrophy (note spherical shape and amorphous laminations); some lie in part or totally within the stroma (arrows) following partial or total loss of epithelium of enclosing glands (×55). (B) Corpora calculi in area of parenchymal atrophy (note angulated contour and tightly concentric dark laminations); most appear to be imbedded in stroma without enclosing glandular epithelium (×88). (C) Dilated prostatic ducts with variable-sized calculi and mostly attenuated lining epithelium (×55). (El-Badawi 1979a).

B. Prolactin

The action of prolactin on the prostate is biphasic. Prolactin levels within the physiological range stimulate prostatic growth in man whereas high levels as in hyperprolactinemic patients are inhibitory (Thomas and Manadhar 1975). There is remarkable synergistic action between androgen and prolactin in the growth promotion of the prostate as judged by biochemical and morphological evidence. In the prostate of the guinea pig, high doses of prolactin can induce a significant decrease in metabolism of testosterone or dihydrotestosterone. Both testosterone and dihydrotestosterone are synergistic with prolactin (Walvoord et al. 1976). Thus, the transformation of testosterone to dihydrotestosterone by the action of 5α reductase is of special significance in androgen action in prostatic tissue. The interactions of prolactin with androgens may involve not only testicular but also adrenal androgens. Prolactin may promote prostatic growth by acting directly at the organ level, or by synergizing with circulating androgens, or by increasing androgen output from the testis and/or adrenals. In patients with pharmacologically induced hyperprolactinemia, an increased rate of conversion of testosterone to dihydrotestosterone was observed (Farnsworth 1976).

C. Hormone receptors

Several polypeptide hormones seem to exert their biological actions, at least in part, without entering the cell, through an interaction with specific receptors located on the external surface of the cytoplasmic membranes. Protein hormone action is mediated by an activation in cyclic AMP, through an enhancement in adenylate cyclase activity. This may be one of the mechanisms of action of these hormones on the prostate. Specific binding sites are present in the prostate glands (Aragona and Friesen 1975, Barkey et al. 1977). There are age-related changes in hormone binding sites to prostatic membranes. For example, prolactin binding sites in the prostate decline progressively during sexual development from high levels in infantile rats to lower levels in adult animals and reaching still lower values in old animals (Negro-Vilar 1980).

III. FUNCTIONAL BIOCHEMISTRY OF THE PROSTATE

The prostatic secretions contain several components of physiological and clinical significance, including acid phosphatase, zinc, prostaglandins, spermine and related aliphatic polyamines. Some of these components have been used as biochemical markers for the functional integrity of the prostate versus that of the seminal vesicles (Table 1). Little is known about the mode of action and physiological mechanisms of their secretory process.

Small molecules and ions in the prostatic secretions include sodium, potassium, calcium, chloride, bicarbonate and phosphate. The calcium content is higher than in blood plasma, but most enzymes and electrolytes are present in concentrations comparable to those found in blood plasma.

A. Acid phosphatase

The prostate contains a high content of acid phosphatase and it has been considered as a physiological and biochemical marker of the development of secondary male sex traits. Its activity is low in childhood, but increases several hundredfold in adulthood.

The crude enzyme (molecular weight 100,000)

Table 1. Some specific biochemical markers and major constituents of secretions of the prostate as compared to that of the seminal vesicles.

Prostate	Seminal vesicle
acid phosphatase	ascorbic acid
albumin	citric acid (traces)
α-Amylase	fructose
β-Glucuronidase	inorganic phosphorous
cephalin	inositol
cholesterol	lactoferrin
choline	phosphorylcholine
citric acid	inositol
diastase	lactoferrin
fibrinolytic enzymes	phosphorylcholine
inositol	prostaglandins
magnesium	protein
plasminogen activator	proteinase inhibitors
phospholipids	sodium
proteolytic enzymes	sorbitol
seminin	uric acid
sodium	
spermine + spermidine	
zinc	

has been separated into two fractions, each of which show heterogeneity on isoelectric focusing due to the presence of N-acetyl neuraminic acid (Ostrowski et al. 1970). One of the acid phosphatases in the prostate differs from any of those found in other tissues (Lam et al. 1973). The isoenzyme found in the semen is a protein of molecular weight of 100,000 with pH optimum of 6.5. Acid phosphatase is active at pH 5-6 toward α and β-glycerophosphate, but not toward fructose diphosphate and pyrophosphate (Ahmed et al. 1979).

In the prostate of the rat, the secretory acid phosphatase has been separated from lysosomal phosphatase, and it is the secretory enzyme which declines readily upon castration (Helminen et al. 1975.

B. Other enzymes

Human prostatic fluid contains diastase, beta glucuronidase, proteolytic enzymes, coagulase and fibrinolysin (Mann 1964, Farnsworth 1976, Hafez 1976, Pontes and Pierce 1977). Coagulase acts upon a fibrinogen-like protein from the seminal vesicles to form a fibrin-like clot, whereas a fibrinolysin cleaves the fibrin clot. It is so active that 2 ml of prostatic fluid can liquefy 100 ml of clotted blood upon incubation overnight at 37 .

Usually less than 1% of the prostatic secretion is protein; and the relative enrichment of prostatic secretion (compared to blood plasma) with free amino acids is thought to be due to the action of proteolytic and transaminating enzymes in the prostatic epithelium.

Several enzymes are involved in the metabolic pathways of the prostate. For example, Δ^4-3 ketosteroid 5α-reductase, 3β-hydroxysteroid oxidoreductase, 3β-hydroxysteroid oxidoreductase and 17β-hydroxy-C_{19}-steroid oxidoreductase are present in varying degrees of activity in the prostate (Liao and Fang 1969, Williams-Ashman and Reddi 1972, Offner et al. 1974, Mainwaring 1977).

C. Zinc

Various histochemical techniques have been employed to demonstrate the presence of zinc in epithelial cells and in prostatic secretion. In the normal prostate, the zinc concentration is much higher in the lateral and dorsal zones than in the inner and anterior zones (Gyorkey et al. 1967). Specific areas have very high zinc levels, e.g. supranuclear and apical portions of the cytoplasm of the epithelial and the basal cells of the hyperplastic acine. Prostatic carcinoma, however, is associated with very little stainable zinc except in the nucleolar portion of the nucleus.

Zinc in the prostate is increased by androgen administration and glandular hyperplasia, and decreased by estrogen administration, castration and prostatic carcinoma (Eliasson and Lindholmer 1971, Mikac-Devic 1970, Polakoski and Zaneveld 1977). In benign prostatic hyperplasia, zinc levels increase with an inverse relationship between the zinc content and the amount of fibromuscular stroma (Byar 1974). Moreover, depletion of zinc in animals following diphenylthiocarbazone injections results in cessation of prostatic secretion as well as severe damage to the viability and morphologic integrity of the prostatic epithelium (Whitmore 1963).

Zinc content of the prostate is associated with a zinc-binding protein (Habib and Stitch 1975). Sites of zinc binding are saturable since there is an inverse relationship between in vivo zinc concentration and in vitro binding capacity (Gyorkey and Sato 1968, Sato and Gyorkey 1969).

Zinc inhibits 5α-reductase activity since in hypertrophic prostate dehydrolectoserone (DHT) its concentration is inversely related to that of zinc (Wallace and Grant 1975, Habib et al. 1976a). It is possible that zinc and androgens may bind to the same protein since, in prostatic cancer, there is an inverse relationship between zinc and testosterone and zinc and DHT.

D. Prostaglandins

Prostaglandins E_1 and E_2 are most abundant in the prostate. In vitro studies show that the human prostate produces, metabolizes and is remarkably affected by prostaglandin $F_{2\alpha}$ ($PGF_{2\alpha}$). When minced human prostate is incubated with radiolabeled testosterone in the presence and absence of concentrations of $PGF_{2\alpha}$ ranging from 4 μg/ml to 40μg/ml, there is a dose-related increase in androgen binding (Cavanaugh and Farnsworth 1977). Assays of a series of surgical specimens of hyperplastic prostate revealed a substantial concentration (Mean 340 ng/gm fresh tissue) of endogenous $PGF_{2\alpha}$ and that this varied according to the concentration of epithelium within the tissue specimen (Farnsworth and Wilks 1975). It is interesting to note that the steroid-peptide hormone (lactogen) complex also stimulates the metabolism of $PGF_{2\alpha}$ to reduction products, most abundant of which is 13, 14-dihydro-15-deto-$PGF_{2\alpha}$.

E. Spermine

The normal human prostate contains high levels of spermine, an aliphatic polyamine. It is formed by combination of citrulline from decarboxylated ornithine (putrescine) and decarboxylated S-adenosylmethionine. Williams-Ashman (1975) advanced several hypotheses as to the function of spermine in the tissue. Direct activation of nuclear RNA polymerase by spermine or spermidine has been demonstrated with prostate preparations in the rat.

F. Prostatic contribution to seminal plasma

Although the prostate may not be absolutely required for reproduction, it contributes a number of substances to seminal plasma which are involved directly or indirectly in capacitation and/or fertilization, and are also involved in coagulase, and probably other coagulum-lysing enzymes (Farnsworth 1976, Pontes and Pierce 1977, Polakoski and Zaneveld 1977). Prostatic fluid safeguards sperm viability by reducing the acidity of the urethra and facilitates and enhances sperm motility by contributing certain factors to seminal plasma that stimulate the motility of epididymal and washed, ejaculated spermatozoa (Eliasson and Lindholmer 1976).

In the ejaculate, free zinc ions are toxic to spermatozoa. However, most of the 100-150 $\mu g/ml$ of zinc in normal prostatic fluid is complexed by a concentration of 1.5 mg/ml albumin (Lindholmer 1974). This combination with protein may regulate sperm metabolism. It is possible that zinc-albumin coating of the cells inhibits the transfer to succinate into the cells and thus keeps them quiescent (Stankova et al. 1976).

Prostatic secretions account for approximately 30% of the seminal fluid or ejaculate. Most of the data on prostatic secretions are based on fluid obtained by prostatic massage. This type of fluid called resting fluid, differs in composition from stimulated secretion that is obtained during ejaculation, since during sexual excitement, certain compounds are secreted at an accelerated rate. For example, resting fluid contains a lower concentration of acid phosphatase than does stimulated secretion (Eliasson and Lindholmer 1976) Debilitating disease is associated with a dramatic decrease in the secretory activity in young and old men.

Components of the early part of the ejaculate differ from those in subsequent fractions. The 'prostatic' contribution is contained within the first fraction whereas the 'vesicular' fluid predominates in the latter part. The majority of spermatozoa are in the first part of the ejaculate and these are the most motile. Those in the latter part generally show poor progressive motility.

IV. PHYSIOPATHOLOGY OF PROSTATIC DISEASES

A. Differentiation of prostatic carcinoma

The malignant prostate may be large, of normal size, or smaller than the normal gland. Some 15-20% of nodular hyperplastic prostates harbor carcinoma in any part of the gland; but mainly in the posterior zone where it begins next to the capsule.

About 96% of malignant neoplasms of the prostate are adenocarcinomas which vary greatly in structure, e.g. differentiated, simple, scirrhous and/or medullary (Anderson 1971).

Atrophic changes are expressed in different form: (a) simple atrophy of the epithelial cells of the acine; (b) sclerotic atrophy associated with characteristic fibrous tissue which replaces the smooth muscle of the acini; and (c) hyalinization of collagen associated with compression of the lumen of the acini.

Diffuse atrophy within a given zone tends to be bilaterally symmetrical and relatively uniform suggesting that general hormonal, constitutional or aging factors are involved (McNeal 1968). The process is initiated after the age of 50 but is not usually advanced until after 70.

Benign proliferative lesions of the prostate include: (a) prostatic epithelial hyperplasia;

(b) nodular prostatic hyperplasia, and (c) prostatic squamous metaplasia (Table 2). Common types of prostatic epithelial hyperplasia include nodular hyperplasia and hyperplasia of the epithelium of the prostatic ducts (prostatoductal hyperplasia) or atrophic prostatic parenchyma (secondary or post-atrophic hyperplasia) (Figures 6-9). Benign nodular hyperplasia originate in the inner paraurethral zone of the prostate gland; this zone has a composite embryological origin which in part can be related to the Müllerian ducts (Gleinster 1962, Mostofi 1970). *1. Ultrastructural differentiation* The cells of prostatic carcinoma show remarkable structural and ultrastructural polymorphism even within a well-formed cancer acinus. The cells may form glands or infiltrate individually. The cells may contain only a few organelles with a definite tendency to imbalance in intracellular organization of the various components. Other cells are well differentiated with the usual number of organelles in orderly relationship as in the epithelial cell of benign prostatic hyperplasia and normal prostate (Brandes et al. 1964; Mao et al. 1965). In some cells, certain organelles may predominate almost to the exclusion of others, such as predominance of mitochondria of ribosomes, and of vesicles or vacuoles. (Mao et al. 1966).

In general, the cells of prostatic carcinoma have several ultrastructural characteristics: (a) absence of basal cells, (b) frequent lack of basement membrane and apposition with smooth muscle cells without the intervention of collagen bundles and fibro-blasts, (c) nuclear irregularity, hyperchromatinism and nucleolar hypertrophy, (d) increase and random distribution of lipid droplets, (e) marked variation of mitochondria in number, size, shape and internal structures, (f) greater amount of free ribosomes and relatively smaller amount of granular endoplasmic reticulum, (g) great variability in the postion and size of the Golgi apparatus and (h)

Table 2. Histologic classification of prostatic carcinoma and of prostatitis (El-Badawi 1979a).

Prostatic Carcinoma	Prostatitis

I. *Prostatoglandular carcinoma*
   1. Tubuloalveolar pattern (Classical carcinoma)
   2. Solid pattern (Encephaloid, medullary or simplex
      carcinoma)
   3. Solid clear-cell pattern (Xanthocarcinoma)
   4. Mucinous pattern (Colloid carcinoma)
   5. Adenocystic pattern (?Origin)
 	
II. *Prostatoductal carcinoma*
  A. Prostatoductal adenocarcinoma
    1. Main duct type
    2. Branch duct type
    3. Main and branch duct type
    4. Endometrioid type (= Endometrial carcinoma of
       uterus masculinus)
  B. Prostatoductal Urothelial-Tube (Transitional)
    Carcinoma
    1. Papillary type
    2. Solid or comedocarcinoma-like type
  C. Prostatoductal Epidemoid (Squamous cell) Carcinoma
 	
III. *Carcinoma of mixed types*
  A. Junctional Carcinoma
  B. Combined Carcinoma
	I. *Acute prostatitis*
	   1. Acute nonspecific prostatitis: usually bacterial
	   2. Prostatic abscess: primary or metastatic
	
	II. *Chronic nongranulomatous prostatitis*
	   1. Chronic bacterial prostatitis: confirmed clinically,
	      microbiologically $\pm$ histologically
	   2. Chronic abacterial prostatitis: confirmed clinically $\pm$
	      histologically
	   3. Chronic interstitial prostatitis in NPH; histological
	      evidence only
	   4. Prostatitis follicularis: histological evidence $\pm$ clinical
	      $\pm$ microbiological confirmation
	
	III. *Chronic granulomatous prostatitis*
	   5. Calculous prostatitis: histological evidence $\pm$ clinical
	      $\pm$ microbiological confirmation
	
	  A. Specific forms: due to a specific microorganism
	    1. Bacterial granulomatous prostatitis: tuberculous;
	      syphilitic
	    2. Mycotic prostatitis: various fungi, most commonly
	      blastomycosis
	    3. Parasitic prostatitis: schistosomal, hydatidosis,
	      metazoal
	  B. Nonspecific forms: due to a nonspecific microorganism
	    or no organism at all:
	    1. Xanthogranulomatous prostatitis: ductal obstruction
	      or repair $\pm$ nonspecific organism
	    2. Eosinophilic granulomatous prostatitis: repair, vascu-
	      litis or allergy
	    3. Malakoplakic prostatitis: nonspecific organism in
	      presence of phagocytic dysfunction

absence of glycogen islets in the basal portion of the cell and absence of apocrine secretion of prostatic cancer cells (Brandes et al. 1964, Fisher and Jeffrey 1965).

B. *Age related changes*

The probability of developing cancer of the prostate increases with age. Death rates appear to be higher in white married men aged 54-74 years than in single white men (Duffield and Jacobson 1975). In certain population groups, mortality rates seems to rise faster in nonwhite males than in white males (Quisenberry 1960). Progressive atrophy of the prostate associated with aging, may begin as early as the fifth decade and is initially focal in distribution. Aging-associated atrophy pursues a parallel but partially independent course in different regions of the prostate. Chronic debilitating disease often produces, in younger men, a degree of atrophy comparable to that seen in normal men 30 or more years older (McNeal 1968). In cases where advanced atrophy has not occurred with aging, there is a progressive, age-related increase in the inci-

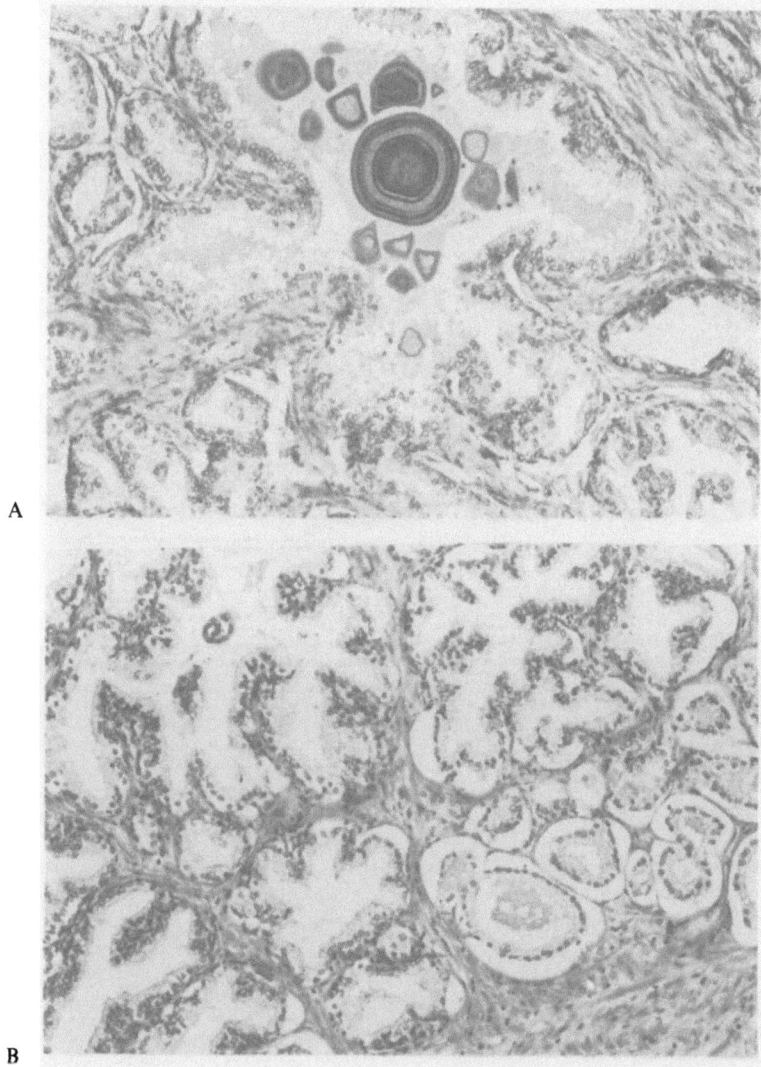

Figure 6. Nodular prostatic hyperplasia. A) Large gland in a mixed nodule with typical convoluted pattern, double-layered epithelial lining and corpora calculi within the lumen (×88). B) Periphery of a mixed nodule: large convoluted glands have papillary infoldings and double-layered epithelial lining; small gland component (lower right corner) consists of acinar structures lined by a single layer of columnar epithelium (×88). (El-Badawi 1979a).

22

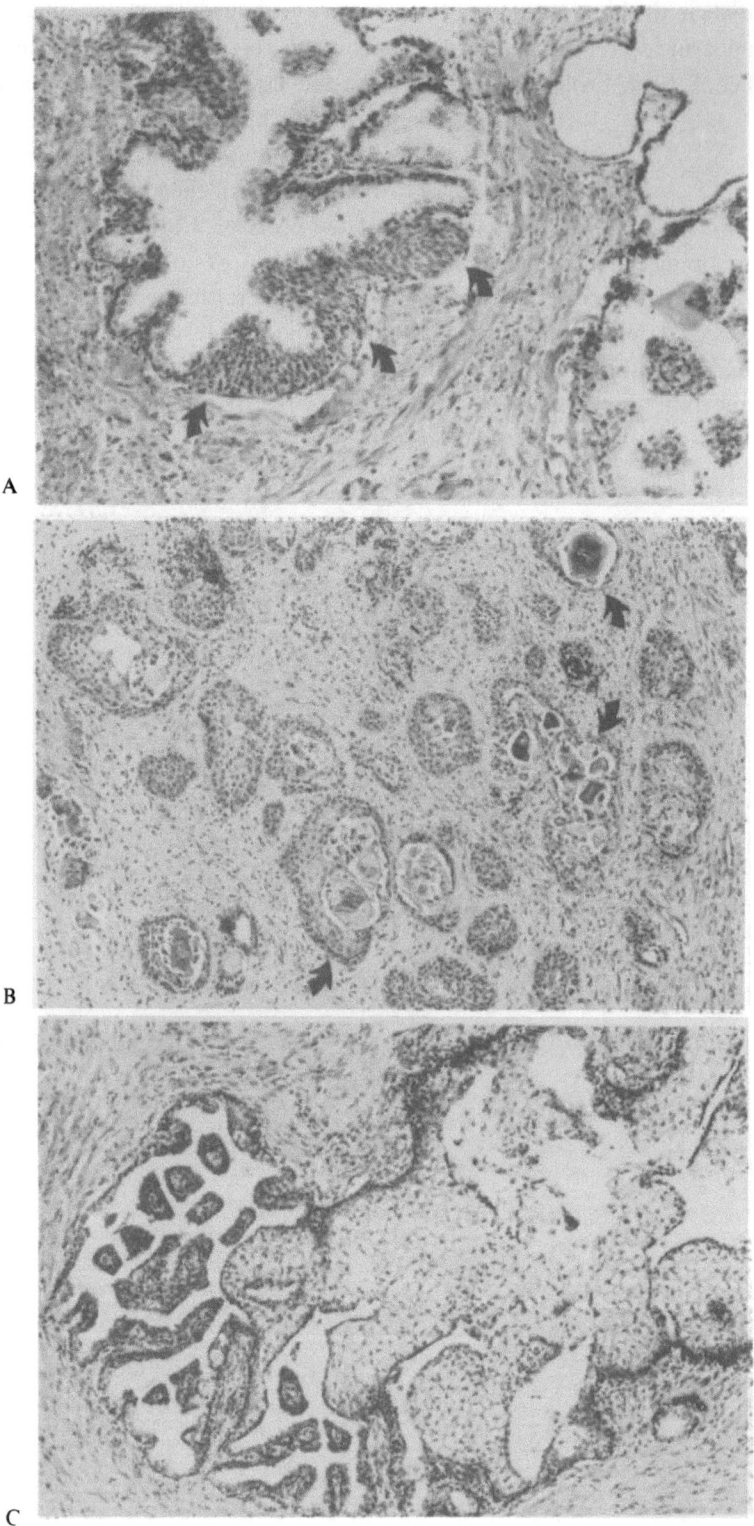

Figure 7. Nodular prostatic hyperplasia, atypical and metaplastic epithelial reactions. **A)** Convoluted gland in mixed nodule has distinct, double-layered epithelial lining, with dark basal and light secretory columnar cell layers; part of lining (arrow) is markedly thickened with a paralumenal layer of columnar cells and several layers of stratified squamous cells (Squamous metaplasia); some glands contain corpora amylacea (arrows) and a few have desquamated cell debris in the lumen (×69). **C)** Main prostatic duct in a gland with NPH; the lining is represented in part by papillary hyperplastic epithelium and largely by squamous metaplastic epithelium consisting of clear cells due to abundant cytoplasmic glycogen content (×55). (El-Badawi 1979a).

dence of a variety of atypical hyperplasia. Age-related changes in the prostate also include neoplasia and nodular hyperplasia. The glandular prostate, the central and peripheral zones, undergoes progessive atrophy with aging. The glandular activity of the prostate declines progressively with age, with great individual variation among men. Testicular production of many steroids decline in normal men after 50 years of age (Vermeulen et al. 1972, Vermeulen and Verdonck 1976).

Since both NPH and prostatoglandular carcinoma are common and have increasing incidence with age, they often co-exist but the relationship between the two syndromes remains controversial. Armenian et al. (1975) have suggested that NPH might be a precursor of prostatoglandular carcinoma.

Corpora amylacea, characteristic of the involuting process and noted as early as the third decade are associated with epithelial atrophy in the immediate area. These formations contain concentric rings probably as the result of successive layers of deposits over several years.

C. Benign prostatic hypertropy (BPH)

Little is known about the exact pathogenesis of benign prostatic hypertrophy (BPH) in man. It seems that BPH is related to some endocrine imbalance rather than to race, marital status or sexual activity, (Chang and Char 1936). However, the incidence of BPH is lower in the Chinese population than in Caucasians.

It seems that the testis plays a primary role in the development of BPH (Zuckerman 1936, Moore 1944), since surgical castration reduces prostate size in most patients with BPH (Huggins and Stevens 1940).

In patients with PBH, there is no change in androgen and estrogen production rates, metabolic clearance rates, and plasma levels (Baynard 1973), but there is an increase in peripheral DHT levels (Siiteri and Wilson 1970, Vermeulen et al. 1972, Horton 1975, Habib et al. 1976b, Krieg et al. 1977a), and a decrease in androstenediols (Geller et al. 1976). The number of receptor binding sites does not appear to be different in BPH vs normal prostates (Shimazaki et al. 1977), whereas enzyme activities which affect the formation and metabolic

degradation of DHT may be abnormal in BPH tissue, e.g. 5α-reductase (Bruchovsky and Lesser 1976, Krieg et al. 1977a) and 17β-hydroxysteroid and dehydrogenase (Morfin et al. 1978). An important clue to the possible elevation of DHT which may be pathogenetic in the BPH, is the level of tissue cofactor concentrations which in turn regulates enzyme directional (oxidation-reduction) activity which in turn regulates tissue DHT concentrations (Bremner 1979). This concept may lead to the ultimate source of elevated DHT and to a rational scheme for its prevention.

D. Prostatitis

In developing countries, the diagnosis of prostatic carcinoma is often confused with that of prostatitis.

Prostatitis is caused by prostatic infection from (a) ascending urethral infection; (b) reflux of infected urine into prostatic ducts that empty into the posterior urethra; (c) invasion by rectal bacteria via direct extension or lymphogenous spread; and (d) hematogenous infection (El-Badawi 1979a). There are several types of prostatitis but acute and chronic bacterial and nonbacterial prostatitis are most common (Table 2).

Prostatitis usually results in focal areas of atrophy, in contrast to the diffuse process characteristic of normal aging. Focal areas of atrophy are usually associated with prostatitis and both show a prominent predilection for the peripheral zone over the central zone. The lymphocytic infiltrate about atrophic glands, often ascribed to aging, is in fact usually a manifestation of chronic prostatitis (McNeal 1968).

In chronic prostatitis there is infiltration around the acini with mononuclear inflammatory cells (Nielsen et al. 1973). Acute prostatitis, an inflammation of the prostate due to bacterial and/or viral infection, often extends to the urethra and urinary bladder.

E. Physiopathological and endocrine mechanisms

The differentation of prostatic carcinoma, a slow-growing tumor, seems to be initiated at a stage of life when androgens are high and may remain quiescent in most men whose androgens decline with advancing age. Any endocrine disturbances of

24

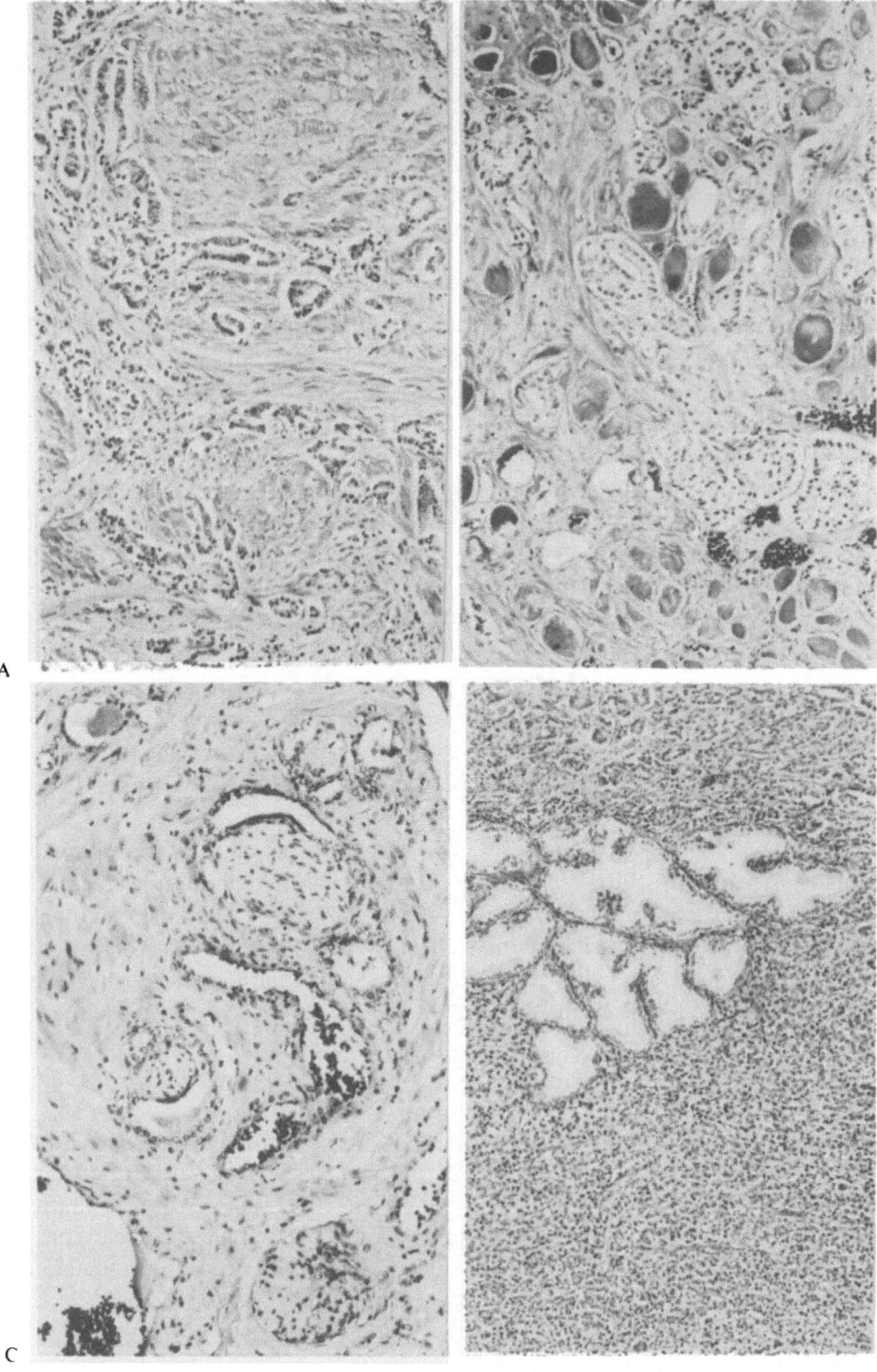

Figure 8. Prostatoglandular carcinoma, invasion. A) Cancer glands and clustered cancer cells infiltrate prostatic fibromuscular stroma (×88). B) Cancer glands infiltrate skeletal muscle of prostatic capsule at apex of gland, focally separating individual muscle fibers (×88). C) Cancer glands surround nerves (N) in prostatic capsule in perineural invasion pattern (×88). D) Predominantly solid cancer growth infiltrates a nodule of NPH but preserves a few convoluted glands in its substance (×55). (El-Badawi 1979).

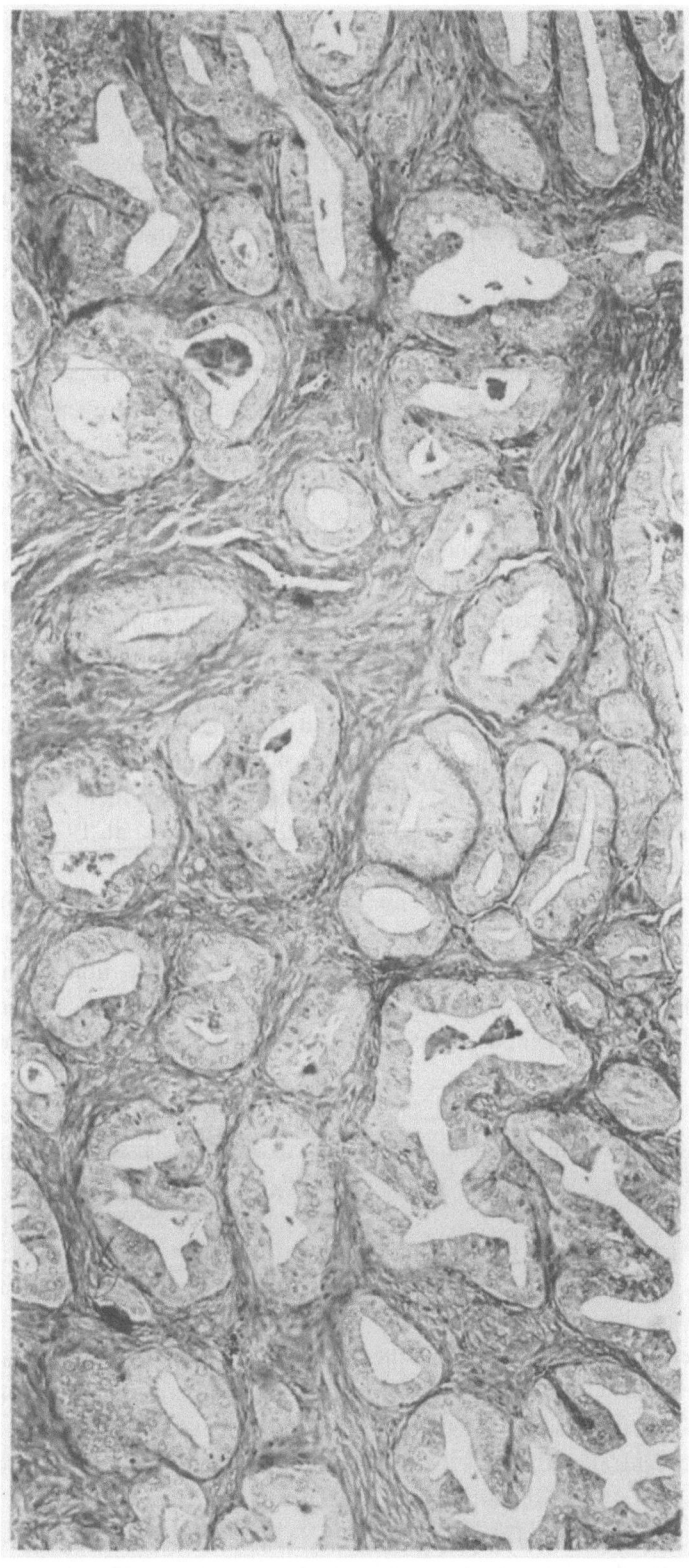

Figure 9. Prostatoductal adenocarcinoma, endometrioid type. This suburothelial tumor infiltrates prostatic stroma as large-sized, irregular and focally branching glands, lined by a tall columnar, focally pseudostratified and focally papillary epithelium with an overall appearance resembling carcinoma of endometrium; apical secretion of lining cells is present in many glands, but cilia are absent (×88). (El-Badawi 1979a).

the hypothalamus pituitary adrenal glands-testis-prostate axis may stimulate the dormant malignant cells to differentiate into prostatic carcinoma. All prostatic functions are regulated by the endocrine system. With the exception of the autonomous tumors of advanced carcinoma, castration or androgen depletion causes the cessation of proliferation and cellular enlargement.

The testes and adrenal glands contribute to the androgen and estrogen pool. With advancing age, there is a remarkable decline in androgen level and a corresponding increase in estrogens. The periurethral inner prostate is responsive to estrogens, whereas the outer prostate and the secondary sex organs are responsive to the androgens.

Anderson (1971) postulated various endocrine relationships of prostatic hyperplasia as follows:

(a) an increase in androgen production by Leydig cells associated with decreased function of tubules and decreased estrogen production

(b) an increase in estrogen production by the increased Sertoli cells in old age associated with decreased androgenic production by Leydig cells

(c) simultaneous stimulation of the prostate by both hormones, the androgens acting on the epithelium and the estrogens on the fibromuscular stroma

(d) structural changes in androgens and/or estrogens

(e) synergistic stimulation of the prostate by both hormones and one or more endogenous or exogenous compounds

(f) change in the response of the endocrine-sensitive target organ, the prostate, brought about by environmental, circulatory or genetic disturbances

(g) nonhormonal stimulation of the prostate, endogenous or exogenous, acting independently of the endocrine system

There has been extensive speculation about the role of estrogens in the genesis of BPH (Mahwinney and Belis 1976). It is possible that there is indirect action via the central nervous system or direct action mediated by estrogen binding macromolecules. In senile or presenile men, there is a shift in the androgen-estrogen ratio. The dominance of estrogens may cause nodular hyperplasia.

1. Androgen receptors There is a functional relationship between intracellular hormone receptor proteins and steroid hormone regulation of target tissue function (Yamamoto and Alberts 1976, Gorski and Gannon 1976). For example in North American (McGuire 1975), European (LeClerg et al. 1975), and Japanese (Nomura et al. 1977), breast cancer patients, 55 to 82 percent of all primary breast cancers and 43 to 72 percent of all metastatic breast tumors are estrogen receptor positive (ER$^+$). Radiolabeled 5α-dihydrotestosterone (5α-DHT) has been employed as a probe to characterize human prostate androgen receptors.

Cytoplasmic androgen receptor content, 4500 receptor sites per cell, represents 75% of the total androgen receptor population per cell of human prostate (Shain et al. 1978). Thus, it would appear that nuclear androgen receptor is not an appropriate index to predict hormone responsiveness. Although cytoplasmic androgen receptor may be measured under certain conditions (Snochowski et al. 1977), it seems that 90% of the total cytoplasmic androgen receptors of the human prostate occur as steroid-occupied receptor which can only be measured by exchange incubation techniques (Rosen et al. 1975, Mobbs et al. 1976). Since androgen receptors occur in normal and hyperplastic human prostate, any diagnostic determination of androgen receptors in primary prostatic adenocarcinoma must account for noncarcinomatous androgen-receptor-containing cells contained in the pathologic specimen. This complication to diagnostic accuracy may be overcome in part by analysis of metastatic foci located in tissues devoid of androgen receptors. The early investigations on the characterization and quantitation of human prostate total androgen receptors, R$_c$ plus R$_c$A, have been hampered by : (a) the necessity to exclude probe binding to plasma SHBG, and (b) the lack of a suitable probe which would not be metabolized during incubation with human prostate preparations at temperatures above 4 °C as would be required for quantitation of endogenous-steroid-occupied receptor sites (Shain et al. 1978).

V. DIAGNOSTIC PROCEDURES

Extensive investigations have been conducted to establish diagnostic procedures for the early detection of lesions: e.g. ultrastructure and surface ultrastructure of carcinoma cells, endocrine profile, hormone receptor assay, radioimmunoassay of acid phosphatase, counterimmuno-electrophoresis of prostatic isoenzymes, identification of tumor markers, and the recognition and quantification of tumor-specific antigens. Several biochemical assays of prostatic tissues and bone marrow have been made in an attempt to explore any possible marker for tumor differentiation. Roentgenologic examinations of the bone for osteoblastic and/or osteolytic lesions have been used for the diagnosis of prostatic carcinoma.

A. Clinical examination

Rectal examination reveals much about the status of the prostate and seminal vesicles (Figure 10). Normally the prostate is widest superiorly near the bladder neck and quite rubbery in consistency. Lack of sexual intercourse and chronic infection produce a mushy texture. Chronic infection with or without calculi causes extreme firmness and advanced carcinoma produces a stony hardness. Elevated nodules, caused by infection, which are hard and indurated in the center, blend into the normal rubbery consistency of the uninvolved gland at their periphery. Carcinomatous lesions, however, are stony hard, sharp-edged, and usually not elevated above the surface of the gland. When pus is absent

from the prostatic secretions and x-ray examination fails to reveal calculi behind or above the symphysis carcinoma should be strongly suspected, especially if an enlargement is felt in the posterior lobe during rectal examination (Tables 3, 4).

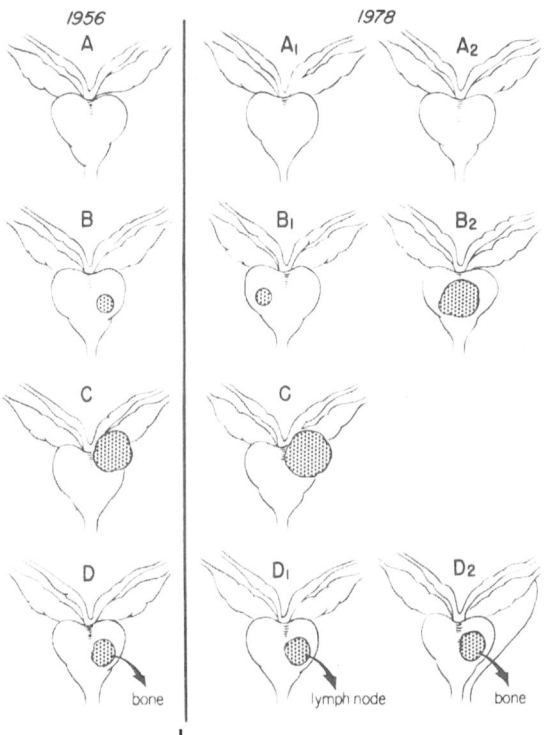

Figure 10. Classification of prostatic carcinoma based on digital rectal examination (Klein 1979).

Table 3. Clinical detection and diagnostic procedures of prostatic carcinoma.

Clinical detection	localized	a. no symptoms
		b. may have obstructive symptoms for associated benign prostatic hypertrophy
		c. incidental binding at time of surgery for benign disease
	advanced	a. obstructive urinary symptoms
		b. metastatic symptoms (bone pain, weight loss, uremia)
		c. hematuria is more often due to benign prostatic disease or malignant disease
Diagnostic procedures	localized	a. rectal examination reveals 50% of prostatic nodules are carcinoma
		b. histologic diagnosis is often made in specimen removed
		c. phosphatases are normal
		d. a needle biopsy (perineal or transrectal) is often adequate
		e. open biopsy may be required in selected cases
		f. negative cytology is useful to rule out carcinoma
		g. bone survey shows no metastases
		h. bone scar (^{85}Sr and ^{18}Fl) may show activity area when skeletal survey is negative
	advanced	a. rectal examination reveals local extension of stony hard tumor
		b. serum acid phosphatase is elevated in some patients with metastatic spread of the tumor
		c. alkaline phosphatase is elevated with bony metastases
		d. bone survey shows common sites of metastases (pelvic are osteoblastic in most patients)
		e. needle biopsy is simple and diagnostic. Open biopsies are rarely required
		f. bone (^{85}Sr and ^{18}Fl) may be positive in a few patients with negative skeletal survey

The mobility of the prostate is restricted in advanced carcinoma because of extension of the tumor through the capsule. This alteration is easily detected during rectal examination. Routine prostatic massage and microscopic examination of the gland's secretion is important for detecting asymptomatic prostatitis and ultimately preventing cystitis and epididymitis. However, prostatic massage is contraindicated in patients suffering from acute urethral discharge, acute prostatitis, acute prostatocystitis, obvious carcinoma, or those with nearly complete urinary retention.

The digital rectal examination has been used exclusively for the screening of asymptomatic patients with potentially curable prostatic carcinoma. Treatment of 'early' tumors detected by routine digital rectal examination results in nearly perfect survival rates. However, in these screening programs, most of the tumors discovered are not 'early.'

B. Clinical staging

Since only 25-35% of prostatoglandular carcinomas have clinical manifestations, the majority being locally silent or latent, the disease has been classified into three biologically different, but histologically similar, forms: clinical, occult and incidental carcinomas (Liavag 1968) (Table 4).

Prostatic carcinomas have been also classified according to site of origin into prostatoglandular carcinoma, prostatoductal carcinoma and carcinoma of mixed types. Prostatoglandular carcinoma is the usual type and arises in glandular (tubuloalveolar) elements of the prostatic parenchyma and their related terminal ductules. Prostatoductal carcinomas are rare, and originate in main (primary) prostatic ducts, which open into the urethra, and their larger (secondary) branches (El-Badawi 1979b).

The four-stage classification of prostatic carcinoma was based on digital rectal examination of the prostate, serum acid phosphatase level and skeletal survey either by bone x-ray study or radioisotope bone scan. The main limitations of this staging procedure is the exclusion of surgical or pathological findings. Three of the four stages have been subdivided so that in reality seven stages were derived. As with the original classification, the new classification is based on clinical and not surgical or pathological data. It is hoped that a modern computerized method will be developed to include other physiopathological parameters, e.g., the status of regional lymph nodes as well as the histological, histochemical and ultrastructural characteristics.

Table 4. Staging of prostatoglandular carcinoma (El Badawi 1979b).

Type of carcinoma and criteria	Staging system		
	TNM	A-D	VACURG (I-IV)
Minimal requirements not met	$T_xN_xM_x$		
Incidental carcinoma	T_o	A	I
Clinical Ca, confined to prostate:	$T_{1-2}N_0M_0$	B	II
No capsular penetration, extraprostatic extension or metastases			
Ca surrounded by normal gland	T_1		
Ca deforms contour: lateral gland and seminal vesicles not involved	T_2		
No lymph node metastasis	N_0		
No distant metastasis	M_0		
Clinical Ca, locally advanced:	$T_{3-4}N_0M_0$	C	III
Capsular penetration and extracapsular spread; no metastasis			
Local extension + involvement of laterial sulci ± seminal vesicle(s) invasion	T_3		
Ca fixed to or invading adjacent structures	T_4		
Disseminated (metastasizing) Ca:	$T_{0-4}N_{1-4}M_1$	D	IV
To lymph nodes			
Single regional group	N_1		
Multiple regional groups	N_2		
Fixed pelvic wall mass with free space from the tumor	N_3	D_1	
Juxtaregional group(s)	N_4	D_2	
And/or distant nonnodal metastases	M_1		

The lymphatic spread of prostatic cancer is still difficult to determine and may account for some of the discrepancy between the clinical stage of the disease and its apparent rapid progression and lack of response to either primary treatment or palliation.

A uniform national and/or international system of classification of prostatic carcinoma will be of great prognostic value for pathologists and clinicians.

C. Histopathology

The common pathohistological characteristics of prostatic carcinoma include: (a) prostatic acini back to back; (b) one single layer of cells lining acini with the absence of a basal layer of cells; (c) prominent eosinophilic large nucleoli (in quickly and properly fixed tissues in formalin or Bouin's solutions); (d) prostatic acini noted as linear infiltrates in the fibromuscular stroma, like boats racing up and down a river; (e) nuclear hyperchromatism (probably due to improper fixation); and (f) perineural invasion in frozen sections (Tannebaum 1975) (Table 5).

In several cases, it may be difficult to evaluate the characteristics of the potential neoplastic activity of the prostate because of the complex configurations within the same zone. One microscopic field of the tumor may include a multitude of patterns such as morphoses as small as an in situ carcinoma, small and large gland carcinomas, 'Indian file' and cribriform patterns.

The growth patterns of prostatic carcinoma are extremely variable (Franks 1954a). Thus, several false therapeutic interpretations are perpetuated due to wrong histopathological data.

There are many long wide-lumened alveoli, not closely spaced. The columnar epithelium forms many thin folds within alveoli. Each is supported by a notably thin plate of stromal tissue. Tangential sections of folds often appear as isolated tissue-islands. Scanning, transmission and immunoelectron microscopy may be very useful tools for histopathological diagnosis of certain syndromes. For example, Takayasu and Yamaguchi (1962) indicated differences in the morphology of mitochondria of prostatic cancer cells when observed by electron microscopy.

D. Cytopathology

In its early stages of development, prostatic carcinoma is identified only with difficulty by the trained cytologist. Tumor cells are best demonstrated after prostatic massage. The neoplastic cells in the smears are pleomorphic and hyperchromatic, the nuclear-cytoplasmic and the nucleolar-nuclear ratios are disturbed, the cells occur in clusters, and cell borders are indistinct but nuclear borders definite. However, neoplastic cells are noted in the bloodstream of 15% of patients with cancer of the prostate who had prostatic massage, and only about 60% to 70% of patients with final diagnosis of cancer give a positive cytology (Anderson 1971). Consequently, this method is of little diagnostic value.

The advanced and undifferentiated adenocarcinoma are characterized by various cylological features e.g. progressive loss of epithelial characteristics which distinguish the advanced, and presence of tall columnar cells in acini enlargement, distortion and vacuolation of the mitochondria, absence of the basal cells, lack of integrity in the basement membrane.

Within the nucleus of the prostatic carcinoma cell there is a tendency to polyploidy e.g. diploid, tetraploid, triploid or hexaploid (Tavares et al. 1973).

E. Biochemical techniques

1. Acid phosphatase Acid phosphatase is present normally in the prostate, blood, urine and saliva. The demonstration of an elevated total serum acid phosphase and prostatic acid phosphatase is a useful diagnostic test for the detection of metastasis even before x-ray films are positive and for evaluating response to therapy.

The serum acid phosphatase is elevated in most patients with prostatic carcinoma or with bony metastasis. Since total serum acid phosphatase is elevated in Paget's and other bone disease, multiple myeloma, Gaucher's disease and hyperparathyroidism, it is advisable to measure the prostatic fraction, prostatic acid phosphatase, which is more reliable than total serum acid phosphatase (Anderson 1971). Prostatic acid phosphatase is also temporarily elevated in cases of digital or operative manipulation of the prostate, and catheterization

Table 5. Summary of some diagnostic and histological characteristics of prostatic carcinoma and other common pathologies of the human prostate. (Data from Randall 1931; Moore 1936, 1943; Franks 1954a; Arias-Stella and Takano-Moron 1958; Shelley et al. 1958; Liavag 1968; Lytton et al. 1968; Scott et al. 1969; Wynder et al. 1971; Chiu and Weber 1974; Higgins 1975; Bagley et al. 1975; Armenian et al. 1975; Belter and Dadson 1970; Makhyoun et al. 1977; El-Badawi 1979b).

Pathology		Diagnostic and histological characteristics
Prostatic carcinoma	Clinical carcinoma	suspected, diagnosed and staged clinically, and the diagnosis is subsequently confirmed histologically; sacral, low back, suprapubic or perineal pain; urinary retention, dribbling; hematuria and metastases; urinary tract infection and constipation from rectal compression may be present; constitutional symptoms, anemia, accompany advanced or metastasizing carcinoma
	Occult carcinoma	no prostate-related symptoms or signs; manifestations of metastases or prostate-related organ invasion; carcinoma is subsequently discovered on clinical workup to detect the primary source
	Incidental carcinoma	unsuspected and undetected clinically, but is discovered incidentally at autopsy or in surgically resected prostate judged clinically to be benign; preoperative rectal findings: benign prostate, commonly with atypical features; difficulty of enucleation during open prostatectomy, with adhesions to surgical capsule
Nodular prostatic hyperplasia (NPH) or benign prostatic hypertrophy or hyperplasia (BPH)		irritative and obstructive lower urinary symptoms comprising pollakiuria with nocturia, difficulty of micturition and abnormal urine stream; hematuria (usually terminal), urinary tract infection and perineal discomfort are common, upper urinary tract symptoms develop in cases with obstructive uropathy; smooth, symmetrical and firm prostatic enlargement; multicentric circumscribed nodules, which differ from normal glands in being estrogen sensitive, but secrete fluid chemically identical to that of normal gland
Prostatoductal hyperplasia		occur alone or in association with hyperplasia or urethral urothelium around orifices of involved ducts; results from epithelial irritation or inflammation, estrogenic stimulation; five histological types of hyperplasia: planophytic, papillary, fibroadenoid, regenerative (inflammatory) and adenomatoid
Prostatoductal planophytic hyperplasia		flat, focal or diffuse thickening of epithelial lining, several basal (reserve) cell layers push surface columnar cell layer toward lumen; basal cells have spherical to ovoid nuclei and scanty eosinophilic, glycogen-free cytoplasm; resemble transitional urothelial cells, particularly beneath paralumenal columnar cell layer; uniform cells, intact ductal basement membrane, absent mitoses, absence of focal necrosis
Prostatoductal papillary hyperplasia		resembles ductal papilloma of female breast; uniform, delicate papillary fronds with thin fibrovascular stalks; epithelium has basal cell and superficial columnar cell layer: duct lumen distended with secretion; presence of a paralumenal columnar cell layer; lesion may be precancerous associated with papillary prostatoductal carcinoma
Prostatoductal fibroadenoid hyperplasia		resembles miniature female mammary fibroadenoma; composed of broad polypoid, fibromuscular cores covered with double-layered ductal epithelium lining enclosing cavity; fibroepithelial masses protrude into lumen, a very early stage of nodular prostatic hyperplasia
Prostatoductal regenerative atypia (atypical hyperplasia or repair)		occurs as a result of acute inflammation or transurethral biopsy; similar to planophytic hyperplasia; paralumenal columnar cell layer may be focally deficient or inconspicuous, epithelium is thickened irregularly and infiltrated by acute inflammatory cells, often with intraepithelial microabscesses; goblet cells secreting acidic and neutral mucins are common; prominent inflammation in surrounding stroma, with focal interruption of epithelial basement membrane
Prostatoductal adenomatoid hyperplasia		common in prostate with ductal obstruction or inflammation; thickening of ductal epithelium, with proliferation into surrounding stroma in form of well-defined, circumscribed cell clusters resembling urothelial nests of von Brunn
Secondary (postatrophic hyperplasia)		hyperplasia of simple acinar atrophy (lobular postatrophic hyperplasia) or sclerotic atrophy (postsclerotic hyperplasia); budding of epithelium from atrophic acini ducts
Lobular hyperplasia		resembles lesion in female breast; small acini bud off periphery of an elongated central duct or alveolus in a clover-leaf pattern; stellate appearance in central lumen; uniformity of epithelial cell proliferation; orderly orientation of surrounding stroma, well-defined periacinar basement membranes, no tissue invasion

Table 5. (continued).

Pathology	Diagnostic and histological characteristics
Postsclerotic hyperplasia	resembles lobular hyperplasia but more irregular, acini surrounded by broad bands of sclerotic stroma, proliferating acini distorted contain mucinous secretion; sclerotic hyperplasia is more similar to carcinoma, than lobular hyperplasia, adenocarcinoma may develop in foci of postsclerotic hyperplasia, particularly those with atypical epithelium

of the prostate. Urine acid phosphatase is of no diagnostic value for it is of renal origin.

Acid phosphatase, secreted by prostatic cancer, can respond to anti-androgen manipulations. Normally, prostatic acid phosphatase is not transported to the bloodstream but may do so transiently as a consequence of prostatic massage or surgery. However, the appearance of the enzyme in blood is particularly remarkable during cancerous growth of the prostate and especially with osteoplastic metastases of prostatic carcinoma (Ahmed et al. 1979). The radioimmunoassay for acid phosphatase may be useful in detecting early stage lesions. The enzyme is further characterized by its virtually total inhibition by L-tartrate. Irrespective of elevation of acid phosphatase level or x-ray evidence of bony metastasis, the clinical diagnosis of prostatic carcinoma is confirmed by removal and pathological diagnosis of a needle or open biopsy.

Bone marrow aspiration, even of sternal bone marrow, in the absence of anemia is an important clinical adjunct in the detection of unexpected tumor dissemination. Bone marrow acid phosphatase may be helpful but its value will increase with frequent use of chemotherapy for advanced states of prostatic carcinoma. Serial evaluations in this instance may also be of value.

In most rodents, there are two acid phosphatases, one lysosomal in origin and the other secretory. Also the secretions of their ventral prostates but not their dorsal or anterior lobes contain alkaline phosphatase activity, as judged by histochemical criteria.

2. Zinc Both normal and hyperplastic human prostates contain approximately 0.8 mg of zinc/gm dry weight. Zinc is localized in the nucleus and cytoplasm of epithelial cells and in the secretion of various regions of the prostate. In hyperplastic prostate, zinc is found in high concentration, in the supranuclear and apical portions of the epithelium, and adjacent to the basement membrane of the basal cells. Except for the nucleolar portion of the nucleus the cells of prostatic carcinoma contain little or no zinc.

3. Hormone receptors The measurement of the estrogen receptors in breast cancer tissue has been used extensively for predicting responsiveness to endocrine or ablative treatment. Similar techniques have not yet been developed for prostate tumors (Geller 1978). A high affinity, low-capacity receptor protein is found in the rat and human prostate cytosol and purified nuclei (Geller et al. 1975, Hansson et al. 1971, Krieg et al. 1977b, Mainwaring and Milroy 1973, Menon et al. 1977, Rosen et al. 1975).

The measurement of androgen receptors in prostatic tissue may help in the treatment of prostatic carcinoma in similar way that measurement of estrogen and progesterone receptors in breast tissue helps predict therapeutic response in breast carcinoma (Menon et al. 1977).

DHT is found in significant amounts only in androgen target tissues. This selectivity is due to the requirements for 5α-reductase and the receptor which are critical for biological activity of androgens as indicated by some of nature's experiments, including male pseudohermaphroditism. Type II and testicular feminization, in which 5α-reductase in the former and cytosol receptor in the latter are virtually absent and prostate and male secondary sex structures are absent or ambiguous have been reported (Geller et al. 1978).

4. Antigen The development of an effective radioimmunoassay for carcinoembryonic antigen may potentially have the ability to identify patients with unsuspected prostatic cancer and help follow their clinical course (Reynoso et al. 1972). For example, CEA can be assayed to a measurable degree in the urine. The decline in this tumor-associated antigen has been clinically associated with chemotherapeutic response in other advanced disease states.

F. Endocrine profile

Serum levels of 5α-dihydrotestosterone and 17α-hydroxyprogesterone are higher in BPH patients than in normal age-matched controls (Chisholm and Ghanadian 1976, Vermeulen and De Sy 1976). This trend is noted in the serum level of progesterone and testosterone in the older PBH patients. There are no differences in the levels of pregnenolone, androstenedione, androsterone and estradiol between normal subjects and patients with BPH or prostatic carcinoma (Hammond et al. 1978).

Tissue dihydrotestosterone and 5α-reductase (^{k4}-3-ketosteroid-5α-oxidoreductase) levels were measured in prostates of patients with cancer and benign prostatic hypertrophy. There was a significant decrease in average values for both of these biochemical parameters in prostate cancer compared to benign prostatic hypertrophy (Geller et al. 1978). Prostate cancer tissue dihydrotestosterone levels appeared to correlate better than did either histological tumor grading or 5α-reductase with the ultimate clinical response to antiandrogen therapy.

5α-dihydrotestosterone which greatly accumulates in BPH tissues (Siiteri and Wilson 1970), may be responsible for the remarkable growth associated with this disease (Gloyna et al. 1970). This accumulation of 5α-dihydrotestosterone in BPH tissues is associated with a decrease in the levels of its further metabolites (Geller et al. 1976, Hammond 1978). 5α-dihydrotestosterone and testosterone also accumulate in prostatic carcinoma tissues when compared to normal controls (Habib et al. 1975). Except for inconsistent changes in prolactin and LH the levels of gonadotropins and steroids are similar in patients with newly diagnosed cancer of the prostate and comparable aged controls (Adler et al. 1968, Shirai et al. 1974, Stearns et al. 1974, Harper et al. 1976, Bartsch et al. 1977, Hammond et al. 1977b).

Serum levels of FSH, LH and testosterone are not affected by benign prostatic carcinoma whereas urinary excretions and serum estrone levels are elevated in BPH patients (Skoldefors et al. 1978).

VI. APPROACHES TO DRUG THERAPY

There have been remarkable advances in the therapeutic approaches to prostatic carcinoma, primarily due to (a) the improvement in the system of classification; (b) the availability of new diagnostic methods and a clearer understanding of the natural history of the tumor; (c) the development of new surgical techniques; and (d) the evolution of hormonal therapy, radiotherapy and chemotherapy. Several accurate but noninvasive staging technics have been also employed, e.g., ultrasonography, computerized tomographic scanning, lymphography and pelvic lymphadenectomy. Hormonal therapy and chemotherapy have been very controversial.

In general some 30 per cent of the new cases are potentially curable when first discovered. Treatment designed to cure these patients is being provided to only a fraction of the potentially curable ones.

A. Hormonal therapy

Since androgens are necessary for the development and maintenance of the prostate and since androgens stimulate the growth of prostatic carcinoma, the removal of the main source of androgen (testes) together with estrogen therapy are beneficial in the control of prostatic carcinoma. If tumors respond, the cells show vacuolization of cytoplasm with 'ballooning' condensation of nuclear chromatin.

Some 60 to 80 per cent of prostate cancer patients will experience improvement of disease status subsequent to orchiectomy and/or estrogen therapy (Shain et al. 1978). However, both the duration and quality of response are unpredictable (Arduino et al. 1967, Fergusson 1972). Medical adrenalectomy (Robinson et al. 1974), surgical adrenalectomy (Mahoney and Harrison 1972, Schoonees et al. 1972) or hypophysectomy (Fergusson and Hendry 1971, Murphy et al. 1971, Silverberg 1977), causes primarily subjective improvement of disease in 35 to 50 per cent of patients in relapse because of failure of primary endocrine therapy

(Shain et al. 1978). In general, the duration of favorable response to secondary endocrine therapy is of limited duration. In a well-controlled investigation by the Veterans Administration Cooperative Urological Research Group on stage D, prostatic carcinoma, placebo was compared to diethylstilbestrol in doses of 0.2, 1.0 or 5.0 mg per day. There was statistically significant improvement in survival among patients receiving 1.0 and 5.0 mg per day, as compared to the groups given placebo or 0.2 mg per day.

The regression of tumor growth due to estrogen treatment is associated with decrease in plasma levels of LH, FSH, and testosterone to a degree and for a period of time that depends upon the drug used, its dosage and duration of treatment. Estrogens increase the entry and uptake of androgens in human prostatic tissue (Giorgi et al. 1972, Giorgi et al. 1974). There is also a rapid, sustained increase in plasma prolactin and GH, hormones that can stimulate testosterone production by the adrenal and testes and can promote the trophic action of testosterone in the prostate. Prolactin increases after estrogen therapy. Variations in clinical course before and after endocrine therapy can be related to the histologic grade of the primary tumor. The failure of endocrine therapy may be due to: (a) the absence of a reliable prognostic index that would identify hormone responsive prostate adenocarcinoma, and (b) insufficient ablation of endocrine function (Fergusson and Hendry 1971, Prout et al. 1976). A rational approach to therapy for endocrine related cancers requires the repeated estimation of the endocrine profile during the course of treatment.

B. Chemotherapy

Several innovative chemotherapeutic agents have been employed to tumors which did not respond to hormonal therapy, e.g. estramustine phosphate, a conjugate of estradiol with nitrogen mustard (mechlorethamine hydrochloride).

Other therapeutic agents are being evaluated under the auspices of the National Prostatic Cancer Project, such as 5-fluorouracil, cyclophosphamide and streptozotocin (streptozocin).

VII. ANIMAL MODELS

The recent development of tumor models in various animal species will lead to significant research into the physical, biochemical and biological processes of prostatic carcinoma.

A. Monkey

There are noted similarities between the physiomorphology of the prostate in man and the nonhuman primate, Macaca mulatta.

In the monkey, Macaca mulatta, the prostate lies entirely on the dorsal aspect of the urethra below the neck of the bladder and two discrete lobes are apparent. The cranial lobe has a lobulated surface and is closely applied to the seminal vesicles; it completely surrounds the vesicular ducts and the distal ends of the deferent ducts in the same way as the central zone of the human prostate (McNeal, 1968). The caudal lobe of the monkey prostate, again located mainly on the dorsal aspect of the urethra, has ducts which connect the urethra caudal to the entrance of the ejaculatory ducts as for the ducts of the peripheral zone in man (McNeal 1972).

B. Dog

Prostatic adenocarcinoma seems to be less common in dogs than in man. This neoplastic condition is strikingly similar in both species (Leav and Ling 1968). Adenocarcinoma of the canine prostate occurs almost exclusively in aged dogs; it arises only in intact animals; and it frequently metastasizes to regional lymph nodes and bone. Meanwhile, human and canine neoplastic prostate cells have similar histochemical characteristics (Leav and Ling 1968).

In spite of the histological and ultrastructural differences, there are several similarities in the development of BPH in the dog and in man (Mahwinney and Belis 1976). In aging dogs as in man, benign and malignant growths develop in the prostate. The dog prostate, but not that of many other animal species, reacts to certain steroids the same as the human prostate.

C. Rat

In rodents, there are regional differences among various lobes of the prostate in the fine structure of cytoarchitectural and enzymorphologic response to hormonal therapy (Brandes and Groth 1963). In the rat, the prostate is less homogeneous and consists of ventral, dorso-lateral and cranio-dorsal entities which cannot be immediately identified with homologous structures in man. The prostate of rodents is similar to the cranial lobe of the monkey, as judged by the anatomical relationship of the cranial-dorsal lobe and its secretion in causing coagulation of seminal vesicular fluid.

In the rat the ventral prostate has exceptionally high galasctosyltransferase activity. Except for the ventral prostate, other accessory organs have much lower fucosyltransferase activity (Reddi et al. 1976). The tissue enzymes are membrane bound from which they are readily activated by non-ionic detergents. Rat and human prostatic secretions contain high activities of these enzymes. In the rat prostate there are synergistic effects of estrogens upon the action of androgens (Grayhack 1965, Karr et al. 1975, Lee et al. 1975, Walvoord et al. 1976).

REFERENCES

Adler A, Burger H, Davis J, Dulmanis A, Hudson B, Sarfaty G, Straffon W: Carcinoma of prostate: Response of plasma luteinizing hormone and testosterone to oestrogen therapy. Br Med J 1: 28, 1968.

Ahmed D, Goueli S, Steer RC, Wilson MJ: Functional biochemistry of male accessory glands. In: Male accessory organs, Spring-Mills E, Hafez ESE, eds. Ann Arbor: Ann Arbor Science, 1979.

Anderson WAD: Pathology, 6th Ed. St. Louis: CV Mosby 1971.

Aragona A, Friesen HG: Specific prolactin binding sites in the prostate and testis of rats. Endocrin 97: 677, 1975.

Arduino LJ, Bailar JC III, Becker LE, et al: Carcinoma of the prostate: treatment comparisons. J Urol 98: 516, 1967.

Arias-Stella J, Takano-Moron J: Atypical epithelial changes in the seminal vesicle. Arch Pathol 66: 761, 1958.

Armenian HK, Lilienfeld AM, Diamond EL, Bross IDJ: Epidemiologic characteristics of patients with prostatic neoplasms. Am J Epidemiol 102: 47, 1975.

Bagley DH, Javadpour N, Witebsky FG, Thomas LB: Seminal vesicle cyst containing mesonephroid tumor. Urology 5: 147, 1975.

Barkey RJ, Shani J, Amit T, Barzilai D: Specific binding of prolactin to seminal vesicle, prostate and testicular homogenates of immature, mature and aged rats. J. Endrocrinol 74: 163, 1977.

Bartsch W, Horst H-J, Becker H, Nehse G: Sex hormone binding globulin binding capacity, testosterone, 5α-dihydrotestosterone, oestradiol and prolactin in plasma of patients with prostatic carcinoma under various types of hormonal treatment. Acta Endocrinol 85: 650, 1977.

Baynard F: Testosterone and 17β-oestradiol production rate in the aging man. Acta Endocrinol 73 (Supp): 121, 1973.

Belter LF, Dodson AI Jr: Papillomatosis and papillary adenocarcinoma of prostatic ducts: a case report. J Urol 104: 880, 1970.

Brandes D, Groth DP: Functional ultrastructure of rat prostatic epithelium. In: National cancer institute monograph, no. 12, biology of the prostate and related tissues, Vollmer EP, Kauffmann G eds. Bethesda, Maryland: Natl Cancer Inst, 1963, pp 47.

Brandes D, Kirchheim D, Scott WW: Ultrastructure of the human prostate: normal and neoplastic. Lab Invest 13: 1541, 1964.

Bremner WJ: Endocrine pathogenesis of BPH. Highlights in Androl 2: 3, 1979.

Bruchovsky N, Lesser B: Control of proliferative growth in androgen responsive organs and neoplasma. In: Cellular mechanisms modulating gonadal hormone action, Singhal RL, Thomas JA eds, Advances in sex hormone research vol. 2. Baltimore: University Park Press, 1976, p 1.

Byar DP: Zinc in male sex accessory organ. In: Distribution and hormonal response in male accessory sex organs: structure and function in mammals, Brandes D, ed. New York: Academic Press, 1974, pp 161.

Cavanaugh AH, Farnsworth WE: Receptor sites on human prostate tissue for prostaglandin $F_{2\alpha}$. Life Sci 21: 83, 1977.

Chang HL, Char GY: Benign hypertrophy of the prostate. Chinese Med J 50: 1707, 1936.

Chisholm GD, Ghanadian R: Comparison between the changes in serum 5α-dihydrotestosterone and testosterone in normal men and patients with benign prostatic hypertrophy. Hamburg: Vth Intl Congress Endocrinol, 1976, Abst 455.

Chiu CL, Weber DL: Prostatic carcinoma in young adults. J Am Med Assoc 230: 724, 1974.

Duffield TJ, Jacobson PH: Cancer mortality and marital status: an analysis of deaths attributed to cancer among the white population of New York City during 1939-1941. J Nat Cancer Inst 6: 103, 1975.

El-Badawi A: Pathology part I: nonproliferative diseases. In: Accessory glands of the male reproductive tract, Spring-Mills E, Hafez ESE, eds. Ann Arbor Michigan: Ann Arbor, Science, 1979a.

El-Badawi A: Pathology part II: Proliferative lesions and neoplasms. In: Accessory glands of the male reproductive tract, Spring-Mills E, Hafez ESE eds. Ann Arbor, Michigan: Ann Arbor Science, 1979b.

Eliasson R, Lindholmer C: Zinc in human seminal plasma. Andrologia 3: 147, 1971.

Eliasson R, Lindholmer C: Functions of male accessory genital organs. In: Human semen and fertility regulation in men. Hafez ESE, ed. St. Louis: CV Mosby, 1976.

Farnsworth WD, Wilks J: Prostaglandin $F_{2\alpha}$ and human prostatic affinity for testosterone. Prostaglandins 9: 67, 1975.

Farnsworth WE: Physiology and biochemistry. In: Scientific foundations of urology. Williams DI, Chesholm GD eds. Chicago: W Heinemann Med Publ, 1976.

Fergusson JD, Hendry WF: Pituitary irradiation in advanced carcinoma of the prostate: analysis of 100 cases. Br J Urol 43: 514, 1971.

Fergusson JD: Castration and oestrogen therapy. In: Endocrine therapy in malignant disease. Stoll BA ed. London: B Saunders Company, 1972, p 247.

Fisher ER, Jeffrey W: Ultrastructure of human normal and neoplastic prostate. With comments relative to prostatic effects of hormonal stimulation in the rabbit. Am J Clin Pathol 44: 119, 1965.

Franks LM: Atrophy and hyperplasia in the prostate proper. J Pathol Bacteriol 68: 617, 1954a.

Franks LM: Latent carcinoma of the prostate. J Pathol Bact 68: 603, 1954b.

Geller J, Cantor T, Albert J: Evidence for a specific dihydrotestosterone binding cytosol receptor in the human prostate. J Clin Endocrinol Metab 41: 854, 1975.

Geller J, Albert J, Lopez D, Geller S, Niwayama G: Comparison of androgen metabolites in benign prostatic hypertrophy (BPH) and normal prostate. J Clin Endocrin Metab 43: 686, 1976.

Geller J, Albert J, Vega D de la, Loza D, Stoeltzing W: Dihydrotestosterone concentration in prostate cancer tissue as a predictor of tumor differentiation and hormonal dependency. Cancer Res 38: 4349, 1978.

Geller J: Differentiation of prostate cancer. In: Steroid receptors and the management of cancer, Thompson EB, Lippman M. eds. Cleveland: CRC Press, 1978.

Geller J, Albert J, Loza D, Geller S, Stoeltzing W: DHT concentrations in human prostate cancer tissue. J Clin Endocrinol Metab 46: 440, 1978.

Giorgi EP, Stewart JC, Grant JK, Shirley IM: Androgen dynamics in vitro in the human prostate gland. Biochem J 126: 107, 1972.

Giorgi EP, Moses T, Grant JK: Androgen dynamics in vitro in the prostate gland. J Endocrinol 61: 17, 1974.

Gleinster TW: The development of the utricle and the so-called 'middle' or 'median' lobe of the human prostate. J Anat 96: 443, 1962.

Gloyna RE, Siiteri PK, Wilson JD: Dihydrotestosterone in prostatic hypertrophy. II. The formation and content of DHT in the hypertrophic canine prostate and the effect of DHT on prostatic growth in the dog. J Clin Invest 49: 1746, 1970.

Gorski J, Gannon F: Current models of steroid hormone action: a critique. Annu Rev Physiol 38: 425, 1976.

Grayhack JT: Effect of testosterone-estradiol administration on citric acid and fructose content on the rat prostate. Endocrinol 77: 1068, 1965.

Gyorkey F, Min K-W, Huff JA, Gyorkey P: Zinc and magnesium in human prostate gland: normal, hyperplastic and neoplastic. Cancer Res 27: 1348, 1967.

Gyorkey F, Sato CS: In vitro ^{65}Zn-binding capacities of normal, hyperplastic, and carcinomatous human prostate gland. Exptl Mol Path 8: 216, 1968.

Habib FK, Stitch SR: The interrelationship of the metal and androgen binding proteins in normal and cancerous human prostatic tissues. Acta Endocrinol Suppl 199: 129, 1975.

Habib FK, Hammond GL, Stitch SR, Dawson JB: Testosterone, dihydrotestosterone, zinc and cadmium in prostatic tissue. J Endocrin 65: 340, 1975.

Habib FK, Hammond GL Lee IR, Dawson JB, Masson MK, Smith PH, Stitch SR: metal-androgen interrelationships in carcinoma and hyperplasia of the human prostate. J Endocrinol 71: 133, 1976a.

Habib FK, Lee IR, Stitch SR, Smith PH: Androgen levels in the plasma and prostatic tissues of patients with benign prostatic hypertrophy and carcinoma of the prostate. J Endocrinol 71: 99, 1976b.

Hafez ESE, ed: Human semen and fertility regulation in men. St. Louis: CV Mosby, 1976.

Hammond GL, Kontturi M, Maattala P, Puukka M, Vihko R: Serum FSH, LH and prolactin in normal males and patients with prostatic diseases. Clin Endocrinol 7: 129, 1977a.

Hammond GL, Ruokonen A, Kontturi M, Koskela E, Vihko R: The simultaneous radioimmunoassay of seven steroids in human spermatic and peripheral venous blood. J Clin Endocrin Metab 45: 16, 1977b.

Hammond GL: Endogenous levels of eight steroids in human prostatic tissues from birth to old age: a comparison of normal and diseased tissues. J Endocrin 1978.

Hammond GL, Kontturi M, Vihko P, Vihko R: Serum steroids in normal males and patients with prostatic diseases. Clin Endocrinol 9: 113, 1978.

Hansson V, Tveter KJ, Attramadal A, Torgersen O: Androgenic receptors in human benign nodular prostatic hyperplasia. Acta Endocrinol 68: 79, 1971.

Harper ME, Peeling WB, Cowley T, Brownsey BG, Phillips MEA, Groom G, Fahmy DR, Griffiths K: Plasma steroid and protein hormone concentrations in patients with prostatic carcinoma, before and during oestrogen therapy. Acta Endocrinol 81: 409, 1976.

Helminen JJ, Ericsson JLE, Rytolluoto R, Vanha-Perttula T: Acid phosphatases of the rat ventral prostate in normal and abnormal growth of the prostate. Goland M, ed. Springfield, Illinois: CC Thomas, 1975, pp 275.

Higgins ITT: The Epidemiology of Cancer of the Prostate. J Chron Dis 28: 343, 1975.

Horton R, Hsieh PC, Barberia J, Pages L, Cosgrove M: Altered blood androgens in elderly men with prostate hyperplasia. J Clin Endocrinol Metab 41: 793, 1975.

Huggins C, Stevens RA: The effect of castration of benign hypertrophy of the prostate in man. J Urol 43: 705, 1940.

Karr JP, Kirdani RY, Murphy GP, Sandberg A: Effects of testosterone and estradiol on ventral prostate and body weights of castrated rats. Life Sci 15: 501, 1975.

King RJB, Mainwaring WIP: Steroid-cell Interactions. Baltimore, MD: Univ Park Press, 1974.

Klein LA: Prostatic carcinoma. New Engl J Med 300: 824, 1979.

Krieg M, Barsch W, Herzer S, Becker H, Voight KD: Quantification of androgen binding, androgen tissue levels, and sex hormone binding globulin in prostate, muscle and plasma of patients with benign prostatic hypertrophy. Acta Endocrinol (Kbh) 86: 200, 1977a.

Krieg M, Bartsch W, Voigt KD: Androgen binding, metabolism and endogenous tissue levels in human benign prostatic hypertrophy (BPH) and normal prostate. Acta Endocrinol 85: 47, 1977b.

Lam KW, LI O, Li CY, Yam LT: Biochemical properties of human prostatic acid phosphatase. Clin Chem 19: 483, 1973.

Leav I, Ling GV: Adenocarcinoma of the canine prostate. Cancer 22: 1329, 1968.

LeClercq G, Heuson JC, Deboel MC, Mattheiem WH: Oestrogen receptors in breast cancer: a changing concept. Br Med J 1: 185, 1975.

Lee DKH, Bird CE, Clark AF In vivo metabolism of ^{3}H-testosterone in adult male rats: effects of estrogen administration. Steroids 26: 137, 1975.

Liao S, Fang S: Receptor-proteins for androgens and the mode of action of androgens on gene transcription in ventral prostate. Vitam and Horm 27: 17, 1969.

36

Liavag I: Carcinoma of the Prostate. Oslo: Universitetsforlaget, 1968. pp. 1-151.

Lindholmer C: Toxicity of zinc ions to human spermatozoa and the influence of albumin. Andrologia 6: 7, 1974.

Lytton B, Emery JM, Harvard BM: The incidence of benign prostatic hyperplasia. J Urol 99: 639, 1968.

Mahoney EM, Harrison JH: Bilateral adrenalectomy for palliative treatment of prostatic cancer. J Urol 108: 936, 1972.

Mahwinney MG, Belis JA: Estrogens in prostatic neoplasia. In: Cellular mechanisms modulating gonadal hormone action. Singhal R, Thomas JA, eds. Adv Horm Res 2: 141, 1976.

Mainwaring WIP, Milroy EJG: Characterization of the specific androgen receptors in the human prostate gland. J Endocrinol 57: 371, 1973.

Mainwaring WIP: The mechanism of action of androgens. New York: Springer-Verlag, 1977.

Makhyoun NA, Veenema RJ, Weshsler M: Microscopic foci of cancer in prostatectomy for benign disease: diagnostic and surgical considerations. Urology 9: 140, 1977.

Mann T: Biochemistry of semen and of the male reproductive tract. New York: John Wiley and Sons, 1964.

Mao P, Nakao K, Bora R, Geller J: Human benign prostatic hyperplasia. Arch Pathol 79: 270, 1965.

Mao P, Nakao K, Angrist A: Human prostatic carcinoma: an electron microscope study. Cancer Res 26: 955, 1966.

Marcus R, Korenman SG: Estrogens and the human male. Ann Rev Med 27: 357, 1976.

McGuire WL: Current status of estrogen receptors in human breast cancer. Cancer 36: 638, 1975.

McNeal JE: Regional morphology and pathology of the prostate. Amer J Clin Path 49: 347, 1968.

McNeal JE: The prostate and prostatic urethra: A morphologic synthesis. J Urol 107: 1008, 1972.

Meares EM Jr: Influence of infections of the male accessory glands on secretory function, sperm viability and fertility. In: Accessory glands of the male reproductive tract, Spring-Mills E, Hafez ESE, eds. Ann Arbor, Michigan: Ann Arbor Science, 1979.

Menon M, Tananis CE, McLoughlin MG, Lippman ME, Walsh PC: The measurement of androgen receptors in human prostatic tissue utilizing sucrose density centrifugation and a protamine precipitation assay. J Urol 117: 309, 1977.

Mikac-Davic D: Methodology of zinc determinations and the role of zinc in biochemical processes. Adv Clin Chem 13: 271, 1970.

Mobbs BG, Johnson IE, Connolly JG: High-affinity binding of androgen by human prostate. Proceedings of the Amer Assoc for Cancer Res 17: 9, 1976.

Moore RA: The evolution and involution of the prostate gland. Am J Pathol 12: 599, 1936.

Moore RA: Benign hypertrophy of the prostate: a morphological study. J Urol 50: 680, 1943.

Moore RA: Benign hypertrophy and carcinoma of the prostate: occurrence and experimental production in animals. Surger 16: 152, 1944.

Morfin RF, DiStefano S, Bercovici JP, Floch HH: Comparison of testosterone, 5α-dihydrotestosterone and 5β-androstane-3β, 17β-diol v metabolism in human normal and hyperplastic prostates. J Steroid Biochem 9: 245, 1978.

Mostofi FK: Benign hyperplasia of the prostate gland. In: Urology, vol 2, 3rd ed, Campbell MF, Harrison JH, eds. Philadelphia, London and Toronto: W.B. Saunders, 1970, p 1065.

Murphy GP, Reynoso G, Schoonees R, Gailani S, Bourke R, Kenny GM, Mirand EA, Schalch DS: Hypophysectomy and adrenalectomy for disseminated prostatic carcinoma. J Urol 105: 817, 1971.

Negro-Vilar AL: Effect of prolactin on male accessory organs. In: Male accessory organs, Spring-Mills E, Hafez ESE, eds. New York: Elsevier – North Holland, 1980.

Nielsen ML, Asnaes S, Hattel T: Inflammatory changes in the non-infected prostate gland: a clinical, microbiological and histological investigation. J Urol 110: 423, 1973.

Nomura Y, Kobayashi S, Takatani O, Sugano H, Matsumoto K, McGuire WL: Estrogen receptor and endocrine responsiveness in Japanese versus American breast cancer patients. Cancer Res 37: 106, 1977.

Offner P, Leav I, Cavzos LF: C$_{19}$-steroid metabolism in male accessory sex glands: correlation of changes in fine structure and radiometabolite patterns in the prostate of the androgen-deprived dog. In: Male accessory sex organs: structure and function in mammals, Brands K, ed. New York: Academic Press, 1974, pp 267.

Ostrowski W, Wasyl Z, Weber M, Guminska M, Luchter E: The role of neuraminic acid in the heterogeneity of acid phosphomonoesterase from the human prostate gland. Biochem Biophys Acta 221: 297, 1970.

Ozols RF, Hilf R: Effect of androgen on glucose-6-phosphate dehydrogenase isoenzyme in rat ventral prostate and seminal vesicles. Proc Soc Explt Biol Med 144: 73, 1973.

Polakoski KL, Zaneveld LJD: Biochemical examination of the human ejaculate. In: Techniques of human andrology, Hafez ESE, ed. Amsterdam: Elsevier – North Holland, 1977.

Pontes JE, Pierce JM Jr: Clinical and biochemical evaluation of the prostate. In: Techniques of human andrology, Hafez ESE, ed. Amsterdam: Elsevier – North Holland, 1977.

Prout GR JR, Kliman B, Daly JJ, MacLaughlin RA, Griffin PO, Young HH, II: Endocrine changes after diethylstilbestrol therapy. Effects on prostatic neoplasm and pituitary-gonadal axis. Urology 7: 148 (1976).

Quisenberry WB: Sociocultural factors in cancer in Hawaii. Ann NY Acid Sci 84: 794, 1960.

Randall A: Surgical pathology of prostatic obstruction. Baltimore: Williams and Wilkins, 1931.

Reddi PRK, Tadoline B, Wilson J, Williams-Ashman HG: Glycoprotein glycosyltransferases in male reproductive organs and their hormonal regulations. Nol Cell Endocrinol 5: 23, 1976.

Reynoso G, Chu TM, Guinan P, Murphy GP: Carcinoembryonic antigen in patients with tumors of the urogenital tract. Cancer 30: 1, 1972.

Robinson MRG, Shearer RJ, Fergusson JD: Adrenal suppression in the treatment of carcinoma of the prostate. Br J Urol 46: 555, 1974.

Rosen V, Jung I, Beaulieu EE, Robel P: Androgen-binding proteins in human benign prostatic hypertrophy. J Clin Endocrinol Metab 41: 761, 1975.

Sato CS, Gyorkey F: Further observations on the in vitro ^{65}Zn-binding sites of human prostatic tissues. Cancer Res 29: 399, 1969.

Schoonees R, Schalch DS, Reynoso G, Murphy GP: Bilateral adrenalectomy for advanced prostatic carcinoma J Urol 108: 123, 1972.

Scott R Jr, Mutchnik DL, Laskowski TZ, Schmalhorst WR: Carcinoma of the prostate in elderly men: incidence, growth characteristics and clinical significance. J Urol 101: 602, 1969.

Shain SA, Boesel RW, Lamm DL, Radwin HM: Characterization of unoccupied (R) and occupied (RA) androgen binding components of the hyperplastic human prostate. Steroids 31: 541, 1978.

Shelley HS, Auerbach SH, Classen KL, Marks CH, Wieder-anders RE: Carcinoma of the prostate: a new system of classification. Arch Surg 77: 751, 1958.

Shimazaki J, Kodama T, Wakisake M, Katayama T: Dihydro-testosterone binding protein in cytosol of normal and hyper-trophic prostates, and influence of estrogen and antiandro-gens on the binding. Endocrinol Japan 24: 9, 1977.

Shirai M, Matsuda S, Mitsukawa S, Nakamura M, Yonezawa K: Changes in plasma levels of FSH, LH and testosterone during anti-androgenic hormone therapy for patients with prostatic cancer. Tohoku J Exp Med 114: 145, 1974.

Siiteri PK, Wilson JD: Dihydrotestosterone in prostatic hyper-trophy. I. The formation and content of dihydrotestosterone in the hypertrophic prostate of man. J Clin Invest 49: 1737, 1970.

Silverberg GD: Hypophysectomy in the treatment of dissemi-nated prostate carcinoma. Cancer 29: 1727, 1977.

Skoldefors H, Blomstedt B, Carlstrom K: Serum hormone levels in benign prostatic hyperplasia. Scand J Urol Nephrol 12: 111, 1978.

Snochowski M, Pousette A, Ekman P, Bression D, Andersson L, Hogberg B, Gustafsson J-A: Characterization and measure-ment of the androgen receptor in human benign prostatic hyperplasia and prostatic carcinoma. J Clin Endocrinol Metab 45: 920 1977.

Stankova L, Drach GW, Hicks T, Zukoski CF, Chvapil M: Regulation of some functions of granulocytes by zinc of the prostatic fluid and prostate tissue. J Lab Clin Med 88: 640, 1976.

Stearns EL, MacDonnell JA, Kaufman BJ, Padua R, Lucman TS, Winter JSD, Faiman C: Declining testicular function with age. Hormonal and clinical correlates. Am J Med 57: 761, 1974.

Strott CA, Yoshimi T, Lipsett MB: Plasma progesterone and 17-hydroxyprogesterone in normal men and children with congenital adrenal phyperplasia. J Clin Invest 48: 930, 1969.

Takayasu H, Yamaguchi Y: An electron microscopic study of the prostatic cancer cell. J Urol 87: 935, 1962.

Tannenbaum M: Diagnostic criteria for histopathologic evalua-tion of prostatic tissue sections. Urology 5: 407, 1975.

Tavares AS, Costa J, Maia J: Correlation between ploidy and prognosis in prostatic carcinoma. J Urol 109: 676, 1973.

Thomas JA, Manandhar MSP: Effects of prolactin and/or testosterone on nucleic acid levels in prostate glands of normal and castrated rats. J Endocrinol 65: 149, 1975.

Vermeulen A, Rubens R, Verdonck L: Testosterone secretion and metabolism in male senescence. J Clin Endocrin Metab 34: 730, 1972.

Vermeulen A, DeSy W: Androgens in patients with benign prostatic hyperplasia before and after prostatectomy. J Clin Endocrin Metab 43: 1250, 1976.

Vermeulen A, Verdonck L: Radioimmunoassay of 17β-hydroxy-5α-androstan-3-one, 4-androstene-3, 17-dione, dehydroepi-androsterone, 17-hydroxy-progesterone and its application to human male plasma. J Steroid Biochem 7: 1, 1976.

Wallace AM, Grant JK: Effect of zinc on androgen metabolism in the human hyperplastic prostate. Biochem. Soc Trans 3: 540, 1975.

Walvoord DJ, Resnick MI, Grayback JT: Effect of testosterone, dehydrotestosterone, estradiol and prolactin on the weight and citric acid content of the lateral lobe of the rat prostate. Invest Urol 14: 60, 1976.

Whitmore WF: Comments on zinc in the human and canine prostates. Natl Cancer Inst Monogr 12: 337, 1963.

Williams-Ashman HG, Reddie AH: Androgenic regulation of tissue growth and function. In: Biochemical action of hor-mone, vol II, Litwack G, ed. New York: Academic Press, 1972, pp 257-294.

Williams-Ashman HG: Introductory overview of the participation of proteinases and their regulators in mammalia reproductive physiology. In: Proteases and biological control. Cold Spring Harbor Laboratory Symposium, 1975, pp 677-681.

Woo SLC, O'Malley BW: Minireview – hormone inducible messenger RNA. Life Sci 17: 1039, 1976.

Wynder EL, Mabuchi K, Whitmore WF Jr: Epidemiology of cancer of the prostate. Cancer 28: 344, 1971.

Yamamoto KR, Alberts BM: Steroid receptors: Elements for modulation of eukaryotic transcription. Annu Rev Biochem 45: 721, 1976.

Zuckermann S: The endocrine control of the prostate. Proc Roy Soc med 29: 1557, 1936.

3. PROSTATIC CYTOLOGY IN THE FOLLOW-UP OF PROSTATIC CARCINOMA

K. Bandhauer, P. Spieler, L. Schmid and H. Toggenburg

The judgement of biological activity of prostatic carcinoma at the time of primary diagnosis is the most important parameter for prognosis and applicability of different forms of therapy. So far there exists no specific test to determine the course of a prostatic carcinoma in advance, although the primary grade of differentiation seems to play an important role for the destiny of the tumor (Bandhauer 1979). Exact progress-checks are therefore necessary including rectal examination, enzyme studies (including radio-immuno-assay for prostatic acid phosphatase) bone scan - 99^m TC.PP. radiological skeletal studies and intravenous pyelography and especially to register the local effect of therapy on the tumor by cytologic studies. In 1960 Franzén et al. reported for the first time on the cytological primary diagnosis of carcinoma of the prostate with transrectal aspiration biopsy. Esposti (1971) found this method useful for the follow-up of hormone treated carcinoma of the prostate.

We were using the transrectal aspiration biopsy for cytological check up of prostatic carcinomas since 1972. 165 patients with Tumor-stage T_1-T_3, without any evidence of metastases, were cytologically followed after either hormonal or radiation therapy. (Not included in this group of patients are 26 patients with radical prostatectomies.) (Table 1)

The following therapies were applied:

1. *Radiotherapy.* Cobalt-60 high-voltage irradiation with crossfire technique. Dosage between 5.000 to 6.000 rad depending on the constitution of the patient and the clinical stage of the tumor.

2. *Hormone Therapy.* Primary orchiectomy followed by stilboestrol-diphosphate-Na (Honvan) from 6 to 12 g during a period of 10 days. After that, at regular intervals of 4 weeks, continuous therapy with 40 mg polyoestradiol-phosphate (Estradurin) i.m. and 1 mg stilboestrol/day. Aspiration biopsies were performed with the Franzén-needle. No anesthesia is necessary for this procedure.

Typical changes due to hormonal therapy were demonstrated in the cytological smear:

1.*Cytoplasm Changes* Whereas the cytoplasm (Figure 1A, B) of the primary carcinoma shows a honeycomb structure, we find in the cytoplasm of treated carcinomas multiple, large, bubble-like, empty vacuoles, which push the nucleus aside. Vacuoles of neighbouring cells melt into one another and the appropriate nuclei are often conglomerated.

2. *Regressive Changes* a) Changes on the Cell Clusters: (Figure 2A,B) Three stages can be differentiated cytologically during the degenerative process. The first stage results in a diminution of the carcinoma cell cluster through shrinkage of the cytoplasm and the nuclei. The cytoplasm tightens and the nucleoli reduce in volume. In the second stage the nuclei are tightly packed together, the chromatin is coarsely condensed and nucleoli can

Table 1. Summary of stage, grade and therapy of 165 patients followed by cytologic studies.

Stage	Grade		Therapy	
T_1 No Mo 18 Pat.	G_1	7	Radiation	No therapy
	G_2	5	15	3
	G_3	6		
T_2 No Mo 41 Pat.	G_1	8	Radiation	
	G_2	19	41	
	G_3	14		
T_3 No Mo 106 Pat.	G_1	18	Radiation hormon	
	G_2	35	54	52
	G_3	53		

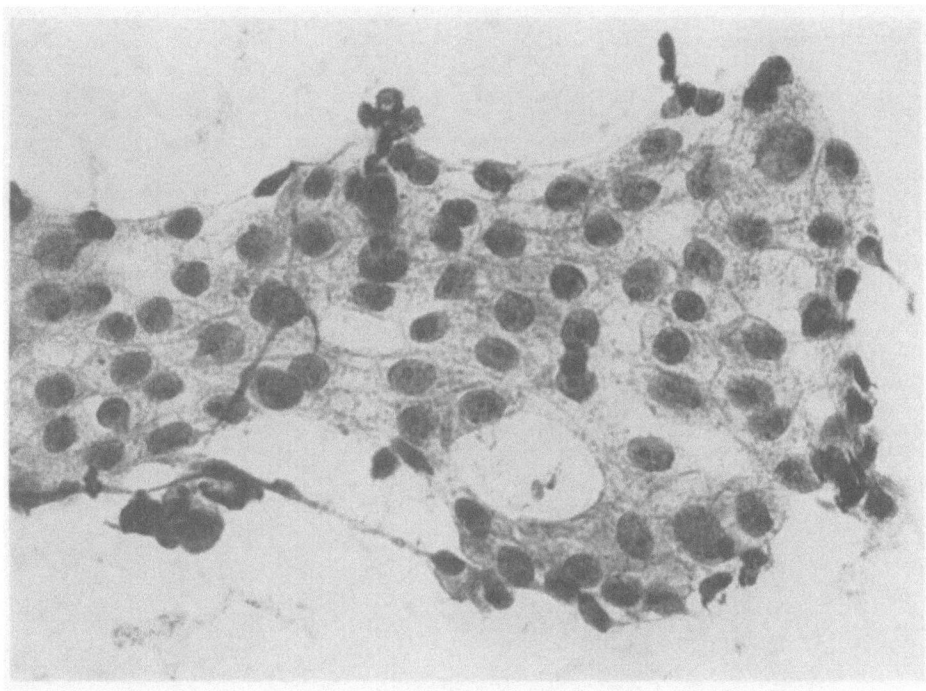

Figure 1A. Large empty vacuoles pushing the nuclei aside. Wet fixed smear, Papanicolaou-stained (× 400).

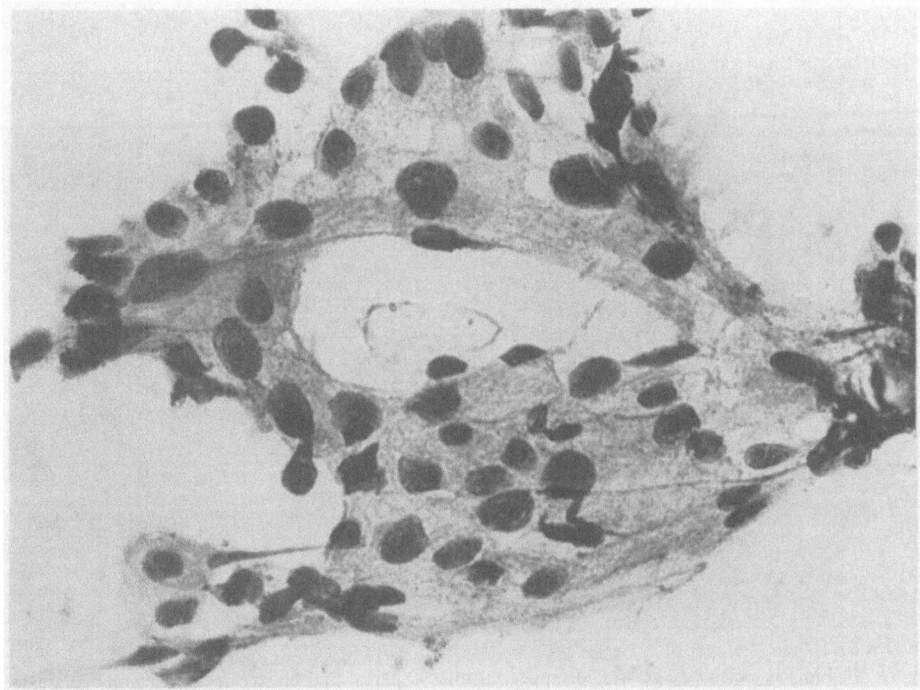

Figure1B. Melting of vacuoles of neighboring cells. Wet fixed smear, Papanicolaou-stained (× 400).

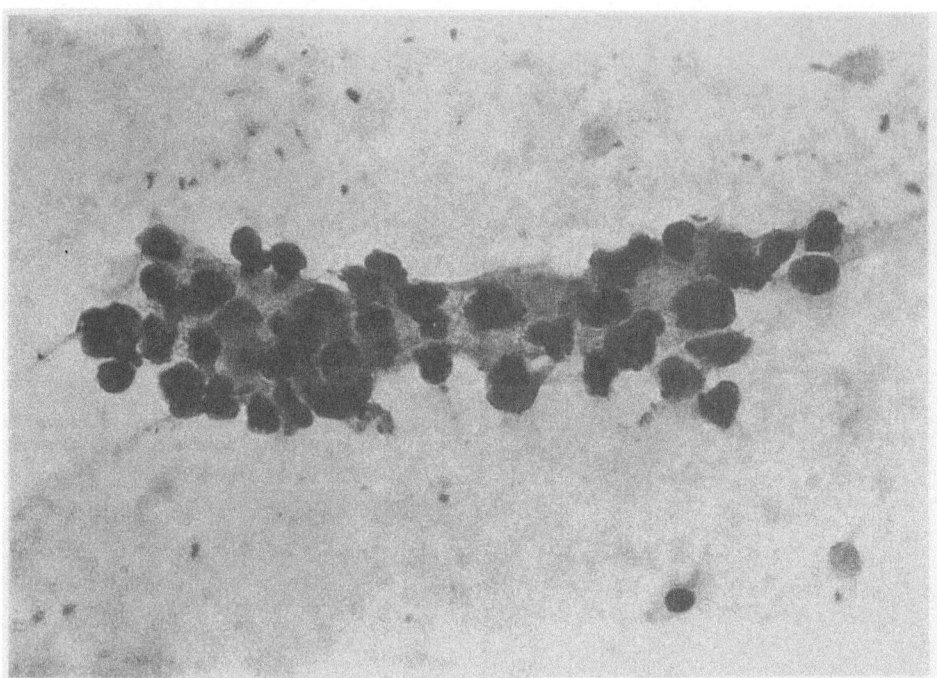

Figure 2A. Beginning regressive stage with shrinking of cytoplasm and nuclei. Wet fixed smear, Pap. stained (×400).

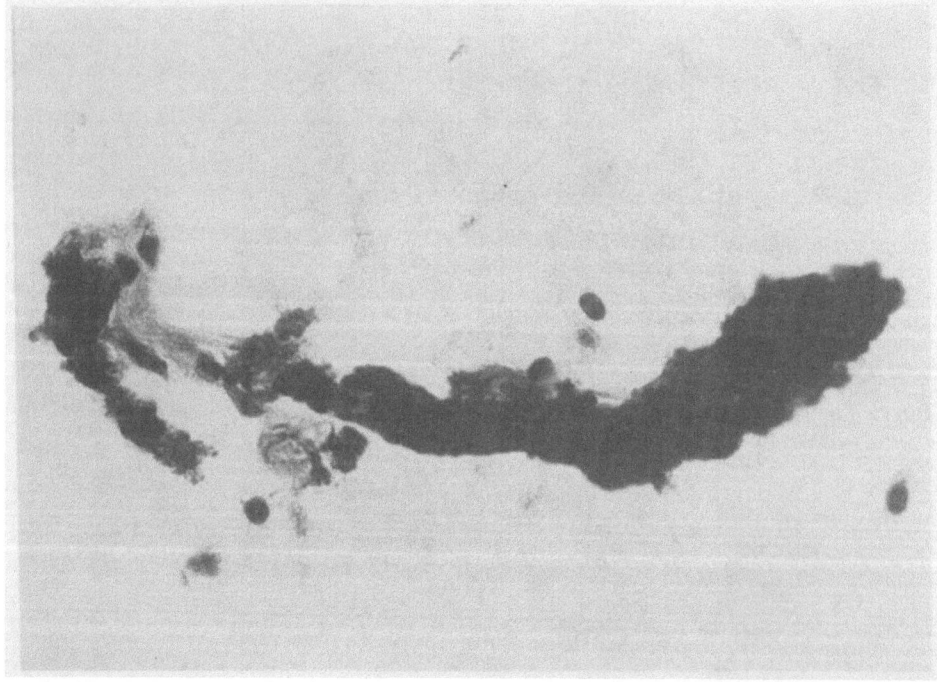

Figure 2B. Final regressive stage with disappearing of cytoplasm and clustering of the homogenously structured and hyperchromatic nuclei. Wet fixed smear, Pap. stained (×400).

only rarely be found. The nuclei are hyperchromatic and enclosed by a homogeneous mass of cytoplasm. In the third stage the greatly shrunken, homogeneous, blue violet-coloured nuclei lie clustered together. The cytoplasm has almost completely disappeared. In the second and third stage the cytological criteria of malignancy are no longer recognizable.

b) Giant Nuclei. (Figure 3) These are greatly enlarged nuclei which have conserved all criteria of malignancy. The nucleus may be lobulated and in the center vacuoles can often be observed.

c) Wasting of Nucleoli. Nuclear shrinkage and nuclear pyknosis take place simultaneously with disappearance of the nucleolus. In some cases changes in the nucleolus are a primary sign of nuclear degeneration. Compared to the findings on the primary tumor, the changes are characterized by diminution and bad coloration of the nucleolus.

3 *Benign Squamous-Cell Metaplasia.* (Figure 4) Squamous-cell metaplasia, as a result of estrogen therapy, is often found in cytological and histological specimens. After *radiation therapy* only karyolysis and karyorrhexis were observed. They practically always appear together with nuclear pyknosis and intact tumor cells.

To correlate the cytological findings and the clinical course after hormonal treatment 3 different types of local response to the different forms of therapy were distinguished:
1. Good response with at least 2 cytological parameters of regression.
2. Moderate response with 1 parameter of regression without signs of progressive malignancy.
3. Poor response without cytologic regression but with progressive malignancy.

After radiation therapy the appraisal of local therapy effect by cytologic studies is more difficult:
1. Good response - No visible tumor cells in the smear 1 year after radiation.
2. Moderate response - karyolysis and karyorrhexis in tumor cells.
3. Poor response - still visible normal tumor cells 1 year after radiation.

For further registration of the clinical course the primary grade of the tumor was recorded and increasing malignancy in the cytological smear gave rise to change of therapy.

For the primary diagnosis of prostatic carcinoma 3 different cytologic grades were distinguished:
Grade 1 = highly differentiated carcinoma (low malignancy)
Grade 2 = moderate differentiated carcinoma
Grade 3 = poorly differentiated carcinoma (high malignancy).

The clinical course which was judged by rectal examination, enzyme-studies, hormone-studies, bone scan and radiological examiniations was in highly significant correlation to the primary grade of the prostatic cancer and the cytological effect of therapy. (Table 2).

Table 2. Relation between cytologic effect and grade.

Stage	Response		
	Good	Moderate	Poor
G_1 (30 pat.)	20 (67%)	8 (26%)	2 (7%)
G_2 (59 pat.)	28 (47%)	16 (27%)	15 (26%)
G_3 (73 pat.)	27 (37%)	14 (19%)	32 (44%)

63% of the group with primarily high differentiated carcinoma showed according to clinical, biochemical and radiological parameters and according to the cytological effect a favorable course and a change of therapy was not necessary during the 3 years of observation. In 37% no or only negligible cytologic regressions were observed. In these cases a change of therapy was required. In this group of patients with primarily highly differentiated tumors the 3 years-death rate was 12%.

In the patient group with grade 2 tumors (moderately differentiated) a good course according to the above mentioned parameters was observed in only 47%, whereas the lack of cytologic regression and the rather poor clinical course required a change of therapy in 53%. The 3 years-death rate ran up to 21%.

In grade 3 tumors (high malignancy) a good course clinically and cytologically appeared in 38%. The death in 3 years of observation was 25%.

42

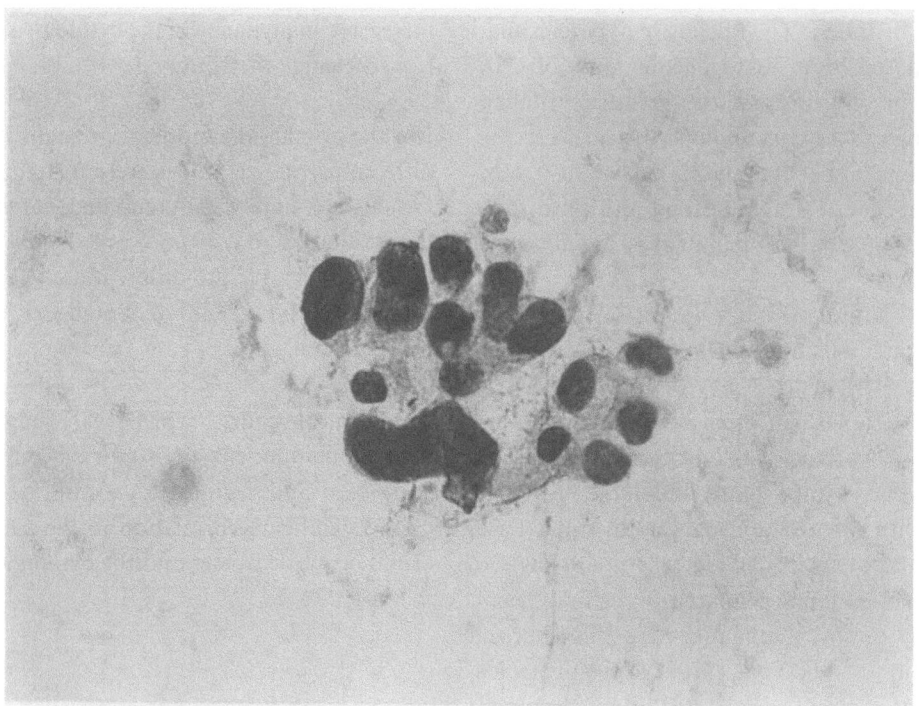

Figure 3. Enlarging, lobulation and vacuolization of nuclei. Criteria of malignancy are well preserved. Wet fixed smear. Pap. stained (×400).

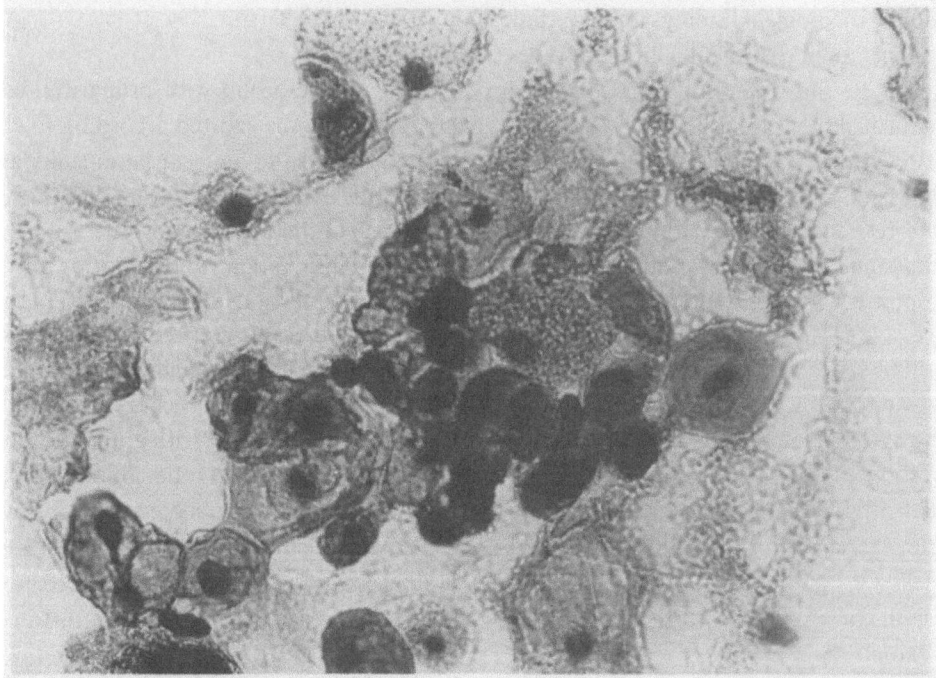

Figure 4. Change of prostatic glandular epithelium into metaplastic squamous epithelium. Wet fixed smear, Pap. stained (×400).

CONCLUSION

The transrectal aspiration biopsy and cytological follow up studies can be considered as a reliable method to judge the local therapeutic effect of hormonal and/or radiological treatment of prostatic carcinomas. The cytological regressive changes due to hormones or high voltage therapy are clearly visible to a trained cytologist.

Because the cytologically observed effect on the tumor cell is according to our studies in rather strong correlation to the further clinical course this evaluation offers important references for therapeutic measures.

Besides these facts the periodic cytologic progress checks gave good evidence that the result of either hormone therapy or high voltage radiation in prostatic carcinomas without metastases depends rather on the grade than on the form of therapy.

The aspiration biopsy and the cytological control is therefore an important and besides a harmless method for progress-checks of carcinoma of the prostate.

REFERENCES

Alken CE, Dhom G, Hohbach M, Sachse D, Schröder FH, Straube W: Therapie des Prostatacarcinoms und Verlaufskontrolle (I). Urologe A (Berl.) 11: 216-220, 1970.

Alken CE, Dhom G, Straube W, Schmidt-Hermes HJ, Moormann JG, Moeller JF: Therapie des Prostatacarcinoms und Verlaufskontrolle (II). Urologe A (Berl.) 12: 191-197, 1973.

Alken CE, Dhom G, Straube W, Braun JS, Kopper B, Rehker H: Therapie des Prostatacarcinoms und Verlaufskontrolle (III). Urologe A (Berl.) 14, 112-116 1975.

Bandhauer K, Spieler P and Egle N: Evaluation of prostatic cytology in primary diagnosis and clinical course of prostatic carcinoma. Prostatic disease-progress in clinical and biological research, Vol 6, Marberger H, Haschek H, Schirmer HKA, Colston JAC, Witkin E, p 329.

Bandhauer K: Histological grading of prostatic carcinoma and its clinical evaluation. Europ Urol 5.4.225, 1979.

Egle N, Spieler P: Zytologische und histologische Verlaufskontrollen beim hochvoltbestrahlten Prostatacarcinom. Helv Chir Acta 43, 337, 1976.

Esposti PL: Cytologic diagnosis of prostatic tumors with the aid transrectal aspiration biopsy. Acta cytol (Philad.) 10, 182-186, 1966.

Esposti PL: Cytologic malignancy grading of prostatic carcinoma by transrectal aspiration biopsy. Scand J Urol Nephrol 5, 199-205.

Faul P: Prostata-Zytologie. Dr. Dietrich Steinkoff Verl, Darmstadt, 1975.

Franzén S, Gierth G, Zajicek J: Cytological diagnosis of prostatic tumors by transrectal aspiration biopsy: a preliminary report. Brit J Urol 32, 193-196, 1960.

Kurth KH, Altwein JE, Skoluda D, and Hohenfellner R: Follow up of irradiated prostatic carcinoma by aspiration biopsy. J Urol 117, 615, 1977.

Leistenschneider W, and Nagel R: Zytologische Verlaufskontrolle beim behandelten Prostatacarcinom. Extr Urol 1,4, 389, 1978.

Spieler P, Gloor F, Egle N, and Bandhauer K: Cytological findings in transrectal aspiration biopsy on hormone- and radio-treated carcinoma of the prostate. Virchows Arch Pathol Anat and Histol 372, 149, 1976.

4. HISTOCHEMISTRY OF PROSTATIC CANCER AND STROMAL INVASION

D. KIRCHHEIM

I. INTRODUCTION

Histochemical techniques have the advantage of localizing enzymes and other important metabolic substances within the tissue and cells. Presently available histochemical methods have shown significant differences in the enzyme profile of the normal, hyperplastic and neoplastic human prostate. (Kirchheim et al. 1964, 1974, Brandes and Kirchheim 1977). Fundamental histochemical work had been done previously on animal prostates (Brandes and Bourne 1954, Brandes 1974). Electronmicroscopic studies have given us further insight into the fine structure of the cytoplasm of prostatic carcinoma in comparison to the normal prostate and benign nodular prostatic hyperplasia (BPH) (Brandes et al. 1964, Fisher and Jeffrey 1965, Mao et al. 1966, Tannenbaum et al. 1967, Kirchheim and Bacon 1969, Kastendieck and Altenähr 1976). Recently published histochemical studies on a rat adenocarcinoma with certain similarities to the human prostatic cancer appears to be a useful animal model for prostatic cancer (Müntzing et al. 1978).

The histological and cytological diagnosis of prostatic cancer does not give us reliable information as to the growth potential and prognosis of a patient with prostatic cancer. The histological incidence of prostatic cancer increases from approximately 10% in the sixth decade to over 40% in the ninth decade (Gaynor 1938, Franks 1954). Clinical prostatic cancer which will metastasize and eventually lead to the death of the patient has a much lower incidence (Ashley 1965, Halpert et al. 1963). Urologists and pathologists have developed a system of staging prostatic cancer according to the extent of the growth and depth of invasion. The American system of staging appears to be most practical as a guideline for the clinician and is summarized in Table 1 (Whitmore 1977). In addition many pathologists use a histological-cytological grading from 1 to 4. Grade 1 prostatic cancer characterizes the most differentiated degree of tumor. At the other end of the scale grade 4 describes a poorly differentiated anaplastic cancer, which shows only a few or hardly any similarities with the normal prostatic cancer cell.

The vast majority of stage A_1 microscopic, well-differentiated grade 1, focal carcinomas, which are only diagnosed *incidentally* by the pathologist at autopsy or in some BPH specimens, do not progress into metastatic cancer within the life span of the host. On the other hand most other stages including A_2 *diffuse* microcarcinoma appear to grow progressively and eventually metastasize. A_2 diffuse microscopic cancer is frequently more aggressive than Stage B nodular cancers. Many prostatic cancers (except Stage A_1) consist of variable aggressive tumor clones and the most aggressive part determines the prognosis (Shelley et al. 1958, Fidler 1978). A more sophisticated pathological evaluation, combining grading and staging, has given better guidelines for prognostication, but still has marked limitations (Mellinger 1977).

The dilemma for the patient and treating clinician is obvious: if the growth potential is misjudged, the patient may be inadequately treated and die from the cancer or undergo unnecessary radical prostatectomy, radiation or hormonal treatments.

The urgent need of reliable adjuncts in tissue diagnosis is evident. This chapter on histochemistry will review our present knowledge. Since patients suffer and die from prostatic cancer, more emphasis will be placed on work which has been or may be useful clinically.

Table 1. Staging of prostatic carcinoma.

Stage	Extent	Grade	Characteristics
A$_1$	Microscopic focal (carcinoma-in-situ)	1	incidentally found by pathologist in both specimens, not palpable, asymptomatic
A$_2$	microscopic, diffuse	1-4	
B$_1$	'palpable nodule' confined to prostate B$_1$ = less than 2 cm	1-3	asymptomatic, palpated rectally during physical exam or annual check-up, potentially curable
B$_2$	B$_2$ = greater than 2 cm usually both sides	rarely 4	by total prostatectomy or high dosage radiation treatment
C$_1$	locally extended into periprostatic region	2-4	rectally palpable, frequently symptomatic, potential control by high dosage radiation treatment.
C$_2$	locally extended and/or into regional (pelvic) lymphnodes	rarely 1	regional spread
D	distant metastases distant nodes, bones, soft tissues and organs	2-4 rarely 1	metastatic systemic disease

II. HISTOCHEMISTRY OF PROSTATIC CANCER CELLS

A. Acid phosphatase

The activity of acid phosphatase is much higher in the secretory cells and secretions of the prostate than in cells such as the tubular cells of the kidney, liver cells, spleen, leukocytes, erythrocytes, platelets and others. The biochemistry, substrate specificities and inhibitions have been extensively investigated (Sodeman and Batsakis 1977). These tissues and the prostate gland contain two or more molecular variants (isoenzymes) of acid phosphatase (Lam 1973, Moncure 1977). Histochemical demonstration of acid phosphatase was one of the first enzyme histochemical techniques (Gomori 1941). Different acid phosphatase techniques were developed later (Table 2). Light and electronmicroscopy histochemistry shows a fine precipitate of acid phosphatase in the supranuclear cytoplasm and luminar secretion of prostate epithelial cells (Figure 1A). The secretion appears to be mediated through the Golgi cysternae, which pinch off Golgi associated vesicles and then migrate as secretory vacuoles towards the lumen, fuse with the membrane (exocytosis) and then secrete their contents into the acinar lumen (Figure 2) by merocrine secretion (Helminen and Ericsson 1971).

Prostatic cancer electronmicroscopic studies show progressive structural and functional disorganization and abnormalities proportional to the degree of de-differentiation (Kirchheim et al. 1974; Kastendieck and Altenähr 1976). Well-differentiated prostatic cancer exhibits high activities of acid phosphatase (Figures 5A, 6B). The secretory vacuoles empty into simple or distorted lumina which do not connect with the excretory ductal system. Less differentiated invasive prostatic cancer cells contain less acid phosphatase, but can still be recognized in metastatic lesions as of prostatic origin due to their positive prostatic acid phosphatase reaction (Figures 1B, 5A, 5D, 6C, 6D).Their secretory vacuoles empty their contents into the surrounding interstitial spaces which are absorbed through lymphatics and get access to the blood stream (Figures 2B through 4). Acid phosphatase was found to be elevated in the serum of patients with metastatic prostatic cancer over 40 years ago (Gutman and Gutman, 1938). This and the pioneer work of Huggins, Hodges and Scott

Table 2. Histochemistry of prostatic acid phosphatase.

A. Frozen sections:
1. lead sulfide (Gomori)
2. azo dye coupling (Burstone, Barka, Rutenburg, Seligman)
3. indirect immunofluorescence (Pontes et al.)
B. Paraffin embedded sections:
   Immuno-histochemistry
1. enzyme-labelled antibody techniques (Nakamura)
2. unlabelled antibody enzyme methods (Mason, Sternberger)

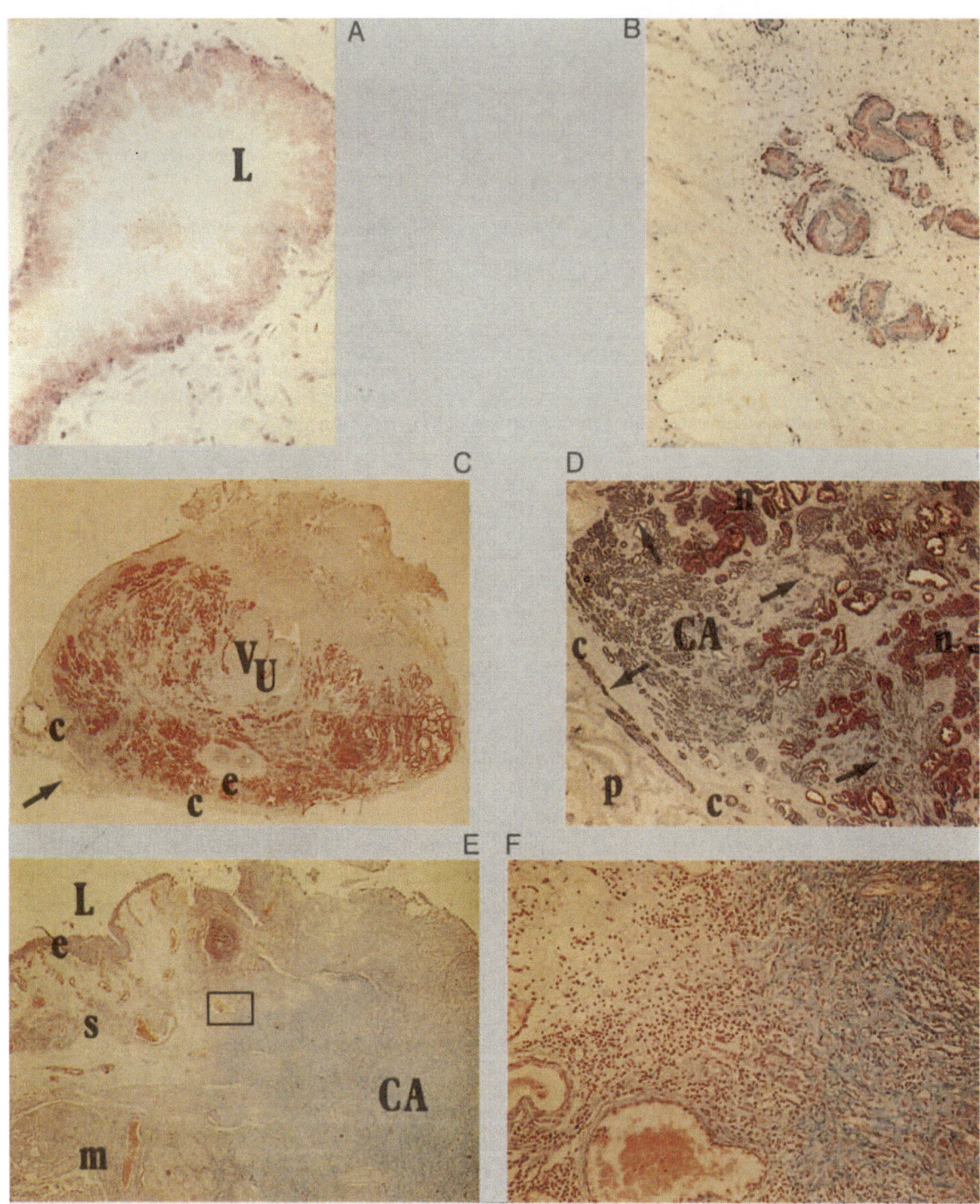

Figure 1A (top, left). Normal prostatic acinus. Acid phosphatase, Burstone method, hematoxylin nuclear counterstain (×690). Fine purple precipitate in cytoplasm of all acinar epithelial cells, predominantly between nucleus and luminar border. Also residual acid phosphatase in acinar lumen (L). No significant staining in surrounding fibromuscular stroma.

Figure 1B (top,right). Invasive grade 2-3 prostatic adenocarcinoma in periprostatic connective tissue. Acid phosphatase, Burstone method, hematoxylin nuclear counterstain (×345). fine purple precipitate present in cytoplasm of all cancer cells, moderate intensity. Prostatic cancer cells can be easily identified by acid phosphatase staining.

Figure 1C (center, left). Complete transverse cryostat section of prostate gland at level of verumontanum (V). Radical Prostatectomy specimen of clinical and pathological stage B_1 cancer. At this level there is only a small cancer area at the left posterior periphery (arrow) adjacent to the true capsule (c) of the prostate gland. U = Urethra. e = ejaculatory ducts. Aminopeptidase, method of Nachlas et al..

introduced hormonal treatment of prostatic cancer (Huggins and Hodges 1941). Until recently only about a third of patients with metastatic prostatic cancer showed serum acid phosphatase elevations by biochemical colorimetric methods (Murphy et al. 1969). Early curable prostatic cancer, which is usually rich in acid phospptase (Fig. 5D), does not show elevated serum acid phosphatase by these conventional colorimetric methods.

Recently developed highly sensitive methods by radioimmuno-assay for serum acid phosphatase have shown elevated values even in localized, curable prostatic cancer (Chu et al. 1978, Foti et al. 1977, Cooper et al. 1978). Similar results have been reported with counter-electroimmunophoresis (Chu et al. 1978, Romas et al. 1978, Drucker et al. 1978, McDonald et al. 1978). These immunological methods are supposed to be specific for prostatic acid phosphatase and much more sensitive than the previous colorimetric methods (Yam 1974, Cooper et al. 1978).

At about the same time, immuno-histochemical methods for acid phosphatase were elaborated (Jöbsis et al. 1978, Pontes et al. 1977, Li et al. 1979). These immunological techniques appear to be specific for prostatic acid phosphatase except for weak reactions of the same enzyme in islet cells of the pancreas and granulocytes. Histochemistry and immuno-histochemistry have found clinical applications and usefulness in diagnosing metastatic cancer tissues of unknown origin. Metastatic pros-

tatic cancers show positive acid phosphatase reaction with the exception of rare anaplastic tumors. Immuno-histochemistry may also become helpful in staging of prostatic cancer. Aspirates of bone marrow can be stained by immuno-histochemistry for acid phosphatase, and if positive tumor cells are found, the patient has metastatic prostatic cancer. This would be very important from the standpoint of treatment (Jöbsis et al. 1978, Li et al. 1979). While histochemical techniques have to be done on frozen sections, immuno-histochemical methods can be done on conventional paraffin embedded tissue (Figures 6A-D).

B. Aminopeptidases

Aminopeptidases are a group of peptidases which act against the terminal amino groups of peptides with the liberation of the amino-acid with a free amino group. Activities of leucine aminopeptidase were first measured by using synthetic substrates, e.g. L-leucyl glycine or L-Leucyl-b-naphthyl-amide (Goldbarg and Rutenberg 1958). The enzymatic reaction is as follows:

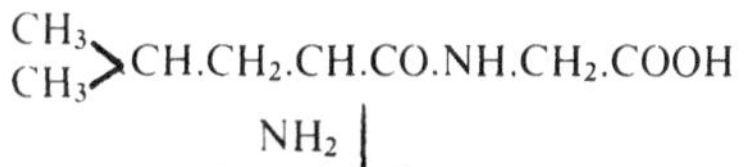

$$\begin{array}{c} CH_3 \\ CH_3 \end{array}\!\!>\!\!CH.CH_2.CH.CO.NH.CH_2.COOH$$
$$NH_2 \,|$$
L-Leucylglycine

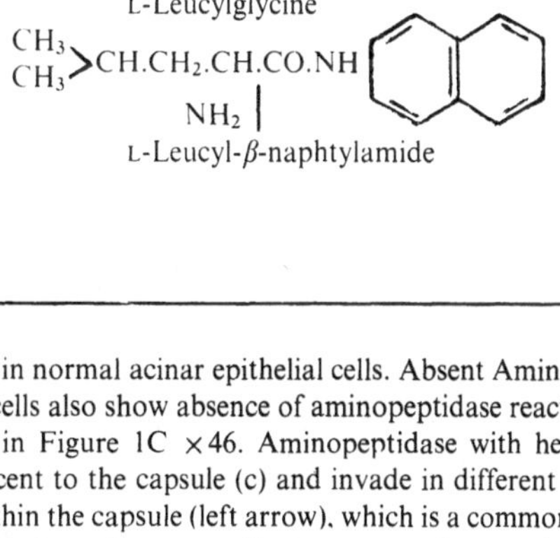

$$\begin{array}{c} CH_3 \\ CH_3 \end{array}\!\!>\!\!CH.CH_2.CH.CO.NH$$
$$NH_2 \,|$$
L-Leucyl-β-naphtylamide

hematoxylin nuclear counterstain. Strong aminopeptidase reaction in normal acinar epithelial cells. Absent Aminopeptidase stain in area of cancer (arrow). Ejaculatory ducts and other non-secretory cells also show absence of aminopeptidase reaction.

Figure 1D (center, right). Area of cancer from specimen shown in Figure 1C ×46. Aminopeptidase with hematoxylin nuclear counterstain as in Figure 1C. The bulk of the cancer cells lie adjacent to the capsule (c) and invade in different directions into the prostate gland (arrows) and have also invaded perineural spaces within the capsule (left arrow), which is a common finding in stage B prostatectomy specimens. The periprostatic connective tissue (p) is free of cancer cells. n = normal prostatic acini with strong aminopeptidase activity.

Figure 1E (bottom, left). Cross-section of bladder wall. L = lumen of bladder, e = transitional cell epithelium, s = submucosa, m = smooth muscle layer. On the right half of this section the bladder wall is densely infiltrated or replaced by grade 3 to 4 bladder cancer. Cystectomy specimen- Alcian Blue (AB) stain without MgCl₂. 1% Alcian Blue in 0.1 molar sodium acetate buffered to pH 2.5. Fixation: 10% formalin in 50% aqueous ethanol. Counterstained with nuclear fast red. Stroma around cancer cells shows strong blue staining (AB) which is enlarged in Figure 1E (black insert). Addition of MgCl₂ to achieve a final concentration of 0.2 molar MgCl₂ or addition of testicular hyaluronidase before AB staining resulted in over 50% reduction of the blue staining. This would suggest that most of the AB staining is due to hyaluronic acid and chondroitin sulfate A and C type of Glycosaminoglycogans. Addition of 0.8 molar MgCl₂ abolished over 90% of the staining (dermatan and keratan sulfate, see Table 3). Addition of 1.3 molar MgCl₂ abolishes all AB staining.

Figure 1F Insert of Fig. 1E enlarged about 115×. Same stain as Figure 1E. On the left side invasive highgrade bladder cancer cells infiltrate in cords and clusters into interstitial spaces and around small vessels. At the margin of the zone of invasion there is an accumulation of lymphocytes. There is no visible AB staining in the tumor free submucosa on the left side of the section. The interstitial tissues (stroma) between the invading cancer cells show strong AB staining (see Figure 1E for further explanations).

48

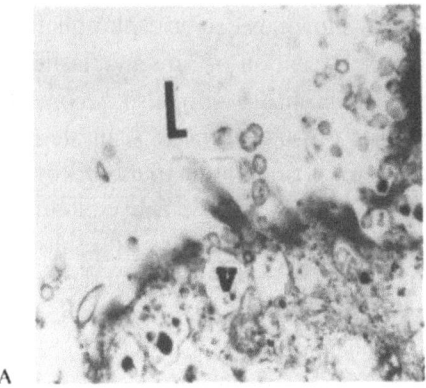

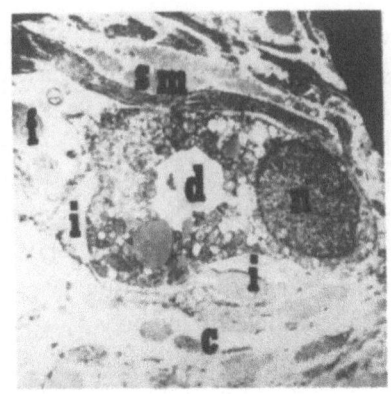

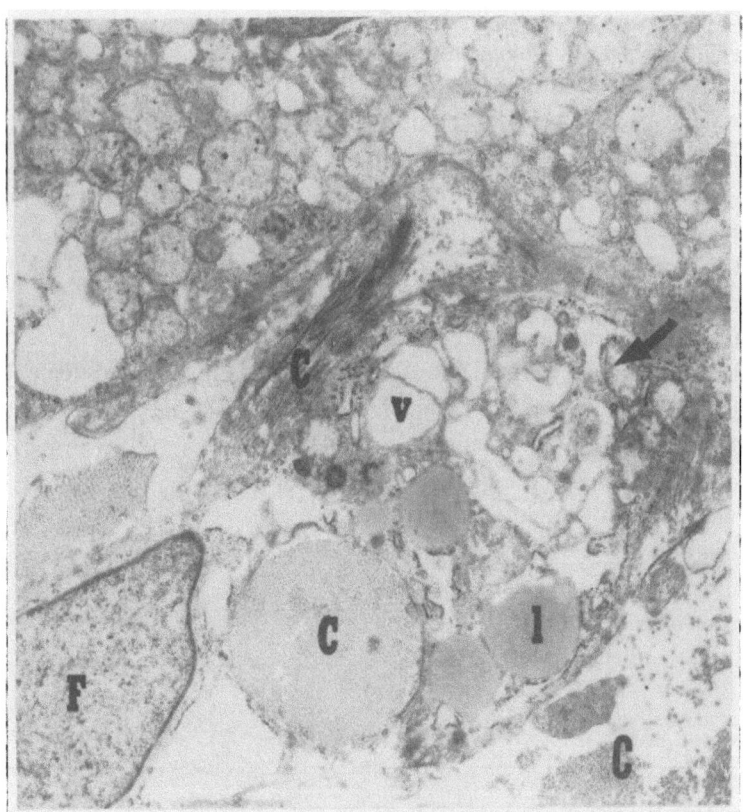

Figure 2A (top, left). Secretory border of normal prostatic acinar cell showing merocrine secretion of enzymes (acid phosphatase et al.) and other secretory products into acinar lumen (L). See text for explanation. v = secretory vacuole migrating towards luminal border. ×16000, electronmicrograph. See diagram Figure 4.

Figure 2B (top, right). Prostatic cancer cell infiltrating along smooth muscle (sm) bundles in stroma. The cytoplasm of the cancer cell is studded with randomly distributed secretory vacuoles and lipid vacuoles. Polarity is lost. The secretory vacuoles excrete their products into pericellular clear spaces (i) and into an intracellular digestive vacuole (d). f = fibroblast, c = collagen. ×8000, electronmicrograph. See diagram Figure 4.

Figure 2C (bottom, center). Prostatic cancer cell infiltrating into surrounding connective tissue. A spherical bundle of collagen fibers (C) adjacent to a fibroblast (F) is partially encircled by the cytoplasm of the cancer cell. Other collagen fibers are cut lengthwise. The disorganized arrangement of secretory (v) and lipid (l) vacuoles and other cell organelles with the cancer cells can be well seen. Arrow = direction of invasion. ×15000, electronmicrograph.

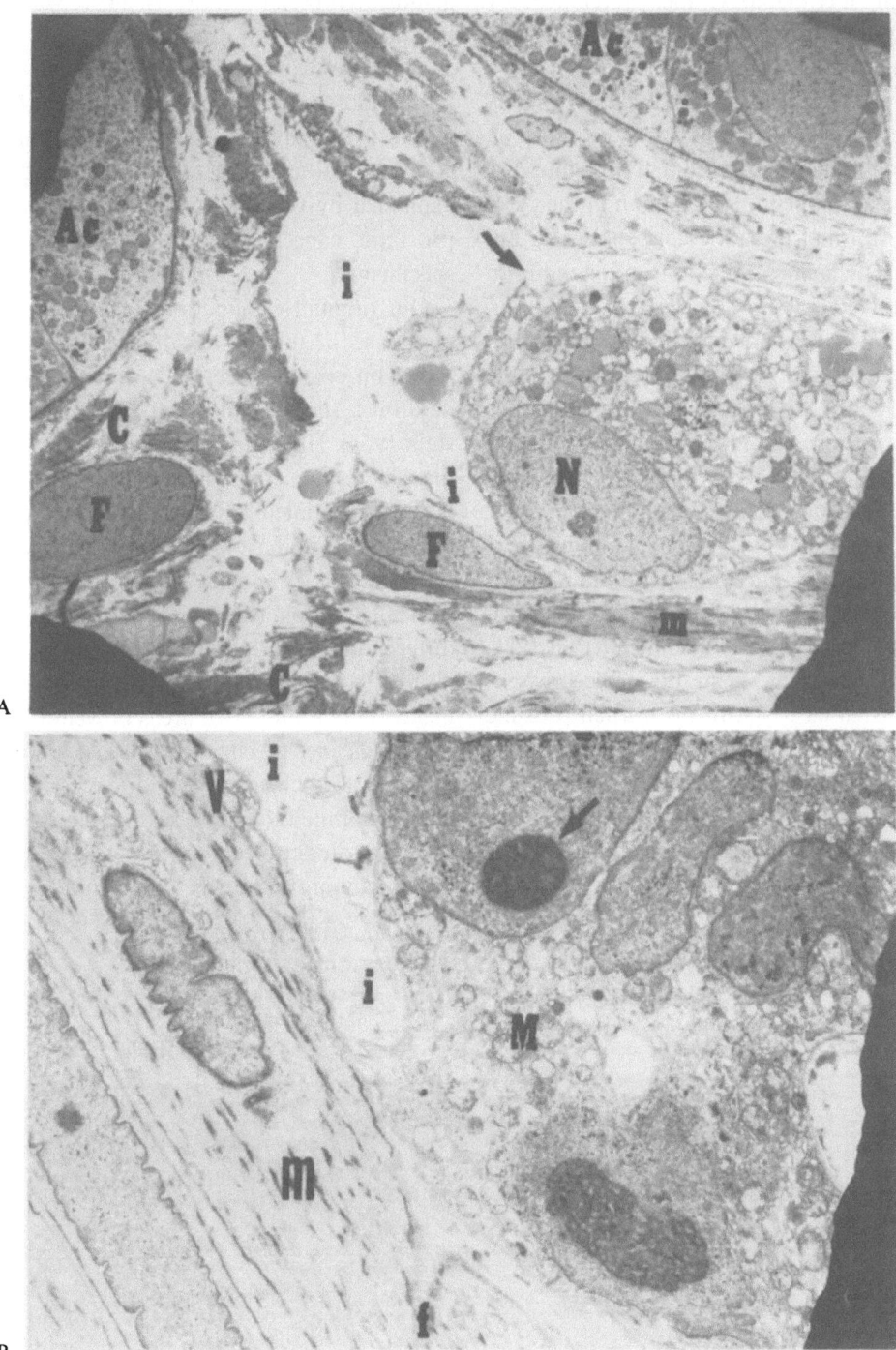

A

B

Figure 3A (top). Prostatic cancer cell infiltrating into stroma showing secretion of products of secretory vacuoles (arrow) into 'clear' spaces (i) around secretion of cancer cell. Edges of small gland forming cancer cells can be seen at upper and left margin of this electronmicrograph (ac). m = smooth muscle, F = fibroblast, C = collagen, N = nucleus of cancer cell with nucleolus. The basement membrane between epithelial cells and stroma is lost or fragmented and the cell membrane of the cancer cell consists of a secretory border with loss of villi (see also diagram, Figure 4).

Figure 3B (bottom). Anaplastic grade 4 prostatic cancer cells infiltrating along and into smooth muscle fibers (m). Cancer cells contain abnormal bizarre nuclei, large nucleoli (arrow), and even more exaggerated disorganisation of cytoplasmic organelles than in Figure 3B. M = abnormal mitochondria, i = interstitial 'clear' spaces with secretory vacuoles, V = vacuolisation in cytoplasm of smooth muscle fiber, f = fraying of muscle fibers at site of invasion.

Histochemical methodology was developed by Seligman's group using similar substrates and azodye coupling for light microscopy visualization (Monis et al. 1959, Nachlas et al. 1962). Applying these histochemical techniques to the normal, hyperplastic and cancerous human prostate, we found intense aminopeptidase reaction in the cytoplasm of the normal prostatic epithelial cells, but absence of histochemical reaction and staining in most prostatic cancer cells (Figures 5B, C) (Kirchheim et al. 1964). The normal prostatic epithelial cell shows intense aminopeptidase reaction chiefly concentrated close to the luminal surface of the cells (Figure 5E). In benign nodular prostatic hyperplasia (BPH), the most frequent benign tumor in men, the localization of aminopeptidase is similar but the intensity is variable and occasional spheroids or areas of BPH show no visible staining. In over forty radical prostatectomy specimens which we studied by step sections (Kirchheim et al. 1966, 1974, Brandes and Kirchheim 1977) the areas of cancer contrasted clearly with the normal prostate by the absence of aminopeptidase staining (Figure 3). The higher magnification of this area of peripherally originating cancer shows the difference between the aminopeptidase negative cancer cells and the surrounding intensely positive normal

glands even better (Figure 4). There were very rare exceptions in which areas of cancer stained histochemically positive for aminopeptidase (Figure 5F). Similar observations were reported by other investigators (Müntzing and Nilsson 1972 and personal communication 1979). This discrepancy may be explained by variable biological behavior of some prostatic cancer clones even within the same specimen.

Our original explanation for absence of aminopeptidase in most clinical prostatic cancers was based on enzyme deletion occurring secondary to de-differentiation and anaplasia of cancer (Greenstein 1954). However, the striking disappearance of histochemical activity of aminopeptidase even in well-differentiated prostatic cancers which still contain good similarities to the polar cytoplasmic organization of normal prostatic epithelial cells is difficult to explain by enzyme deletion due to de-differentiation and anaplasia. It would be of great interest to do aminopeptidase histochemistry on incidentally found focal areas of well-differentiated prostatic cancers. The difficulty has so far been the fact that histochemical techniques for aminopeptidase are limited to frozen section material and such focal histological cancers are usually only found after scanning many sections of BPH specimens,

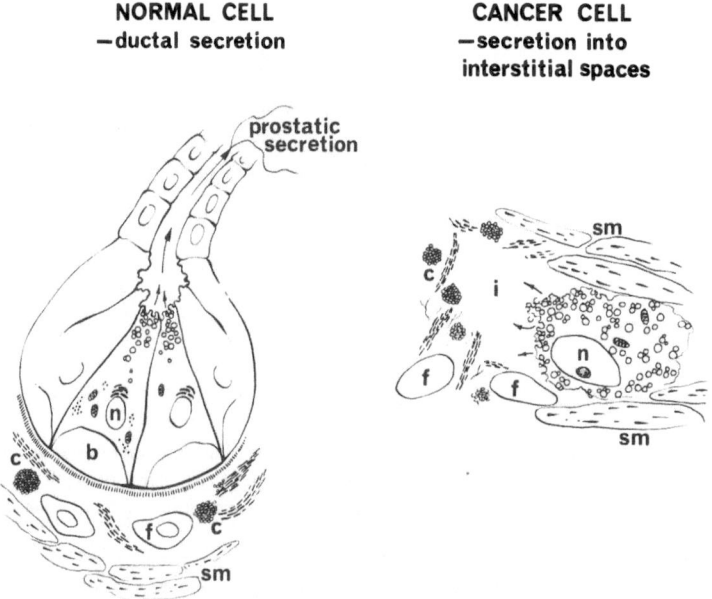

Figure 4. Diagrammatic sketch of mode of acid phosphatase secretion in normal prostatic acinar cells into prostatic ducts and abnormal phosphatase secretion of invasive prostatic cancer cells into surrounding interstitial spaces (see also Figures 2A-3B).

(Denton et al. 1965). This Stage A$_1$ (focal, well-differentiated cancer) prostatic cancer has a completely different prognosis than the other stages of prostatic cancer (Table 1) and most urologists follow these patients carefully, but do *not* treat them (Lehman et al. 1968, Montgomery et al. 1961).

Immuno-histochemistry opens new avenues to tackle this problem. Since the prostate gland is very rich in proteolytic enzymes and in aminopeptidases, immunological methods have been applied to 'prostate' and other tissue aminopeptidases (Mattila 1969, Moncure 1977). Isolation of prostatic aminopeptidase and production of specific antisera against it would permit immunohistochemical evaluation of aminopeptidase on paraffin embedded tissue and simultaneous aminopeptidase evaluation of A$_1$ focal prostate cancer when found incidentally in hematoxylin eosin sections. The development of immunologic techniques will help to differentiate various isoenzymes of aminopeptidases and may explain why a few prostate cancer cells react positively for aminopeptidase and give us further insights. Most likely, the prostate gland contains a number of proteolytic enzymes and possibly also several isoenzymes of aminopeptidase. In contrast to the human prostatic adenocarcinoma our presently most promising animal model, the Dunning R-3327 rat prostatic cancer, was reported to show high histochemical activity for aminopeptidase both in well and poorly differentiated cancer (Müntzing et al. 1978).

C. Beta-glucuronidase and glycosidases

An increase in beta-glucuronidase has been reported in many tumors (Fishman and Bigelow 1950, Fishman et al. 1959). We also found increased beta-glucuronidase activity in many prostate cancer cells and this was confirmed biochemically (Müntzing and Nilsson 1972). Since many tumors and active tissue growth shows elevated beta-glucuronidase activity, there has been so far no clinical usefulness for this finding. The Dunning R-3327 rat prostatic cancer also showed high beta-glucuronidase (Müntzing et al. 1978). Various other glycosidases and beta-glucuronidase were examined in the human prostate, BPH and prostatic cancer (Sinowatz et al. 1978). They found variable amounts of N-acetyl-beta-glucosaminidase (beta-Nag) and betaglycyronidase (beta-Glu) depending upon the degree of differentiation. They found little difference between normal and well-differentiated prostatic cancer cells. In solid and cribriform cancer greatly differing reactions within tumor areas were found. Actively invasive cords of tumor cells showed the highest concentration of beta-Glu and beta-Nag. A strong reaction for both these glycosidases was found in invasive anaplastic cancer cells and also in the surrounding degenerating stroma (Sinowatz et al. 1978).

D. Esterases

Esterases are enzymes which catalyze the hydrolysis of esters to acids and alcohols. Several histochemical methods are available and have been applied to the human prostate and BPH and cancer (Kirchheim et al. 1964). We found a decrease in activity in cancers (Figures 6E, F). Little is known about the nature of these enzymes in the human prostate and present techniques for esterases are probably nonspecific for many ester linkages.

E. Alkaline phosphatase

This enzyme was not found in the epithelial cells of the human prostate (Brandes and Bourne 1956, Kirchheim et al. 1964). It is chiefly found in the walls of small blood vessels in the stroma.

Elevated serum alkaline phosphatases in certain patients with prostatic cancer with bone metastases is produced by activated osteoblasts in the areas of prostatic osteoblastic metastases.

F. Oxidative enzymes

Succinic dehydrogenase (SDH), isocitrate-dehydrogenase (ICDH), beta-hydroxy-butyrate-dehydrogenase (beta-BDH), glucose-6-phosphate-dehydrogenase (G-6-PDH), glutamate-dehydrogenase (GDH) and lactate-dehydrogenase (SDH) have been investigated in the human normal, hyperplastic and neoplastic prostate gland (Feustel et al. 1970, 1971). They found presence of all these oxidative enzymes in the normal and malignant prostate with the exception of G-6-PDH, 'indicating failure of energy gain via the pentose phosphate cycle'. Other investigators found uniform staining of G-6-PDH with only moderate variation in intensity in the fetus, infant and adult normal and neoplastic prostatic gland. At the present no definite differences in the energy metabolism between the normal and neoplastic human prostate gland are proven. Ultrastructural studies show marked deformities and changes of the mitochondria (Kirchheim and Bacon 1969) where oxidative enzymes are localized.

G. Golgi region associated enzymes

Certain nucleoside-diphosphatases are thought to

be associated with the Golgi apparatus of cytoplasm. The Golgi apparatus can also be demonstrated by DaFano's silver impregnation method and its ability to react with osmium tetroxide. Work on prostatic cancer is limited and no relevant differences have been reported. DPH and TPN-diaphorases stained strongly in the normal and neoplastic human prostate.

H. Zinc

The prostate gland, testicles and spermatozoa of

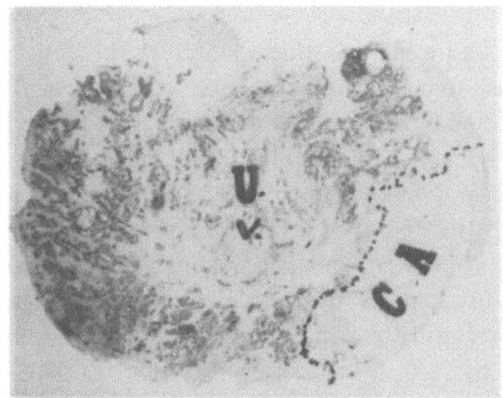

Figure 5A. Invasive prostatic cancer cells around nerve (N) along perineural space. Acid phosphatase, Burstone method. hematoxylin nuclear counterstain. (×300). Acid phosphatase reaction product is seen as fine precipitate within cytoplasm of invasive prostatic adenocarcinoma.

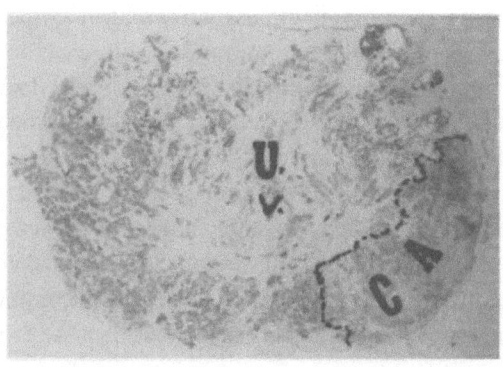

Figure 5B. Well-differentiated prostatic adenocarcinoma on left side of section, normal prostate glands on right side. Aminopeptidase, method of Nachlas et al., hematoxylin nuclear counterstain. The normal prostatic acinar epithelium shows strong aminopeptidase reaction, (arrow) there is complete absence of aminopeptidase staining in the adjacent prostatic adenocarcinoma. ×300.

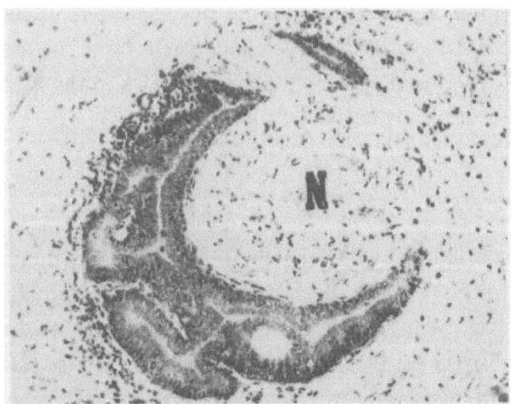

Figure 5C. Complete transverse cryostat section of prostate gland close to level of verumontanum (v). Radical prostatectomy specimen of clinical and pathological stage B$_1$ prostatic cancer. CA = area of cancer (also marked by dotted line). U = Urethra. Aminopeptidase, method of Nachlas et al., *no* nuclear counterstain. Area of cancer is clearly visible by its lack of aminopeptidase staining in contrast to the normal secretory prostatic epithelium.

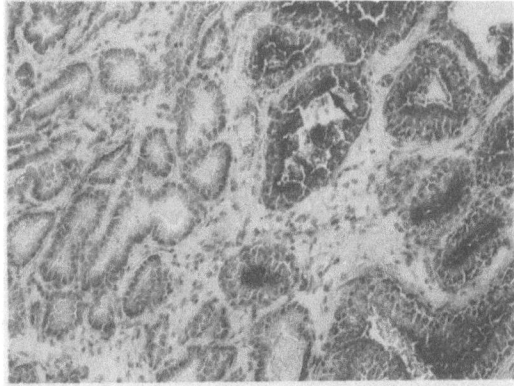

Figure 5D. Adjacent prostatic cross-section to specimen shown in Figure 5C. Acid phosphatase, Burstone method, *no* nuclear counterstain. The area of cancer cells (CA) shows decreased (in comparison to normal acini) but moderately strong acid phosphatase reaction.

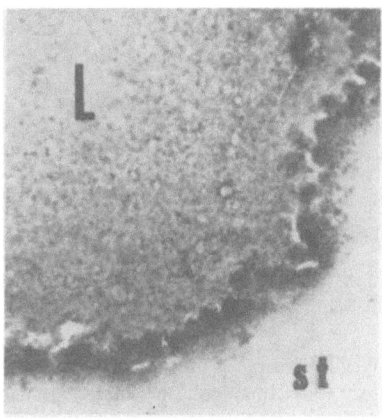

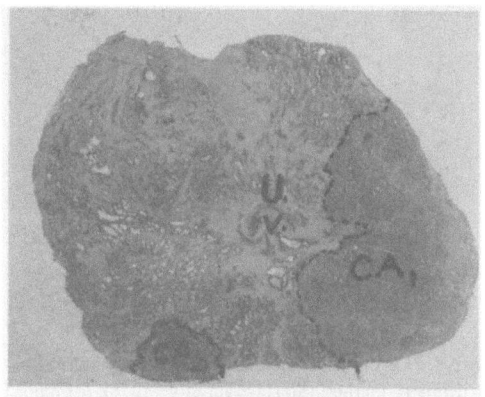

Figure 5E. Portion of normal secretory prostatic acinus. Aminopeptidase, method of Nachlas et al., *no* nuclear counterstain. ×800. Strong aminopeptidase reaction in supranuclear cytoplasm with highest intensity close to luminal secretory border of prostatic cells. Also strong reaction in luminal secretion (L). Practically no reaction in surrounding stroma (st). Unstained nuclei stand out as pale ghosts.

Figure 5F. Complete transverse cryostat section of prostate gland at level of proximal verumontanum (v). Radical prostatectomy specimen of clinical stage B_1 but pathological stage C_1. CA_1 = clinically palpated area of cancer. Since cancer had extended anteriorly, the induration appeared by palpation smaller. CA_2 = smaller second area of cancer, only found at time of histological examination. U = urethra. Aminopeptidase, method of Nachlas et al., hematoxylin nuclear counterstain. The larger palpable area of cancer, CA_1, shows no aminopeptidase staining, only the hematoxylin staining of closely packed adenocarcinoma. The smaller area of cancer in the left posterior area, CA_2, shows strong aminopeptidase reaction similar to the normal secretory acini of the prostate gland.

men and other animals contain much more zinc than other tissues (Byar 1974, Daniel et al. 1956, Mawson and Fisher 1952). Histochemical techniques for zinc have been applied using the dithizone method (Mager et al. 1953). We found decrease in activity in cancer with the dithizone method (unpublished data). Other investigators reported a multifold increase in BPH and histochemical absence of staining in prostatic cancer. Most work on zinc in the prostate has been done by biochemical and radioisotope uptake studies and has been extensively reviewed.

III. HISTOCHEMISTRY OF CONNECTIVE TISSUE INVADED BY CANCER CELLS

A. Connective tissue stroma in general

Invasion and metastasis are the cardinal features of malignancy. Even fast growing huge benign prostatic hyperplastic (BPH) tumors do *not* invade into other tissues or metastasize, they just keep expanding and frequently cause urinary retention by obstructing the urethra and bladder neck.

With the exception of carcinoma-in-situ (stage A_1), other stages of prostatic cancer traverse the basement membrane of the acinus and invade into the surrounding stroma (Figures 2B,C, 3A, B). The normal prostatic acinus is surrounded by an inner layer of connective tissue and an outer layer of smooth muscle similar to the bladder, urethra and other genital organs, only in a concentric fashion. The peri-aciniar connective tissue layer is the first zone of cancer-host interaction. Bio- and histochemical studies of connective tissues have been difficult because of their complex chemistry. Ultrastructural studies of prostatic cancer have suggested destructive lytic changes of invaded stromal tissues (Kirchheim and Bacon 1969, Brandes and Kirchheim 1977). Histological sections with evidence of active malignant invasion showed in adjacent section high collagenolytic activity (Strauch 1972). Protease inhibitors have inhibited malignant cell invasion 'in-vitro' (Lather et al. 1973). Ultrastructural observations show evidence of excretion of secretory vacuoles into the invaded stroma (Figures 2C, 3B). There is considerable evidence for the involvement of degradative enzymes in invasion by many different tumors (Fidler et al. 1978). These

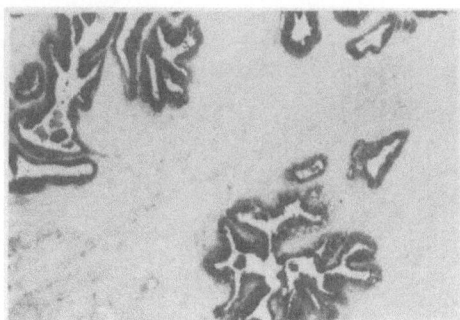

Figure 6A. Normal prostatic acini. Acid phosphatase, Immuno-histochemistry method (Sternberger et al. 1976), formalin fixed, paraffin embedded. Strong acid phosphatase reaction in cytoplasm of secretory prostatic epithelium similar to cryostat section in Figure 1A. Practically no staining in nuclei and stroma.

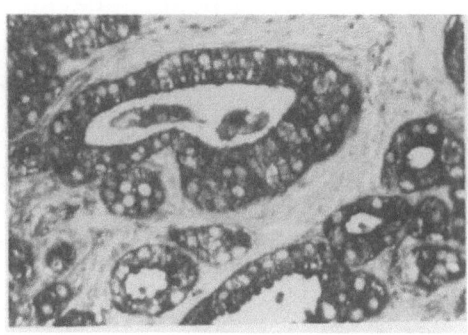

Figure 6B. Well-differentiated prostatic adenocarcinoma, grade 2. Acid phosphatase, Immunohistochemistry as in figure 6A × 400. Moderately strong reaction in cytoplasm of prostatic adenocarcinoma cells. Nuclei stand out as unstained.

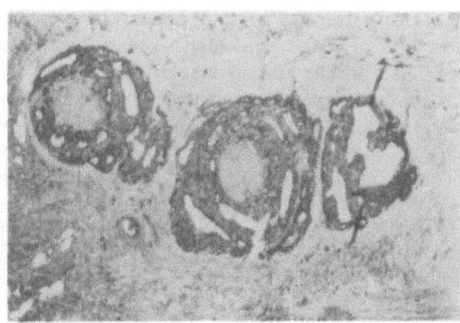

Figure 6C. Cribriform prostatic carcinoma infiltrating along perineural spaces. Acid phosphatase, Immunohistochemistry as in figure 6A × 100. Decreased acid phosphatase reaction in cribriform invasive prostatic cancer.

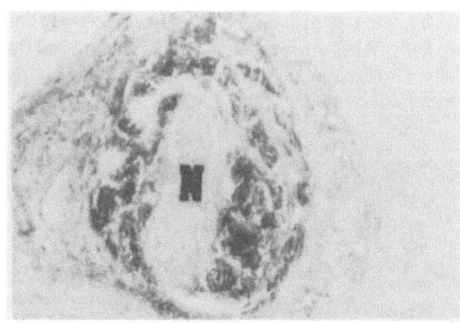

Figure 6D. Adenocarcinoma of prostate, grade 2-3, invading around perineural space. N = nerve. Acid phosphatase, Immunohistochemistry as in Figure 6A × 200. Moderately strong reaction in cytoplasm of prostatic adenocarcinoma.

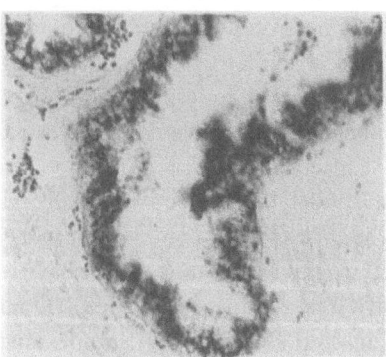

Figure 6E. Normal prostatic acinus. Non-specific esterase. Gomori method (naphthyl acetate). No nuclear counterstain. × 150. Strong precipitate in cytoplasm of secretory prostatic cells.

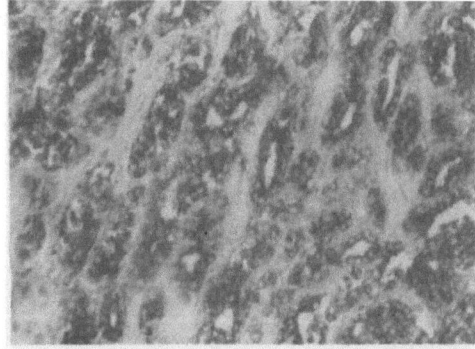

Figure 6F. Prostatic adenocarcinoma, grade 2-3. Non-specific esterase as in Figure 6E. Some decrease in esterase activity in comparison to the normal in Figure 6E, but still moderately active esterase staining in cytoplasm of prostatic adenocarcinoma cells. × 200.

enzymes, either soluble or cell surface bound, are thought to destroy the tissue of the host so that the multiplying tumor cells can infiltrate the areas of destruction (Dresden 1973, Hashimoto et al. 1973, Strauch 1972, Sylven 1972).

B. Glycosaminoglycans (muco-polysaccharides)

Histochemical investigations have chiefly concentrated on the study of glycosaminoglycans (mucopolysaccharides). The fibroblasts of connective tissue produce extracellular collagen and the so-called ground substance which is chiefly made up of different glycosaminoglycans (GSG). The glycosaminoglycans of connective tissue comprise a group of protein carbohydrate complexes or proteoglycans, the carbohydrate parts of which have been relatively well characterized. By contrast relatively little is known regarding the structure of the protein moiety. The carbohydrate chains of glycosaminoglycans are composed of repeating dissacharides units containing uronic acid and then amino sugar. As seen in Table 3 this generalization holds with the exception of keratan sulfate which contains galactose in place of uronic acid. Glycosaminoglycans (GSG) are found in differing amounts in all connective tissues, but the types of GSG present vary greatly from tissue to tissue. For example: cartilage contains large amounts of the chondroitin sulfate isomers together with keratan sulfate while the major GSG of skin are hyaluronic acid and dermatan sulfate. These tissue differences have been reviewed (Jackson and Bentley 1968).

The association of large amounts of 'mucoid' material with many different tumor types is well documented and has been reviewed (Sylven 1965, Hukill and Vidone 1967). Differential staining of acid glycosaminoglycans by alcian blue in salt solutions and its molecular biological basis has been elaborated (Scott and Dorling 1965, Scott 1968, 1972). The technique of alcian blue staining in the presence of varying concentrations of electrolytes has permitted to distinguish histochemically between various alcianophilic mucopolysaccharides on the basis of the type of negative charges present (Quintarelli 1964, 1968). We applied this technique to thirty human prostate and bladder cancers (Kirchheim et al. in preparation). The invaded stroma of high grade invasive bladder cancers show more intense staining with alcian blue than slower growing prostatic adenocarcinoma. There appeared to be a direct relationship between the degree of alcianophilia and the invasiveness of the tumor. Figures 1E, F show the significant increase of alcian blue staining around high grade bladder cancer cells in contrast to minimal staining in the normal bladder wall of the same section.* Most of the increase of GSG is due to hyaluronic acid and poorly charged mucines. To a lesser extent there is also an increase in sulfated GSG, such as chondroitin-4- and -6-sulfates and possibly dermatan sulfates (see Table 3). The stroma around normal glands or benign tumors (BPH) did *not* show a significant increase in GSG staining.

Changes in GSG in other tumor tissues have been reported applying biochemical methods on tissue homogenates: Glycosaminoglycans (GSG) were markedly increased in human lung carcinoma, predominantly chondroitin-4- and/or -6- sulfates and hyaluronic acid (Hatae et al. 1977). These findings were consistent with investigations in human hepatic carcinoma (Kojima et al. 1975). Biochemical tissue extractions contain the GSG from connective tissue matrix plus GSG from plasma and nuclear membranes. Our above described histochemical

* Invasive prostatic cancers show similar findings, but because of the more intense staining of the invaded stroma, a bladder cancer was chosen for the color plate.

Table 3. Mucopolysaccharides of connective tissue.

	Synonyms	Disaccharide repeating unit
chondroitin	—	glucuronic acid + galactosamine
chondroitin 4 sulfate	chrondroitin sulfate a	glucuronic acid + 4 sulfo galactosamine
chondroitin 6-sulfate	chondroitin sulfate c	glucuronic acid + 6 sulfo galactosamine
dermatan sulfate	chondroitin sulfate b β heparin	iduronic acid + 4 sulfo galactosamine
hyaluronic acid	—	glucuronic acid + glucosamine
keratan sulfate	kerato sulfate	galactose + 6 sulfo glucosamine

studies referred only to matrix GSG.

In over 100 examined human cancers significant variations in the GSG pattern in comparison with the normal tissues were found (Chiarugi et al. 1978). They concluded that heparan sulfate (HS) and dermaton sulfate (DS) are positive elements for cell adhesion and tissue homeostasis while chondroitin sulfate C and hyaluronic acid could interfere in mechanisms disrupting recognition sites. Other data also suggested a regulative role for surface polysaccharides of eukaryotic cells in cellular recognition and tissue homeostasis (Dietrich et al. 1976. Takeuchi 1968). Recently a new histochemical technique for GSG has been described (Green and Pastenka 1974, Green 1978). This simple staining method using a metachromatic cationic carbocyanine dye gave information concerning the types of macromolecules present in connective tissue and in secretions within cells, alveolar lumina and ducts. Enzymatic digestion with streptomyces hyaluronidase showed variable amounts of haluronic acid in the connective stroma of several types of breast cancer (Green 1978). Further work is needed to better identify chemically the various connective tissue substances. Comparison of these substances in cancer with benign tumors and various inflammatory tissues may shed some light on the mecha- nism of invasion and the interaction between cancer cells and host tissues.

IV. CONCLUSIONS

Histochemical techniques have the great advantage of localizing enzymes and other substances and permit comparisons between neoplastic invasive areas and normal tissue on the same slide (Figures D-F). The number of available techniques and lack of specificities have slowed progress. Immunochemistry opens many new possibilities. Several clinical applications are now available. Differences in the enzyme profiles of the normal tissues and various degrees of malignancies have been discovered and further knowledge and clinical usefulness can be expected. Histochemical methodology and identification of connective tissue components, especially of glycosaminoglycans, is making steady progress and is a useful adjunct in the study of the mechanism of malignant tumor invasion.

ACKNOWLEDGEMENTS

The author wishes to thank Dr. Kenneth L. Partlow for the acid phosphatase immunohistochemistry sections of our surgical material, Mrs Judith Smith for medical illustration work and Mrs. Lorilie Steen for secretarial work.

REFERENCES

Ashley DJB: On the incidence of carcinoma of the prostate J Path Bact 90: 217, 1965.

Barka T, Anderson PJ: Histochemical methods for acid phosphatase using hexazonium pararosanilin as coupler. J Histochem Cytochem 10: 741, 1962.

Brandes D, and GH Bourne. The histochemistry of the prostate in normal and in castrated and hormone-treated mice and of prostatic homografts exposed to 20-methylcholanthrene. Brit J Exp Path 35: 577, 1954.

Brandes D and Bourne GH: Histochemistry of the human prostate; normal and neoplastic J Path Bact 7: 33, 1956.

Brandes D, Kirchheim D, and Scott WW: Ultrastructure of the human prostate: normal and neoplastic. Lab Invest 13: 1541, 1964.

Brandes D: Fine struture and cytochemistry of male sex accessory organs. In: Male accessory sex organs. Brandes D. ed. New York: Academic Press, 1974, pp 17-113.

Brandes D, and Kirchheim D: Histochemistry of the prostate. In: Urologic pathology: the prostate. Tannenbaum M. ed. Philadelphia: Lea and Febiger. 1977. pp 99-128.

Burstone MS: Histochemical demonstration of phosphatases in frozen section with naphthol-AS-phosphates. J Histochem 9: 146. 1961.

Byar DP: Zinc in male accessory sex organs In: Male accessory sex organs, Brandes D. ed. New York: Academic Press, 1974, pp 161-171.

Chiarugi VP, Vannucchi S, Cella C, Fibbi G, Del Rosso M, Cappelletti R: Intercellular glycosaminoglycosans in normal and neoplastic tissues. Cancer Res 38: 4717, 1978.

Cooper JF and Foti A: A radioimmuno-assay for prostatic acid phosphatase. I Methodology and range of normal male serum values. Invest Urol 12: 98, 1974.

Cooper JF Foti HH, Hershman and Finkle W: A solid phase radioimmuno-assay for prostatic acid phosphatase. J Urol 119: 388, 1978.

Chu TM, Wang MD, Scott WW, Gibbons RP, Johnson DE, Schmidt JD, Loening SA, Prout GR, and Murphy GP: Immunochemical detection of serum prostatic acid phosphatase. Invest Urol 15: 319.

Daniel O, Farid H, Prout G, and Whitmore WF: Some observations on the distribution of radioactive zinc in prostatic and other human tissues. Brit J Urol 28: 271.

Denton SE, Choy SH, Valk WL: Occult prostatic carcinoma diagnosed by the step section technique of the surgical specimen. J Urol 93: 296, 1965.

Dietrich CP, Sampais LO, Toledo OMS: Characteristic distribution of sulfated mucopolysaccharides in different tissues and in their respective mitochondria. Biochem Biophys Res

Commun 71: 1, 1976.

Dresden MH, Heilman SA, and Schmidt JD, Collagenolytic enzymes in human neoplasm. Cancer Res 32: 993, 1972.

Drucker JR, Moncure CW, Johnson CL, Smith MJV, and Koontz WW: Immunologic staging of prostatic carcinoma: three years of experience. J Urol 119: 94, 1978.

Feustel A, Schönfelder M, and Wohlrab F: Fermenthistochemische Untersuchungen an Prostatakarzinomen unter Therapieeinfluss. Urol int 26: 77, 1971.

Feustel AM, Schönfelder M, and Wohlrab F: Fermenthistochemische Untersuchungen zur Differenzierung benigner und maligner Wachstumsprozesse in der menschlichen Prostata. Urol Int 25: 86, 1970.

Fidler IJ, Gersten DM and Hart IR: The biology of cancer invasion and metastasis. In: Advances in cancer research, Vol. 28, Klein G, Weinhouse S, eds. New York: Academic Press, 1978, pp 150-236.

Fischer ER, Jeffrey W Ultrastructure of human normal and neoplastic prostate. Amer J Clin Path 44: 119, 1965.

Fishman WH, Bigelow R: A comparative study of the morphology and glucoronidase activity in 44 gastrointestinal neoplasm. J Nat Cancer Inst 10: 1115, 1950.

Fishman WH, Baker JR, and Borges PRF: Localization of B-glucoronidase in some human tumors. Cancer 12: 240, 1959.

Foti AG, Herschman H, Cooper JF: Comparison of human prostatic acid phosphatase by measurement of enzymatic activity and by radioimmunoassay. Clin Chem 23: 96, 1977.

Franks LM: Latent carcinoma of the prostate. J Path Bact 68: 603, 1954.

Gaynor EP: Zur Frage des Prostatakrebses. Virchows Arch path Anat 301: 602, 1938.

Goldbarg JA, and Rutenberg AM: The colorimetric determination of leucine aminopeptidase in urine and serum of normal subjects and patients with cancer and other diseases. Cancer 11: 283, 1958.

Gomori G: Distribution of acid phosphatase in the tissues under normal and under pathologic conditions. Arch Path 32: 189, 1941.

Green MR, and Pastenka JV: Simultaneous differential staining by a cationic carbocyanine dye of nucleic acids, proteins and conjugated proteins. II. Carbohydrate and sulfated carbohydrate containing proteins. J Histochem Cytochem 22: 774, 1974.

Green MR: Simultaneous differential staining of phosphoproteins, sialoglycoproteins, hyaluronic acid, sulfated glycosaminoglycans, proteins, and nucleic acids in human breast tissue with a cationic carbocyamine dye. J Natl Cancer Inst 61: 351, 1978.

Greenstein JP: Biochemistry of cancer, ed 2. Academic press, New York, 1954, p 575.

Gutman AB, and Gutman EB: Acid phosphatase occurring in the serum of patients with metastasizing carcinoma of the prostate. J Clin Invest 17: 473, 1938.

Györkey F, Min K, Huff J, Györkey P: Zinc and magnesium in human prostate gland: Normal, hyperplastic and neoplastic. Cancer Research 27: 1348, 1967.

Halpert B, Sheehan EE, Schmalhorst WR, and Scott R, Jr: Carcinoma of the prostate, a survey of 5000 autopsies. Cancer 16: 737, 1963.

Hashimoto K, Yamanishi Y, Moeyeus E, Dabbous MK, and Kauzaki T: Collagenolytic activities of squamous cell carcinoma of the skin. Cancer Res 33: 2730, 1973.

Hatae Y, Atsuta T, and Makita A: Glycosaminoglycans in human lung carcinoma. Gann 68: 59, 1977.

Helminen HJ, and Ericsson JLE: Evidence for a Golgi-mediated,

merocrine type of secretion of acid phosphatase in prostatic epithelium. J Ultra Res 36: 532, 1971.

Huggins C, and Hodges CV: Studies on prostatic cancer. I. The effect of castration of estrogen and of androgen injection on serum phosphatases in metastatic carcinoma of the prostate. Cancer Res 1: 293, 1941.

Hukill PB, and Vidone RA: Histochemistry of mucus and other polysaccharides in tumors. Lab Invest 16: 395, 1967.

Jackson DS, and Bentley JP: Collagen Glycosaminoglycan interactions. In: Treatise on collagen, vol 2a, Gould B, ed. New York: Academic Press, 1968.

Jöbsis AC, Devries GP, Anholt RRH, Sanders GTB: Demonstration of the prostatic origin of metastases. Cancer 41: 1788, 1978.

Kastendieck H, and Altenähr E: Cyto- and histomorphogenesis of the prostatic carcinoma. Virchows Arch A Path Anat and Histol 370: 207, 1976.

Kirchheim DF, Györkey F, Brandes D, and Scott WW: Histochemistry of the normal, hyperplastic and neoplastic human prostate gland. Invest Urol 1: 403, 1964.

Kirchheim D, Niles NR, Frankus E, and Hodges CV: Correlative histochemical and histological studies on thirty radical prostatectomy specimens. Cancer 19: 1683, 1966.

Kirchheim D, Bacon RL: Ultrastructural studies of carcinoma of the human prostate gland. Invest Urol 6: 611, 1969.

Kirchheim D, Brandes D, and Bacon RL: Fine structure and cytochemistry of human prostatic carcinoma. In: Male accessory sex organs, Brandes D, ed. New York: Academic Press, 1974, pp 597-423.

Kojima J, Nakamura N, Kahatani M, and Ohmari K: The glycosaminoglycans in human hepatic cancer. Cancer Res. 35: 542 1975.

Lam KW: Biochemical properties of human prostatic acid phosphatase. Clin Chem 19: 483, 1973.

Latner AL, Longstaff E, and Pradhau K: Inhibition of malignant cell invasion in vitro by proteinase inhibitor. Brit J Cancer 27: 460, 1973.

Lehman T, Kirchheim D, Braun E, Moore R: An evaluation of radical prostatectomy for incidentally diagnosed cancer of prostate. J Urol 99: 646, 1968.

Li CY, Lam KW, Yam LT: Immunohistochemical evaluation for identification of metastatic prostatic carcinoma. Arch Androl 2, suppl 1: 90, 1979.

Mager M, McNary WF, and Lionetti F: The histochemical detection of zinc. J Histochem Cytochem 1: 493, 1953.

Mao P, Nakao K, and Angrist A: Human prostatic carcinoma: An electronmicroscopic study. Cancer Res 26: 955, 1966.

Mattila S: Further studies on the prostatic tissue antigens. Separation of two molecular forms of aminopeptidase. Invest Urol 7: 1, 1969.

Mawson CA, and Fisher MI: The occurrence of zinc in the human prostate gland. Can J Med Sci 30: 336, 1952.

McDonald I, Rose NR, Pontes EJ, and Choe BK: Human prostatic acid phosphatase. Counterimmunoelectrophoresis for rapid identification. Arch Androl 1: 235, 1978.

Mellinger GT: Prognosis of prostatic carcinoma. Recent Res Cancer Res 60: 61, 1977.

Moncure CW: Isoenzymes in prostatic carcinoma. In: Urologic pathology: the prostate, Tannenbaum M, ed. Philadelphia: Lea and Febiger, 1977, pp 141-155.

Monis B, Nachlas MM, and Seligman AA: Study of leucine aminopeptidase in neoplastic and inflammatory tissues with a new histochemical method. Cancer 12: 601, 1959.

Montgomery TR, Whitlock GF, Mohlgren JE, Lewis AM: What becomes of the patient with latent or occult carcinoma of the prostate. J Urol 86: 655, 1961.

Müntzing J, and Nilsson T: Enzyme activity and distribution in the hyperplastic and cancerous human prostate. Scand J Urol Nephrol 6: 107, 1972.

Müntzing J, Saroff J, Sandberg AA, and Murphy GP: Enzyme activity and distribution in rat prostatic adenocarcinoma. Urology 11: 278 1978.

Murphy GP, Reynoso G, Kenny GM, and Gaeta JF: Comparison of total and prostatic fraction serum acid phosphatase levels in patients with differentiated and undifferentiated prostatic carcinoma. Cancer 23: 1309, 1969.

Nachlas MD, Goldstein TP, and Seligman AM: An evaluation of aminopeptidase specificity with seven chromogenic substrates. Arch Biochm Biophys 97: 223, 1962.

Nakamura RM: Immunoenzyme histochemical methods. In: Immunopathology: clinical laboratory concepts and methods. Boston: Little, Brown, 1974. p 650.

Pontes JE, Choe B, Rose N, and Pierce JM, Jr. Indirect immunofluorescence for identification of prostatic epithelial cells. J Urol 117: 459, 1977.

Quintarelli G, and Dellovo MC: The chemical and histochemical properties of alcian blue IV. Histochemie 5: 196, 1965.

Quintaretti G: Methods for the histochemical identification of acid mucopolysaccharide: a critical evaluation. In: The chemical physiology of mucopolysaccharides. Quintarelli G, ed. Boston: Little, Brown, 1968.

Romans NW, Hsu KC, Tomashefsky P, and Tannenbaum M: Counterimmunoelectrophoresis for detection of prostatic acid phosphatase. Urology 12: 79, 1978.

Rutenburg AM, and Seligman AM: The histochemical demonstration of acid phosphatase by a postincubation coupling technique. J Histochem Cytochem 3: 455, 1955.

Scott JE: Histochemistry of Alcian blue. III the molecular biological basis of staining by Alcian blue 8GX and analogous phthalocyanins. Histochemie 32: 191, 1972.

Scott JE, and Dorling J: Differential staining of acid glycosaminoglycans (mucopolysaccharides) by Alcian blue or salt solutions. Histochemie 5: 221, 1965.

Scott JE: Patterns of specificity in the interaction of organic cations with acid mucopolysaccharides. In: The chemical physiology of mucopolysaccharides. Quintarelli G, ed. Boston: Little, Brown, 1968.

Shelley HS, Auerbach SH, Classen KL, Marks CH, and Wiederanders RE: Carcinoma of the prostate - New system of classification. AMA Arch Surg 77: 751, 1958.

Shnitka TK, and Seligman AM: Role of esteratic inhibition on localization of esterase and the simultaneous cytochemical demonstration of inhibitor sensitive and resistant enzyme species. J Histochem Cytochem 9: 504, 1961.

Sinowatz F, Weber P, Gasser G, Mössig H, and Skolek-Winnisch R: A histochemical study of glycosidases in benign prostatic hyperplasia and in prostatic carcinoma in the human. Urol Research 6: 103, 1978.

Sodeman TM, and Batsakis JG: Acid Phosphatase In: Urologic pathology: the prostate, Tannenbaum M, ed. Philadelphia: Lea and Febiger, 1977, pp 129-139.

Sternberger LA: Electronmicroscopic immunocytochemistry: a review. J Histochem Cytochem 15: 139, 1967.

Sternberger LA: Some new developments in immunocytochemistry. Mikroskopie 25: 346, 1969.

Sternberger LA: An immunohistological Study of Follicular Lymphoma, Reticulum Cell Sarcoma and Hodgkin's Disease. Europ J Cancer 126: 75, 1976.

Strauch L: The role of collagenases in tumour invasions. In: Tissue interactions in carcinogenesis, Tarin D, ed. New York: Academic Press, 1972, pp 399-434.

Sylven B: Biochemical and enzymatic factors involved in cellular detachment. In: Chemotherapy of cancer dissemination and metastasis, Garattini S, Frauchi G, eds. New York: Raven Press, 1973, pp 129-138.

Sylven B: Aminosugar containing compounds in tumors. In: The amino sugars, Balazs E, Heanloz RW, eds. New York: Academic Press, 1965.

Takeuchi J, Sobue M, and Sato E: Variation in GSG components of breast tumors. Cancer Res. 36: 2133, 1976.

Takeuchi J: Effect of chondroitin sulphate on the growth of solid Ehrlich Ascites tumor under the influences of other intestinal components. Cancer Res 28: 1520, 1968.

Tannenbaum M, Spiro D, and Lattimer J: Biology of the prostate gland: the electronmicroscopy of cytoplasmic filamentous bodies in human benign prostatic cells adjacent to cancer cells. Cancer Res 27: 1415, 1967.

Taylor CR: Immunoperoxidase techniques. Practical and theoretical aspects. Arch Pathol Lab Med 102: 113, 1978.

Whitmore SF: Retropubic implantation of I^{125} in the treatment of prostatic cancer. In: Progress in clinical and biological research, vol 6, Prostatic disease, Marberger H, ed. New York: Alan R. Liss, 1977, pp 223-233.

Yam LT: Clinical significance of the human acid phosphatases – a review. Am J Med 56: 604, 1974.

5. ENDOCRINE ASPECTS AND STEROID RECEPTORS IN PROSTATIC CARCINOMA

G. CONCOLINO and F. DI SILVERIO

I. INTRODUCTION

The treatment of prostatic carcinoma, the most common cancer arising in the male urogenital tract, is controversial with regard to the pathogenesis and the natural history of the disease. The hormone dependence of the carcinoma of the prostate, known since 1939, has received biochemical support from the demonstration of steroid receptors in human prostatic tissue and from the knowledge of the mechanism of action of steroid hormones. In vitro studies of steroid metabolism and steroid receptors in benign prostatic hyperplasia (BPH) and in prostatic cancer (PC), together with studies on the hormonal status of patients, have shed some light on certain aspects of these diseases. The results obtained with endocrine treatment not only in patients with BPH, but also in patients with PC have further emphasized the role of the hormonal status and of the effects of the hormonal manipulations in the *etiopatho*genesis of the disorders. The endocrine treatment employed in patients with PC, either ablative (orchiectomy, adrenalectomy, hypophysectomy) or additive with estrogens, progestins or antiandrogenic compounds has been often correlated with the histological staging and with different grades of the disease. Attempts have been made to correlate the response to hormonal manipulation of prostatic carcinoma patients with the steroid receptor content of the tumor, but the results are still controversial and a longer follow-up is required in order to draw definitive conclusions.

II. ENDOCRINE THERAPY

Huggins and Hodges (1939) introduced endocrine therapy for PC in 1941, based on the hypothesis of hormone-dependence of prostatic tumors resulting from their experiments. In view of the growth promoting action of androgens on prostatic tissue, efforts have been made to remove the main source of androgens in man, i.e. performing orchiectomy in patients with PC. More than 95% of plasma testosterone can be abolished and plasma testosterone concentrations fall to levels comparable to those of normal women (Sciarra et al. 1973). After orchiectomy, adrenal hyperfunction may be responsible for an increased production of weak androgen (Bracci et al. 1977), susceptible to be transformed by the prostatic tissue into more active compounds (Di Silverio et al. 1976). In order to remove the extratesticular sources of androgens and to suppress the release from the pituitary of adrenocorticotrophic hormone (ACTH) or of prolactin (PRL) that is able to interfere with androgen metabolism in the prostate (Grayhack 1963, Thomas and Manandhar 1975), more agressive forms of ablative endocrine therapy like adrenalectomy or hypophysectomy have been proposed. Such surgical procedures, besides being more harmful for the affected patients, do not always give the expected results, despite relief of bone pain (Fergusson and Hendry 1971, Murphy et al. 1971). The hazard of such major surgery can be avoided by adrenal suppression with dexamethasone or chemical hypophysectomy by means of estrogens to suppress luteinizing hormone (LH) or by means of antiprolactinemic drugs to suppress PRL. The endocrine therapy for PC is usually orchietomy and/or different forms of additive endocrine treatments: administration of estrogens, of progestational compounds or anti-androgens.

Although estrogens at high concentrations (3-5 mg per day of diethylstilbestrol: DES) directly inhibit testicular steroidogenesis and androgen metabolism in the prostatic cells (Yanaihar and Troen 1972) and shrink the prostatic glands) as demonstrated by Scott and Schirmer 1966 in the intact rat, the high incidence of cardiovascular complications and mortality (Veterans Group 1967) with high doses has led to the use of small amounts of estrogen (1 mg per day of DES): effective in patients with PC although not through the suppression of testosterone levels (Kent et al. 1973). Unfortunately, according to Scott and Schirmer's experience (1966), estrogens always synergize with exogenous androgens in the rat, and are also able to stimulate prolactin release from the pituitary (Mertes and Niccol 1966). Progestational compounds devoid of estrogenic and androgenic activity, such as cyproterone acetate (CPA) or hydroxyprogesterone caproate are able to decrease plasma testosterone levels and to reduce the size of the prostate and have been employed in the treatment of benign and malignant prostatic diseases (Geller et al. 1965, 1967). The compounds can act to lower the plasma levels of testosterone, as well as display peripheral antiandrogenic activity. Progesterone and gestonorone caproate inhibit the uptake of testosterone into prostatic cells (Orestano et al. 1975), medroxyprogesterone acetate (MPA) interferes with intracellular metabolism of testosterone (Orestano et al. 1975, Corvol et al. 1975), while other synthetic progestational compounds, such as CPA, act at receptor levels (Hansson and Tveter 1971), and prevent the formation of a dihydrotestosterone-protein-chromatin complex in the nucleus of the effector cell (Geller and McCoy 1974, Walsh and Korenman 1971).

Wein and Murphy (1973), reported that CPA therapy for untreated carcinomas of the prostate is as good as conventional estrogenic treatment. CPA may offer a better chance for improvement than conventional estrogenic therapy for those patients who have had a relapse following another form of hormonal treatment. Similar favorable results with CPA have been reported by other authors (Smith et al. 1973, Bracci and Di Silverio 1973).

Despite the favorable results of endocrine therapy, the primary treatment of prostatic cancer is still a matter of debate between clinicians. The controversy is mainly due to the natural history of the disease: only 5-15% of cases are diagnosed incidentally at the time of prostatectomy for obstruc-tion, while many patients are known to have a focus in the prostate when they die for other causes. Should local treatment be preferred to hormonal treatment, it would be essential to confirm that the tumor has not yet spread to either bones or nodes. Staging investigations should be equally performed with use of endocrine treatments. Moreover, do asymptomatic patients require any treatment or do early tumors need to be treated with hormonal manipulation, or should no treatment be preferred?

In a study done on a heterogeneous group of elderly men whose one common feature was a tumor that was undiagnosed upon clinical examination (in the laboratory and on x-ray studies), it was possible to identify two major factors that related to tumor progession and patient survival: tumor differentiation and endocrine therapy. The 5 and 10 year survival rates of patients with a well-differentiated tumor is comparable to the expected rate for an age-matched population (67 vs. 72 and 41 vs. 49 percent, respectively). The 10 years survival rate for patients with moderately to poorly-differentiated tumors was less than the expected rate (25 vs. 49 percent) (Heaney et al. 1977). Although many patients respond symptomatically and objectively to endocrine therapy, there is no evidence that their survival is lengthened and perhaps it would be wise to reserve therapy for use as a palliative agent. Tveter et al. (1978) reported an objective improvement in 3, a reduced size of the gland in 7, and subjective relief of dysuria and frequency in 4 out of 16 patients, but could not recommend CPA as the only kind of hormonal treatment of PC. Synthetic gestagens, like 17α-hydroxy-19-Nor-progesterone caproate, may cause an incomplete suppression of plasma testosterone (compared to that observed after orchiectomy) not reflected in a concomitant clinical improvement, although this compound interferes with 5α-reductase activity in the prostate and therefore may inhibit the growth of an androgen-dependent PC (Sander et al. 1978).

In a large-scale clinical study of endocrine therapy for PC on 1818 cases with and without metastases, Nesbit and Baum (1950) suggested that endocrine treatment in any form prolonged patient survival. In contrast, the Veterans Administration Cooperative Urological Research Group demonstrated: 1) the over-all survival among patients given a placebo was not diminished with respect to other forms of therapy; 2) in stages III and IV, 1 mg of DES was as effective as the 5 mg dose and was better than a placebo; and 3) in stages III and IV, 30 mg of MPA; 1.25 mg of premarin daily for one month followed by 2.5 mg daily, or 30 mg of MPA plus 1 mg of DES daily, were not superior to 1 mg of DES daily alone in terms of survival or cancer mortality (Blackard 1975).

There are other important questions to be answered: 1) whether a patient orchiectomized for PC should receive any other form of endocrine treatment; and 2) when the endocrine therapy should be initiated (early in the disease to obtain a longer time-free interval, or late to obtain long-term palliation once the patient has become symptomatic) (Catalona and Scott 1978).

Although a significant correlation exists between tumor grade and prognosis, irrespective of tumor stage (Jewett 1975, Bauer et al. 1960), effort should be made to detect as early as possible a failure of response to therapy. The study of hormonal environment of the patient as well as recent techniques for estimating prostatic metabolism, and particularly steroid receptors, may be helpful in predicting the response to endocrine therapy. The patient hormonal status has been recognized as an important factor since prostatic carcinoma remains, at least for a time, androgen-dependent. Androgens are produced by interstitial cells of the testis and the adrenal cortex. The pituitary interferes with prostatic growth through the secretion of LH which stimulates the interstitial cells, and PRL which stimulates the metabolism of testosterone (T) in the prostate. Bramble and Jacobs (1975) hypothesized that patients with PC could be divided into three groups: normal LH and T plasma levels, high LH and normal T plasma levels, and high LH and low T plasma levels. The last group has interstitial cell failure and an unlikely response to orchiectomy since the tumor is androgen-independent. In choosing treatment, however, one must be aware that approximately 80 per cent of patients respond to hormonal manipulation for some time, suggesting that this should be the first line of attack (Smith et al. 1976). This responsiveness could be related to the presence of steroid receptors in the neoplastic cells that make low circulating hormones available for tissue action. The presence of two populations of cells, one with receptor content, and the other

without, should also be considered. Data is now accumulating in the literature on the relationship between steroid receptors and response to endocrine therapy.

III. STEROID RECEPTORS IN PROSTATIC CARCINOMA

This topic will be discussed elsewhere in the present book. However, for a better understanding of the linkage between endocrine treatment and response to therapy it is useful to draw some conclusion from the results obtained on steroid receptor studies in the carcinoma of prostatic gland.

After the identification of the steroid receptor molecules and the knowledge of the mechanism of action, androgen receptors (AR) have been demonstrated in the cytosol and in the nuclei of normal prostatic tissue as well as in the benign and malignant prostatic carcinoma. More recently, the presence of estrogen receptors (ER) in the prostatic tissue with both benign or malignant transformations has also been reported (Wagner et al. 1975, Bashirelahi et al. 1976, 1979, Hawkins et al. 1976, Marklana et al. 1978, Concolino et al. 1978). Furthermore, the occurrence of a progestin receptor (PR) in the cytosol from hyperplastic and carcinomatous human prostate has been demonstrated by some authors (Cowan et al. 1977, Gustafsson et al. 1978, Concolino et al. 1979).

In view of the reports concerning the treatment of BPH and of PC with progestational compounds, the study of PR together with AR and ER in prostatic diseases appears to be extremely important. These receptors, in fact, may represent the biochemical support of the hormone-dependence of prostatic carcinoma and therefore, receptor studies could be useful not only to determine the treatment of choice, but also to predict the response to endocrine treatment in the patients with a tumor growth still under the influence of hormonal factors. Two points must be stressed on this: first, the different distribution of the receptors in the prostatic gland (AR being mainly localized in the epithelial cells and ER and PR in the stromal compartment of the prostate (Bashirelahi and Sanefugi 1979, Cowan et al. 1977, Wagner and Jungblut 1979) with a consequence of different morphological tissue changes in response to estrogenic, anti-androgenic or progestational treatment; second, the possibility that a correlation between endocrine treatment and steroid receptors could be found particularly when hormonal manipulation is related to a specific receptor molecule that is affected by endocrine modification produced in the patient.

In order to examine these peculiar aspects of the problem, the results obtained in the experimental animals are reported: they could help us to better understand in which way the prostatic tissue responds to hormonal manipulation.

IV. PROSTATIC CARCINOMA IN EXPERIMENTAL ANIMALS

Carcinoma of the prostate can be produced in rats only by direct application of chemical carcinogens to the gland (Dunning et al. 1946, Kallen and Rohl 1960, Gupta et al. 1971). However, the induction of prostatic carcinomas in the Nb strain of rats by prolonged administration of sex hormone was recently reported by Noble (1977) who was able to increase the low spontaneous incidence of grossly recognizable prostatic carcinoma in these rats from 0.45% to 20% by prolonged treatment with testosterone propionate pellets.

In 1963, Dunning described the R-3327 transplantable prostatic adenocarcinoma, arising spontaneously in 1961 in a Copenhagen male rat, line 2331, which has been preserved by subcutaneous transplantation into the same inbred line, retaining its well-differentiated histology. This tumor is androgen responsive because differences in the growth rate of the tumor were found after it was transplanted into intact male rats or male rats previously castrated (Voigt and Dunning 1975). Furthermore, AR and ER could be detected in this tumor (Voigt et al. 1975) Cell kinetic studies have indicated that 70 to 90 percent of the total tumor cells are hormonally sensitive and 8-30 per cent are insensitive. The tumor attains a larger size in the presence of androgens, and some growth was also observed in the castrated animals. The therapeutic relapse to androgen deprivation represented the continued growth of the hormone-insensitive cells (Smolev et al. 1977).

Markland et al. (1978) have characterized several histological variations of transplantable R-3327 prostatic carcinoma. One type, an adenocarcinoma, is hormone-responsive (grows better in male than female rats) and contains substantial amounts of both AR and ER. Another histological type, a fibroadenoma, is hormone-insensitive (grows rapidly in female and in intact and castrated male rats) and does not contain either AR or ER. A third histological variant, carcinosarcoma with elements of the other two types, is hormone-sensitive but has lower receptor levels than the adenocarcinoma. In normal prostate of Copenhagen rats, low levels of AR are present, but no ER can be measured. These animal prostatic tumors show the existence of a correlation between the presence of steroid receptors and hormonal responsiveness of the neoplasia. The combined effects of testosterone and estradiol on explants of rat ventral prostate have also been reported. In the absence of testosterone, prostatic epithelium regresses and the non-epithelial component increases. Estradiol did not change this picture, whereas testosterone maintained the epithelial cells and prevented the increase of the perialveolar sheath and interstitial stroma. Estradiol, in any concentration, was effective in counteracting the androgen-induced inhibition of the stroma when combined with physiological (but not with supraphysiological) concentration of testosterone. In animal studies, DES, which does not mimic estradiol action (Feyel-Cabanes et al. 1978) does not have an inhibitory effect on the cytoplasmic binding of 5α-dihydrotestosterone (DHT) to the receptor, while equimolar doses of CPA, chlormadinone acetate, SC 9022 and flutamide inhibited the binding of DHT to the receptor complex in vivo by 44 to 50 per cent (Ghanadian et al. 1977).

As reported recently for BPH (Symes et al. 1978), the development of tissue culture lines from human prostatic carcinoma, together with in vitro techniques to assess the potency of putative anti-androgens could help to define clones of hormone-sensitive cells and correlate the presence of steroid receptors with the hormonal treatment employed.

V. CORRELATION BETWEEN THE CLINICAL RESPONSE AND STEROID RECEPTORS

The hormone dependence and hormone-responsiveness of human prostatic carcinoma is at present well established. Sixty to 80 per cent of the patients with PC respond to hormonal manipulations (Bracci and Di Silverio 1973, Smith et al. 1976), with the lack of responsiveness being mainly related to a poorly differentiated tumor (Heaney et al. 1977). Besides the histological grade, the age of the tumor is also important in the response to endocrine treatment. In an early phase, in fact, the tumor may be constituted almost entirely by clones of hormone-sensitive cells. The presence of steroid receptors in the hormone-responsive PC is now accepted although the correlation between the response to hormonal treatment and the presence of steroid receptors remains to be established. It is not yet known whether the effects of some therapeutic procedures like orchiectomy or administration of estrogens, progestins or antiandrogens act through a receptor-activated process at the nuclear level or through receptor independent events at the cytoplasmic level. These receptor-independent events could be inhibited by a decrease in available levels of plasma steroids, or in the uptake or metabolism of T. Nevertheless, receptor determination will always be useful in establishing the hormone dependence of the tumor and its hormone responsiveness regardless of the way the therapeutic drugs are active.

Orchiectomy is effective through a decrease in the levels of circulating T, but a decrease in the amount of cytoplasmic androgen receptors, presumably as a result of protein degradation, has also been demonstrated between the days 1 and 5 after orchiectomy (Van Doorn et al. 1972).

Administration of estrogens is as effective as orchiectomy in lowering plasma T by reducing T secretion by the testis. The effects of 1 mg of DES are comparable to those of 5 mg dose whithout the risk of cardiovascular complications (Mackler et al. 1972). Since estrogens are able to shrink the prostatic gland (Scott and Schirmer 1966), it can be hypothesized that they act through the specific ER present in the non epithelial part of the gland. Hyperplasia of interstitial stroma under estrogen stimulation could explain the shrinking of the tumor during estrogen treatment which counteracts the androgen-induced inhibition of the stroma (Feyel-Cabanes et al. 1978). Jungblut et al. (1971) showed that AR has a considerable affinity for

estradiol and that it can be blocked in vitro by excessive amounts of the steroid. Thus, the effect of estrogens on prostatic carcinoma could be explained by a blockage of AR, with suppression of the growth-promoting effect of endogenous androgens. However, from the data of Wagner and Schulze (1978) and Wagner (1978) on 11 patients, treated with high doses of DES for advanced PC, it was concluded that no correlation existed between AR and ER content in the tumor, and response to DES treatment. In fact, of the 5 tumors which regressed with DES only, 3 contained measurable amounts of AR. In 3 tumors, unchanged by the treatment, neither AR nor ER could be detected. The remaining 3 carcinomas were not influenced at all by DES and grew progressively, although considerable amounts of AR were found in them. These results counter the hypothesis that DES could act via the AR system. This was further demonstrated with competition experiments performed on AR binding site where estradiol and CPA compete for AR, while DES does not (Wagner 1978, Ghanadian et al. 1977). A correlation between DES and ER in prostatic carcinoma is also unexpected since DES does not mimic estradiol action on rat ventral prostate (Feyel-Cabanes et al. 1978). Therefore, the objective remission of over 70 per cent of the prostatic carcinoma treated with DES may be related to the suppression of androgen production by the testis or the increased serum levels of SHBG with decreased free T levels and a direct antiproliferative action of DES (Mangan et al. 1967).

Other investigators, however, claim that receptor studies can be a valuable diagnostic tool in choosing the most appropriate form of therapy for PC and report a high correlation between the presence of AR in the tumor and the response to hormonal treatment (Snochowski et al. 1977, Mobbs et al. 1974, Gustaffson et al. 1978). From preliminary correlations with response to endocrine treatment, Mobbs et al. (1974) reported that in patients with low endogenous androgens and tumors with a high degree of malignant involvement, androgen insensitivity may be reflected by a low binding capacity of AR. Patients whose tumors had an androgen binding capacity of 0.4-1.0 fmol/mg showed at least a partial response to hormonal manipulation under the same conditions. According to Gustaffson et al. (1978) a good correlation exists between the short-term response to estrogen treatment (polyestradiol phosphate, ethynylestradiol or estramustine phosphate) and the presence of AR in the prostatic cancer. He reported 16 patients investigated for receptor content and randomized for the endocrine treatment (the choice of therapy was in no case influenced by receptor analysis). Of the 12 patients whose tumors contained measurable amounts of AR, one died before initiation of hormonal treatment, and 9 of the remaining 11 patients (82°_0) showed a good response to estrogen treatment. The 2 receptor-positive non responders had the lowest measured amounts of receptors. Of the 4 patients whose tumors lacked measurable amounts of AR, only one had a remission from estrogen therapy, and 3 did not respond to hormonal treatment.

Taking into consideration that tissue DHT levels depend upon plasma T (DHT precursor), 3-hydroxysteroid dehydrogenase, 5α-reductase and steroid receptors, Geller et al. (1978) demonstrated that prostate cancer tissue DHT levels appeared to correlate better than did either histological tumor grading or 5α-reductase with the clinical response to antiandrogen therapy (either orchiectomy, diethylstilbestrol or megestrol acetate).

Although some authors reported that CPA is the least effective method for androgen suppression while both DES and orchiectomy produce a significantly greater suppression of T (O'Donoghue et al. 1979) a good correlation between the presence of AR, ER or PR and the response to CPA and/or orchiectomy was found in our patients with prostatic cancer (Concolino et al. in press). Ekman (in press) reported a study on 8 patients with PC whose steroid receptor content was measured and the response to estrogen treatment correlated with the presence of steroid receptor. Seven out of 8 tumors investigated had an AR, 3 had a PR, 5 had a glucocorticoid receptor and none had ER. The correlation between AR and the response to endocrine treatment was 86 per cent.

In a more detailed study, Bashirelahi and Sanefugi (in press) reported the distribution of AR, ER and PR in the epithelial and stromal cells of human prostate. They claimed to have found a better correlation between ER and antiandrogen treatment than between AR and estrogen therapy.

From the data reported by Teulings et al. (in press) it has become clear that, although MPA & CPA compete for steroid receptors in metastatic lymph nodes of prostatic cancer patients, no results could be obtained with MPA on the involved lymph nodes of prostatic carcinoma.

Recently De Voogt and Dingjan (in press) used a computerized method to evaluate the correlation between AR and ER in the prostatic tumor and estrogen treatment. Tumor size, patient complaints and laboratory assessments were used to obtain the final evaluation of the response. The study was done on 3 groups of patients with PC: 27 untreated patients, 20 patients treated with estrogens for 38 months, and 15 patients of the first group after 8 months of estrogen treatment. The last group only showed a correlation between the clinical response and the presence of AR and ER. No correlation was found between the binding capacity of the steroid receptors and the histological grading, nor between the binding capacity and the amount of stromal and epithelial cells, except in the patients treated with estrogens for 38 months. Here, the binding capacity of ER was in fact found to be greater in the stromal than in the epithelial cells.

It is reasonable to believe that the importance of the steroid receptors, relative to the endocrine treatment employed may become more evident if the hormonal treatment is made with compounds which effectively compete for such receptors. CPA and flutamide, or its hydroxilated derivative (Symes et al. 1978), are compounds which actively compete for AR sites (Orestano et al. 1975, Hansson and Tveter 1971, Geller and McCoy 1974). Therefore, the use of antiandrogenic compounds such as CPA seems a suitable treatment for prostatic carcinoma. This compound, with its progestational activity, could act through a progesterone binding component which is absent in the epithelium (Cowan et al. 1977), and could act to induce a response in the stroma.

From these considerations, AR, ER and PR were studied by our group as predictive parameters of the hormone dependence of human PC, and the response to orchiectomy and administration of CPA evaluated on the basis of receptor studies. The clinical follow-up of 11 patients examined is reported in Table 1. It is of interest to notice the PR found in patients N 8 and N 10 whose tumors were devoid of AR.

For evaluation of response, *remission* was considered when only subjective and clinical criteria were used, *partial objective regression* and *objective stable* tumor refer to the use of objective criteria including changes in bone metastases, tumor mass, and prostatic acid phosphatase.

There was no tumor progression, but there were 2 favorable subjective responses and 9 objective responses to orchiectomy plus CPA treatment, regardless of the TNM of the patients examined. Whether CPA acts in these patients with hormone-responsive cancers only as an antiandrogen, blocking the formation of DHT-receptor complex, or as a progestational compound able to interfere with tumor growth when PR are present, cannot be stated.

(plasma testosterone and LH levels), endogenous androgen concentration and steroid receptor assays may help to predict the response to endocrine treatment. Recurrence of carcinoma of the prostate in castrated patients or hormone-treated patients may be due to a selection of a clone of hormone-insensitive cells. These cells may be present, although in small amounts, at an early stage of the disease. Therefore the association of endocrine therapy with a specific non-hormonal treatment for the insensitive cells should, perhaps, be initiated in the earliest phase of the disease. Further studies and longer follow-up will help to better define the correlation between steroid receptors and response to the endocrine treatment in human prostatic carcinoma.

VI. CONCLUSIONS

Prostatic carcinoma is a hormone-dependent and hormone-responsive tumor. Some useful parameters, such as endocrine status of the patients

ACKNOWLEDGEMENT

This work was supported in part by a grant of the Italian Research Council – CNR – special project "Control of Neoplastic Growth."

Table 1. Steroid receptors and clinical response to hormonal therapy.

Patients	Initials	Age	TNM[a]	AR	ER	PR	Treatment	Mos. of	Response
1	G.M.	74	$T_2N_0M_0$	+	−	n.d.	O.[d]+TVR[b]+CPA[c]	84	Remission
2	C.F.	70	$T_3N_0M_0$	+	−	n.d.	,,	24	Partial objective regression
3	V.V.	63	$T_3N_0M_1$	+	−	n.d.	,,	25	Objectively stable
4	C.C.	71	$T_4N_1M_1$	−	+	n.d.	,,	9	Objectively stable
5	B.O.	64	$T_0N_0M_0$	+	−	n.d.	,,	24	Objectively stable
6	D.M.	74	$T_3N_0M_0$	+	−	n.d.	,,	12	Remission
7	C.F.	72	$T_2N_0M_1$[a]	+	−	+	,,	8	Partial objective regression
8	C.G.	77	$T_2N_0M_0$	−	−	+	,,	7	Objectively stable
9	F.S.	59	$T_1N_0M_0$	+	+	−	,,	17	Objectively stable
10	M.G.	62	$T_4N_0M_0$	−	+	+	,,	22	Objectively stable
11	Z.L.	68	$T_3N_0M_0$	+	−	+	,,	28	Partial objective regression

[a] = Tumor- nodes metastases classification (Union Internationale contre Cancrum, Geneva 1974). [b] = Trans Vesical Resection, [c] = Cyproterone - acetate, [d] = orchiectomy, n.d. = not detected.

REFERENCES

Barnes R, Hirst A, Rosenquist R: Early carcinoma of the prostate: comparison of stages A and B. J Urol 115: 404, 1976.

Bashirelahi N, O'Toole JH, Young JD: A specific 17B-estradiol receptor in human benign hypertrophic prostate. Biochem Med 15: 254, 1976.

Bashirelahi N, and Sanefugi H: Androgen and progestagen receptors and their distribution in epithelial and stromal cells of human prostate. In: Steroid receptors, metabolism and prostatic cancer, Workshop of the European Prostatic Cancer Research Group, Amsterdam, 27-28 april 1979. Excerpta Medica (in press).

Bauer WC, McGavran MH, and Carlin MR: Unsuspected carcinoma of the prostate in suprapubic prostatectomy specimens: a clinicopathological study of 55 consecutive cases. Cancer 13: 370, 1960.

Blackard CE: The Veterans Administration Cooperative Urological Research Group studies of carcinoma of the prostate: a review. Cancer Chemother Rep 59: 225, 1975.

Bracci U, and Di Silverio F: Il cancro della prostata: nostro attuale orientamento terapeutico. Il Progresso Medico 29: 779, 1973.

Bracci U, Di Silverio F, Sciarra F, Sorcini G, Piro C, and Santoro F: Hormonal pattern in prostatic carcinoma following orchiectomy: 5 year follow up Brit J Urol 449: 161,

1977.

Bramble FJ, and Jacobs HS: Hormones, elderly testes and carcinoma of the prostate Brit Med J 3: 307, 1975.

Catalona WL, and Scott WW: Carcinoma of the prostate: a review. J Urol 119: 1, 1978.

Concolino G, Di Silverio F, Marocchi A, and Tenaglia R: Recettori steroidei nel carcinoma prostatico umano. Atti della Soc Ital Biochim Clin 7: 512, 1978.

Concolino G, Marocchi A, Ricci G, Liberti M, Di Silverio F, and Bracci U: Steroid receptors and endocrine therapy of prostatic carcinoma. In: Steroid receptors, metabolism and prostatic cancer. Workshop of the European Prostatic Cancer Research Group, Amsterdam, 27-28 April 1979, Excerpta Medica (in press).

Concolino G, Marocchi A, Iacobelli S, Liberti M, Di Silverio F, and Bracci U: Binding and biological activity of androgens in prostatic carcinoma: clinical response to therapy. Archives of Andrology 2, suppl 1: 82, 1979.

Correa RJ Jr, Anderson RG, Gibbons RP, and Mason JT: Latent carcinoma of the prostate - Why the controversy? J Urol 111: 644, 1974.

Corvol P, Michaud A, Menard J, Freifeld M, and Mahoudeau J: Antiandrogenic effect of spironolactones: mechanism of action. Endocrinology 97: 52, 1975.

Cowan RA, Cowan SK, and Grant JK: Binding of methyltrienolone (R1881) to a progesterone receptor-like component of human prostate cytosol. J Endocrinol 74: 281, 1977.

Davies P, and Griffiths K: Similarities between 5-alpha-dihydrotestosterone receptor complexes from human and rat prostatic tissue: effect on RNA polymerase activity. Molecular and Cellular Endocr 3: 143, 1975.

de Voogt HJ, and Dingjan PJ: Is there a place for the assay of cytoplasmic steroid receptors in the treatment of prostatic cancer? In: Steroid receptors, metabolism and prostatic cancer, Workshop of the European Prostatic Cancer Research Group, Amsterdam 27-28 April 1979, Excerpta Medica (in press).

Di Silverio F, Gagliardi V, Sorcini G, and Sciarra F: Biosynthesis and metabolism of androgenic hormones in cancer of the prostate. Investigative Urology 13: 286, 1976.

Dunning WF, Curtis MR, and Segaloff A: Methylcholanthrene squamous cell carcinoma of the rat prostate with skeletal metastases and failure of the rat liver to respond to the same carcinogen. Cancer Res 6: 256, 1946.

Dunning WF: Prostate cancer in the rat. Nat Cancer Inst Monogr 12: 351, 1963.

Ekman P: Clinical significance of steroid receptor assay in human prostate. In: Steroid receptors, metabolism and prostatic cancer, Workshop of the European Prostatic Cancer Research Group, Amsterdam, 27-28 April 1979, Excerpta Medica (in press).

Fergusson JD, and Hendry WF: Pituitary irradiation in advanced carcinoma of the prostate: analysis of 100 cases. Brit J Urol 43: 514, 1971.

Feyel-Cabanes T, Secchi J, Robel P, and Baulieu EE: Combined effects of testosterone and estradiol on rat ventral prostate in organ culture. Cancer Res 38: 4126, 1978.

Geller J, Bora R, Roberts T, Newman H, Lin A, and Silva R: Treatment of benign prostatic hypertrophy with 17-alpha-hydroxyprogesterone caproate. JAMA 193: 121, 1965.

Geller J, Fruchtman B, Newman H, Roberts T, and Silva R: Effects of progestational agents on carcinoma of the prostate. Cancer Chemother Rep 51: 41, 1967.

Geller J, and McKoy K: Biological and biochemical effects of antiandrogens on rat ventral prostate. Acta Endocr (Kbh) 75: 385, 1974.

Geller J, Cantor T, and Albert J: Evidence for a specific dihydrotestosterone-binding cytosol receptor in the human prostate. J Clin Endocrinol Metab 41: 854, 1975.

Geller J, Albert J, de la Vega D, Loza D, and Stoeltzing W: Dihydrotestosterone concentration in prostate cancer tissue as a predictor of tumor differentiation and hormonal dependency. Cancer Res 38: 4349, 1978.

Ghanadian R, Smith CB, Williams G, and Chisholm GD: The effect of antiandrogens and stilbestrol on the cytosol receptor in rat prostate. Brit J Urol 49: 695, 1977.

Ghanadian R, Auf G, Chaloner PJ, and Chisholm GD: The use of methyltrienolone in the measurement of the free and bound cytoplasmic receptors for dihydrotestosterone in benign hypertrophied human prostate. J Steroid Biochem 9: 325, 1978.

Grayhack JT: Pituitary factors influencing growth of the prostate. Nat Cancer Inst Monogr 12: 189, 1963.

Gupta SK, Mathur IS, and Kar AB: Chemical induction of prostatic tumours in random-bred rats. J Exp Biol 9: 296, 1971.

Gustafsson JA, Ekman P, Pousette A, Snochowski M, and Hogberg B: Demonstration of a progestin receptor in human benign prostatic hyperplasia and prostatic carcinoma. Investigative Urol 15: 361, 1978.

Gustafsson JA, Ekman P, Snochowski M, Zetterberg A, Pousette A, and Hogberg B: Correlation between clinical response to hormone therapy and steroid receptor content in prostatic cancer. Cancer Res 38: 4345, 1978.

Hansson V, and Tveter KJ: Effect of the androgens on the uptake and binding of androgen by human benign nodular prostatic hyperplasia in vitro. Acta Endocr (Kbh) 68: 69, 1971.

Liao S, Liang T and Tymoczko JL: Structural recognition in the interactions of androgens and receptor proteins and in their association with nuclear acceptor components. J Steroid Biochem 3: 401, 1971.

Lieskovsky G, and Bruchovsky N: Assay of nuclear androgen receptor in human prostate. J Urol 121: 54, 1979.

Lubaroff DM: Development of an epithelial tissue culture line from human prostatic adenocarcinoma. J Urol 118: 612, 1977.

Kallen B, and Rohl L: Tissue culture studies on a rat-prostatic cancer, induced with 20-methylcholantrene. Acta Path Microb Scand 20: 283, 1960.

Kent JR, Bishoff AJ, Arduino LJ, Mellinger GT, Byar DP, Hill M, and Kozbur X: Estrogen dosage and suppression of testosterone levels in patients with prostatic carcinoma. J Urol 109: 858, 1973.

Jewett HJ: The present status of radical prostatectomy for stages A and B prostatic cancer. Urol Clin N Amer 2: 105, 1975.

Jungblut PW, Hughes SF, Gorlich L, Gowers U, and Wagner RK: Simultaneous occurrence of individual oestrogen and androgen receptors in female and male target organs. Hoppe Seyler's Z Physiol Chem 352: 1603, 1971.

Hansson V, Tveter KJ, Unhjem O, Djosland O, Attramadal A, Reusch F, and Torgersen O: Androgen binding in the male sex organs, with special reference ot the human prostate. In: Golan M, Thomas CC, (eds), Normal and abnormal Growth of the Prostate, Springfield, Illinois, 1975, p 676.

Hawkins EF, Nijs M, and Brassinne C: Steroid receptors in the human prostate. II. Some properties of the estrophilic molecule of benign prostatic hypertrophy. Biochem Biophys Res Comm 70: 854, 1976.

Heaney JA, Chang HC, Daly JJ, and Prout GR Jr: Prognosis of clinically undiagnosed prostatic carcinoma and the influence of endocrine therapy. J Urol 118: 283, 1977.

Huggins C, Masina NH, Eichelberger L, and Warton JD: Quantitative studies of prostatic secretion: characteristics of the normal secretion; influence of thyroid, suprarenal and testis extirpation and androgen substitution on prostatic output. J Exper Med 70: 543, 1939.

Huggins C, and Hodges CV: Studies on prostatic cancer. I. The effect of castration, of estrogen and androgen injection on serum phosphatases in metastatic carcinoma of the prostate. Cancer Res 1: 293, 1941.

Mackler MA, Liberti JP, Vernon Smith MJ, Koontz WW Jr, and Prout GR Jr: The effect of orchiectomy and various doses of stilbestrol on plasma testosterone levels in patients with carcinoma of the prostate. Invest Urol 9: 423, 1972.

Mainwaring WIP The binding of (1,2-³H)-testosterone within nuclei of rat prostate. J Endocr 44: 323, 1969.

Mainwaring WIP, and Milroy EJG: Characterization of the specific androgen receptors in the human prostate gland. J Endocr 57: 371, 1973.

Mangan FR, Neal GE, and Williams DC: The effects of diethylstilboestrol and castration on the nucleic acid and protein metabolism of rat prostate gland. Biochem J 104: 1075, 1967.

Markland FS, Chopp RT, Cosgrove MD, and Hovard EB: Characterization of steroid hormone receptor in the Dunning R-3327 rat prostatic adenocarcinoma Cancer Res 38: 2818, 1978.

Mertes J, and Niccol CS: Adenohypophysis: prolactin. Ann Rev Physiol 28: 57, 1966.

Mobbs BG, Johnson IE, Conolly JG: Hormonal responsiveness of prostatic carcinoma. Urology 3: 105, 1974.

Mobbs BG, Johnson IE, Conolly JG and Clark AF: Evaluation of the use of cyproterone acetate competition to distinguish between high-affinity binding of ³H-dihydrotestosterone to human prostate cytosol receptors and to sex hormone binding globulin. J Steroid Biochem 8: 943, 1977.

Mobbs BG, Johnson IE, Conolly JG, and Clark AF: Androgen receptor assay in human benign and malignant prostatic tumor cytosol using protamine sulphate precipitation. J Steroid Biochem 9: 289, 1978.

Murphy JP, Reynoso G, Schoonees R, Gailani S, Bourke R, Kenny GM, Mirand EA, and Schalch DS: Hypophysectomy and adrenalectomy for disseminated prostatic cancer. J Urol 105: 817, 1971.

Nesbit RM, and Baum WC: Endocrine control of prostatic carcinoma: clinical and statistical survey of 1818 cases. JAMA 143: 1317, 1950.

Noble RL: The development of prostatic adenocarcinoma in Nb rats following prolonged sex hormone administration. Cancer Res 37: 1929, 1977.

O'Donoghue EPN, Ghanadian R, and Puah CM: Serum Di-hydrotestosterone and testosterone after endocrine manipulation in carcinoma of the prostate. Archives of Andrology 2, suppl 1: 89, 1979.

Orestano F, Altwein JE, Knapstein P, and Bandhauer K: Mode of action of progesterone, gestonorone capronate (Depostat) and cyproterone acetate (Androcur) on the metabolism of testosterone in human prostatic adenoma: in vitro and in vivo investigation. J Steroid Biochem 6: 845, 1975.

Sander S, Nissen-Meyer R, and Aakvaag A: On gestagen treatment of advanced prostatic carinoma. Scand J Urol Nephrol 12: 119, 1978.

Sciarra F, Sorcini G, Di Silverio F, and Gagliardi V: Plasma testosterone and androstenedione after orchiectomy in prostatic adenocarcinoma. Clin Endocr 2: 101, 1973.

Scott WW, and Schirmer HKA: A new oral progestational steroid effective in treating prostatic cancer. Transaction of American Association of Genito-Urinary Surgeons 58: 54, 1966.

Smith PH, Robinson MRG, and Cooper EH: Prospective in cancer research. Carcinoma of the prostate: a focal point for divergent disciplines. Europ J Cancer 12: 937, 1976.

Smith RB, Walsh PC, and Goodwin WE: Cyproterone acetate in the treatment of advanced carcinoma of the prostate. J Urol 110: 106, 1973.

Smolev JK, Coffey DS, and Scott WW: Experimental models for the study of prostatic adenocarcinoma. J Urol 118: 216, 1977.

Snochowski M, Pousette A, Ekman P, Bression D, Andersson L, Hogberg B, and Gustaffson JA: Characterization and measurement of the androgen receptor in human benign prostatic hyperplasia and prostatic carcinoma. J Clin Endocr Metab 45: 920, 1977.

Symes EK, Milroy EJG, and Mainwaring WIP: The nuclear uptake of androgen by human benign prostate in vitro: action of antiandrogens. J Urol 120: 180, 1978.

Teulings FAG, Alexieva-Figusch J, Henkelman MS, Portengen H, and Van Gilse HA: Steroid receptors in metastases of prostatic cancer. In: Steroid receptors, metabolism and prostatic cancer, Workshop of the European Prostatic Cancer Research Group, Amsterdam, 27-28 April 1979. Excerptia Medica (in press).

Thomas JA, and Manandhar M: Effects of prolactin and/or testosterone on nucleic acid levels in prostatic glands of normal and castrated rats. J Endocr 65: 149, 1975.

Tveter KM, Unhjem O, Attramadal A, Aakvaag A, and Hansson N: Androgenic receptors in rat and human prostate. Advances in Biosciences 7: 193, 1970.

Tveter KJ, Otnes B, and Hannestad R: Treatment of prostatic carcinoma with cyproterone acetate. Scand J Urol Nephrol 12: 115, 1978.

Voigt W, and Dunning WF: In vivo metabolism of testosterone-³H in R-3327, an androgen sensitive rat prostatic adeno-carcinoma. Cancer Res 34: 1447, 1974.

Voigt W, Feldman M, and Dunning WF: 5α-dihydrotestos-terone-binding proteins and androgen sensitivity in prostatic cancers of Copenhagen rats. Cancer Res 35: 1840, 1975.

Wagner RK, Schulze KH, and Jungblut PW: Estrogen and androgen receptors in human prostate and prostatic tumor tissue. Acta Endocr (Kbh) 78, suppl 193: 52, 1975 (Abstr).

Wagner RK: Extracellular and intracellular steroid binding proteins. Properties, discrimination, assay and clinical applications. Acta Endocr (Kbh) 88: 1, 1978.

Wagner RK, and Schulze KH: Clinical relevance of androgen receptor content in human prostate carcinoma. Acta Endocr (Kbh) 87: 139, 1978.

Wagner RK, and Jungblut PW: Lack of correlation between androgen receptor content and clinical response to treatment with diethylstilboestrol in human prostatic carcinomas. In: Steroid receptors, metabolism and prostatic cancer, Workshop of the European Prostatic Cancer Research Group, Amsterdam, 27-28 April 1979. Excerpta Medica (in press).

Walsh PC, and Korenman SG: Mechanism of androgen action: effect of specific intracellular inhibitors. J Urol 105: 850, 1971.

Wein AJ, and Murphy JJ: Experience in the treatment of prostatic carcinoma with cyproterone acetate. J Urol 109: 68, 1973.

Van Doorn E, Craven S, and Bruchovsky N: The relationship between androgen receptors and the hormonally controlled responses of rat ventral prostate. Biochem J 160: 11, 1976.

The Veterans Administration Cooperative Urological Research Group: Treatment and survival of patients with cancer of the prostate. Surg Gynec Obstet 124: 1011, 1967.

Yanaihara T, and Troen P: Studies of the human testis. III Effect of estrogen on testosterone formation in human testis in vitro. J Clin Endocr Metab 34: 968, 1972.

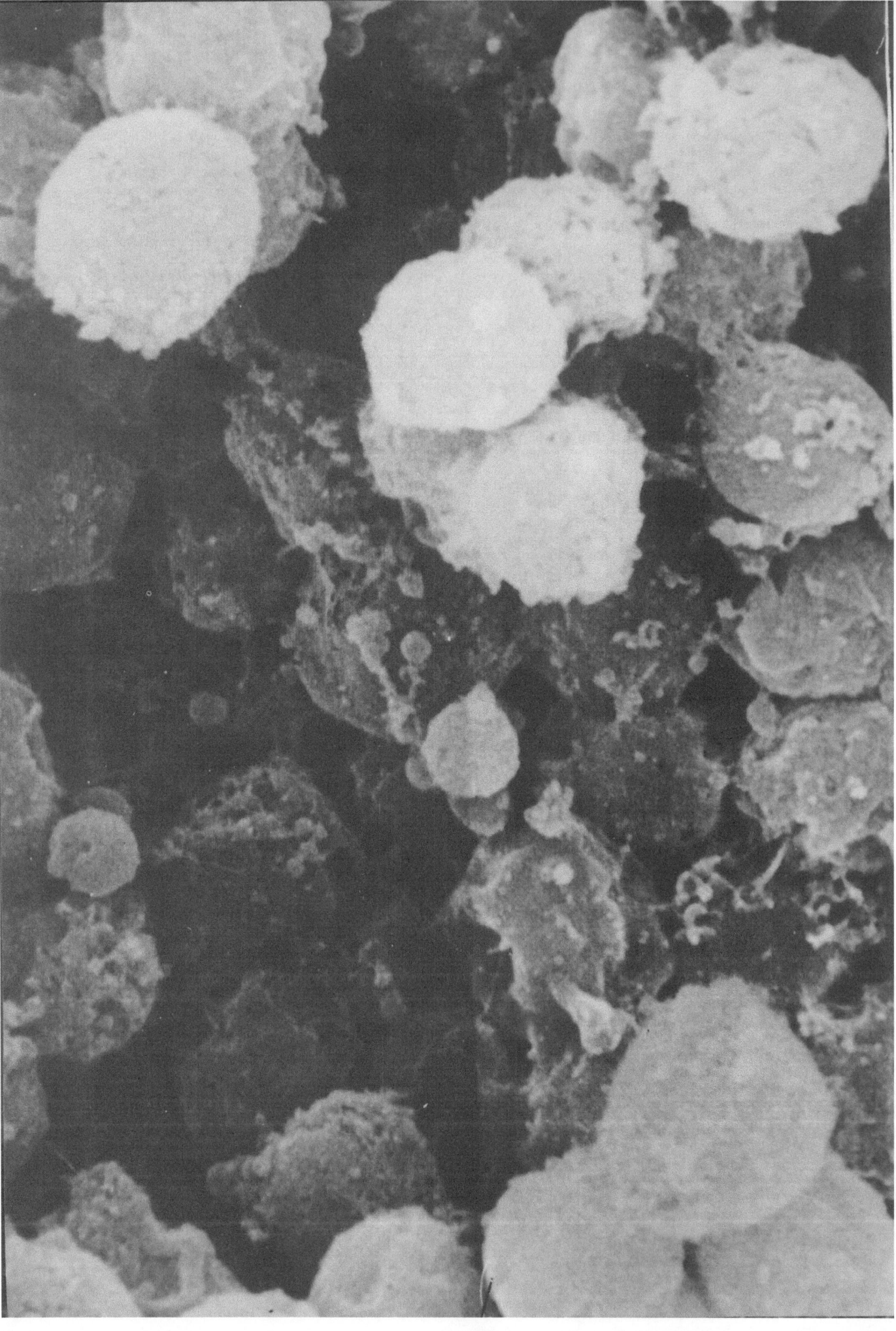

II. DIAGNOSTIC PROCEDURES

6. MASS SCREENING OF PROSTATIC DISEASES

H. WATANABE, T. MISHINA and H. OHE

I. INTRODUCTION

In 1967, Watanabe developed transrectal ultrasonotomography to show the anatomic structure of the prostate in the form of an easily comprehensible cross-section map (Watanabe 1971, 1974, 1975). According to our surveys the false negative rate of this examination in the diagnosis of clinically manifest prostatic cancer was 0.3 per cent (Watanabe et al. 1978a) (Table 1). Transrectal ultrasonotomography is suitable as a screening test for prostatic cancer because of its low false negative rate and of its non-invasive procedure. We began the development of a new mass screening system for prostatic diseases 4 years ago, using transrectal ultrasonotomography as the primary study (Watanabe et al., 1977a).

Table 1. Ultrasonic and final diagnosis of prostatic cancer (June 1976-May 1978, Kyoto Prefectural University of Medicine).

Ultrasonic diagnosis		PC	Suspicion of PC	Other prostatic diseases
Final diagnosis	PC (+)	36(100%)	6(5.9%)	2(0.3%)
	PC (−)	0	95 (94.1%)	606 (99.7%)
Total		36	101	608

II. METHOD

Our system for the mass screening program was made up of a primary and a secondary study. In the primary study, a questionnaire (Table 2) about history was completed by subjects and transrectal ultrasonotomography was performed. After the examination all examinees were asked for their impressions about the test by another questionnaire (Table 3).

Along with the history card, obtained by the first questionnaire, a number of recorded tomograms which were usually taken for each subject was evaluated carefully by senior urologists. All subjects who show any pathological findings on the sonograms, however slight, were submitted to a secondary study. The secondary study, which consisted of general urological examinations including prostatic biopsy, was performed by senior urologists. The final diagnosis was made after the secondary study and appropriate urological treatment begun. The special chair-type scanner developed by Watanabe for transrectal ultrasonotomography as used in the primary study is shown in Figure 1. When the patient sat on the chair, the anus was positioned

Table 2. Questionnaire before transrectal ultrasonotomography.

Name   , Age   , Occupation
Final academic career   , No.   , No of echo

Have you ever complained of the following symptoms? Please check, yes or no.

1. dysuria		yes, no
2. retardation		yes, no
3. protraction		yes, no
4. more than three times' urination over a night		yes, no
5. dysuria after drinking		yes, no
6. pollakisuria in day time		yes, no
7. micturition pain		yes, no
8. sense of residual urine		yes, no
9. macrohematuria		yes, no
10. sense of dullness in the perineal region		yes, no
11. backache		yes, no
12. lumbago or pain in the leg		yes, no
13. urinary incontinence		yes, no
14. contusio in the back and lumbar region		yes, no
15. epileptic seizure		yes, no
16. nocturnal enuresis during school children		yes, no
17. gonorrhea		yes, no
18. syphilis		yes, no
19. diseases of the urinary bladder		yes, no
20. nephropathy		yes, no

over a hole in the seat and a specially designed transducer tube was pushed up into the rectum (Figure 2). Horizontal sections of the intrapelvic organs around the rectum, including the prostate, the bladder or the seminal vesicles were obtained by radial scanning with the automatic rotation of an oscillating disc inside the transducer (Figure 3).

Table 3. Questionnaire after transrectal ultrasonotomography.

Name   , Age   , Occupation
Final academic career

Thank you very much for your cooperation with us in this mass screening program for prostatic diseases. Please choose and check your impression from the following.
1. Comments on ultrasonic examination:
   Had heard about it
   Had heard but had no interest
   Had never heard of it
2. Comments on insertion of transducer:
   Painful
   Not painful but discomfort
   No pain and no discomfort
3. Comments during examination:
   Painful

   Felt faint
4. Comments on this mass screening
   Good idea
   Better than nothing
   Bad idea

III. MODEL EXPERIMENT

The first model mass screening program for prostatic diseases was performed for limited groups at the Cancer Detection Center of the Miyagi Cancer Society from January 20 to 31, 1975 (Watanabe et al. 1977b). According to data for the incidental ages of prostatic cancer, subjects are usually more than 55 years of age (Hirayama 1978). For our first model experiment, however, 132 males surveyed in the primary study were from 40 to 76 years of age, with an average age of 55.0.

According to the answers given in the first questionnaire frequent urination and a sense of residual urine were present in 27 per cent, various disturbances of urination in 25 per cent and nocturia in 15 per cent. Of the 132 cases clear tomograms of the prostate were recorded in 127. The examination was interrupted in 2 cases because of slight dizziness in one and pain from hemorrhoids

in the other. In 3 further cases the tomogram failed to record because of a camera malfunction. A total of 1,990 minutes was required for the over-all tests, including 1,044 minutes for the preparation, 816 minutes for the examination, 77 minutes for preparing mechanical troubles and 53 minutes for idle time. The average time per case inclusive of all factors was 5.3 minutes (Table 5). Tomograms were evaluated and in 48 of 127 cases (37.8 per cent) it was thought necessary to do secondary studies. Almost all subjects showed an affirmative reaction to the examination and a positive interest in the mass screening program at the second questionnaire.

Secondary urological examinations were performed from March 6 to 24, 1975. Of the 48 cases for which secondary studies were considered necessary 46 were evaluated. Benign prostatic hypertrophy in the 1st stage (BPH 1) was detected in 9 cases, BPH in the second stage in 9, prostatitis in 5, prostatic tuberculosis in 1 and no prostatic diseases in the other 22 (Table 4). These patients have all been successfully treated.

The second model mass screening program was

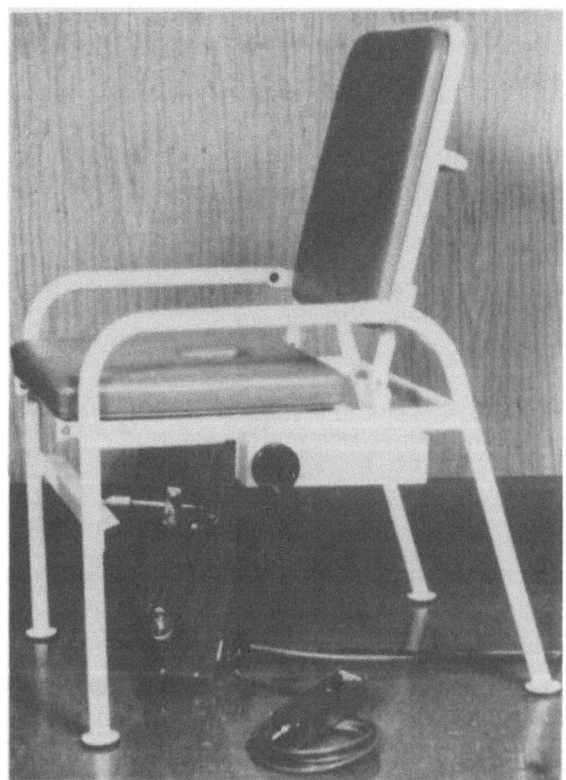

Figure 1. A special chair-type scanner for transrectal ultrasonotomography.

performed at two old people's homes in Ichihara and Arashiyama, Kyoto, from February 14 to 18, 1977 (Watanabe et al. 1977b). The 48 males surveyed in the primary study were from 62 to 88 years of age, with an average age of 77.3.

The first questionnaire revealed frequent urination and a sense of residual urine was present in 52 per cent, various disturbances of urination in 35 per cent and nocturia in 54 per cent of the examinees. Clear tomograms of the prostate were recorded in 46 of 48. The examination was interrupted in 2 cases because of some reluctance in one and of a camera malfunction in the other. The average time per case inclusive of all factors was 15.9 minutes as shown in Table 5.

The secondary studies were needed in 21 of 48 cases (43.8 per cent). Among them, BPH in the first stage was detected in 5 cases, BPH in the second stage in 6, prostatitis in 1, prostatic stone in 1 and no prostatic diseases in the other 8.

In these 2 model experiments, there were 3 persons, including a doctor, a medical assistant and a technical assistant, usually concerned with the test daily. According to a rough estimate the cost per subject for the primary test was ¥1.500 or $7.50, including personal expenses ¥850 or $4.25, repayment for equipment (¥400 or $2.00) and cost of disposable goods (¥250 or $1.25).

IV. FIELD EXPERIMENT

It was presumed from these 2 model experiments that our mass screening program was inexpensive, excellent and useful to detect prostatic diseases. As the next step, a field experiment of mass screening program for general people living in a limited area was carried out in order to develop this system.

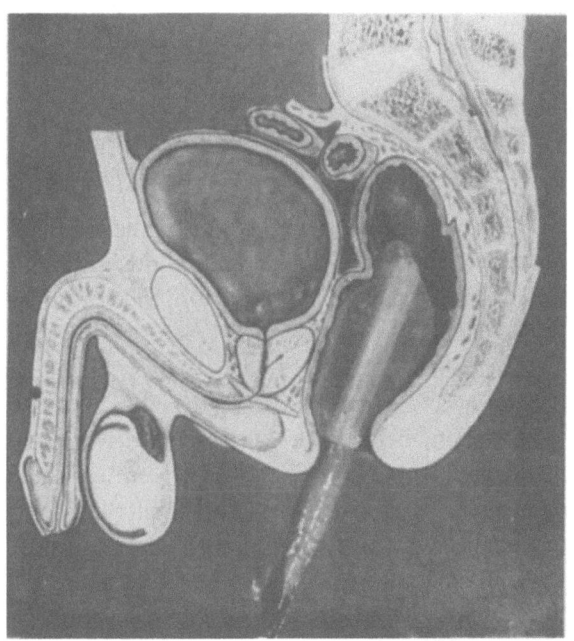

Figure 2. A specially designed transducer tube which is pushed up into the rectum.

Table 4. Experiments of mass screening for prostatic diseases I.

	Model experiments		Field experiments		Total
	First	*Second*	*First*	*Second*	
Location	The cancer detection center of the Miyagi cancer society	2 old-age homes in Kyoto Prefecture	Keihoku-cho Kyoto Prefecture		
Date	Jan.—Mar., 1975	Feb.—Apr., 1977	Dec.—Oct., 1977	Jul., 1978	
Volunteers of primary study	132	48	58	37	275
Average age of volunteers	55.0 y.o.	77.3 y.o.	71.2 y.o.	72.3 y.o.	64.6 y.o.
Cases of secondary studies					
necessary	48 (36.4%)	21 (43.8%)	25 (43.1%)	16 (43.2%)	110 (40.0%)
evaluated	46 (34.8%)	21 (43.8%)	25 (43.1%)	15 (40.5%)	107 (38.9%)
BPH 1	9 (6.8%)	5 (10.4%)	9 (15.5%)	8 (21.6%)	31 (11.3%)
BPH 11	9 (6.8%)	6 (12.5%)	6 (10.3%)	4 (10.8%)	25 (9.1%)
Prostatic cancer	0	0	2 (3.4%)	0	2 (0.7%)
Prostatitis	5 (3.8%)	1 (2.1%)	0	1 (2.7%)	7 (2.5%)
Prostatic stone	1 (0.8%)	1 (2.1%)	0	2 (5.4%)	4 (1.5%)

(Final diagnosis)

Table 5. Experiments of mass screening for prostatic diseases II.

Experiments		Model experiments		Field experiments		Total
		First	Second	First	Second	
Volunteers of primary study		132	48	58	37	275
No performance of primary study		2 (1.5%)	1 (2.1%)	0	0	3 (1.1%)
No performance of recording		3 (2.3%)	1 (2.1%)	0	0	4 (1.5%)
Average number of pictures		9.9	8.2	6.9	9.2	8.9
	Preparation	1.044 min.	274 min.	207 min.	137 min.	1662 min.
Total	Examination	816	258	271	206	1551
time	Repairing	77	187	2	0	266
	Idle time	53	0	28	49	130
	Average	15.3 min.	15.9 min.	8.8 min.	9.6 min.	13.3 min.

The Keihoku-cho town located to the north of Kyoto was chosen as the target area. According to the census of the population in 1975, this town had 7,774 persons, 638 of whom were more than 60 years old in age. The first field mass screening program was carried out from November 28 to 30, 1977 (Watanabe et al. 1978), and the second one from July 3 to 4, 1978. 95 (14,9 per cent of whole men more than 60 years old) underwent the test at the town office and another meeting place. Exceptionally, one case was 56 years old, therefore the patients ranged in age from 56 to 85, with an average of 71.6 (Table 4). Clear tomograms of the prostate were recorded in all cases. On the average 7.8 pictures were taken per case. The average time per case inclusive of all factors was 9.5 minutes (Table 5). Though field experiment was performed just like as model experiment, the average time per case was shorter than in model experiments because there were only few mechanical troubles and the examinees were highly intelligent, taking up a positive attitude. 41 (43.2%) cases were picked up for the secondary studies. The 40 cases were evaluated from November 20 to 22, 1977. BPH in the first stage was detected in 17 cases (17.9 per cent), BPH in the second stage in (10.5 per cent), prostatic cancer in 2 (2.1 per cent) and no prostatic diseases in 8 (8.4 per cent) (Table 4).

It is very surprising that 2 cases of prostatic cancer were detected in this mass screening program. These patients have been treated successfully. In our two model and two field mass screening programs, the 275 males were surveyed in the primary study and of the 110 cases for which the secondary studies were considered necessary 107 were evaluated.

BPH in the first stage was detected in 31 cases (11.3 per cent), BPH in the second stage in 25 (9.1 per cent), prostatic cancer in 2 (0.7 per cent), prostatitis in 7 (2.5 per cent), and prostatic stone in 4 (1.5 per cent) (Table 4). We had 10 (3.6%) drop out cases who did not visit the secondary studies.

V. CASE REPORT

Case 1. A 56-year old man had complained of macrohematuria two or three times a year for these 3 years and of pollakisuria for these 4 weeks. Transrectal ultrasonotomography revealed prostatic cancer, showing slightly enlarged prostate, asymmetric prostatic contour, irregular prostatic capsule and not-homogeneous internal-echoes (Figure 4). Rectal examination revealed almost normal prostate, showing walnut size, smooth surface, almost normal consistency but slight hardness in the right lobe, with a symmetrical and well bordered contour. Transperineal needle biopsy was performed on December 20, 1977, and adenocarcinoma of the prostate was confirmed by histological study (Figure 5).

The value of serum acid phosphatase was elevated and no bone metastasis was found by rectogenologic examination. Clinical diagnosis was adenocarcinoma of the prostate, stage D. Castration was performed under lumbar anesthesia on January 13, 1978, and diethylstilbesterol was administered. Postoperative and following courses were uneventful.

Case 2. A 82-year old man had complained of nocturia, small urinary stream and micturition pain for a month. Transrectal ultrasonotomography revealed prostatic cancer, showing asymmetricity and non-homogeneous internal echoes (Figure 6). Rectal examination revealed prostatic cancer, showing hen's egg size, uneven surface, stony hard, asymmetric and ill border. Transperineal needle biopsy was performed on December 20, 1977, and adenocarcinoma of the prostate was confirmed by histological study (Figure 7).

The value of serum acid and alkaline phosphatase was normal and no bone metastasis was found. Clinical diagnosis was adenocarcinoma of the prostate, stage B. Castration was performed under lumbar anesthesia on January 13, 1978, and diethylstilbesterol was administered. Postoperative and following courses were uneventful.

VI. DISCUSSION

Almost no report on mass screening program for prostatic cancer has been published except for Raasch et al. They performed rectal palpation for the screening of prostatic diseases on males more than 45 years old in Worbis, East Germany. Of 5,951 cases studied, 1,734 cases (29.1 per cent) and 134 cases (2.3 per cent) were suspected of BPH and prostatic cancer, respectively, and 44 cases (0.74 per cent) were diagnosed as prostatic cancer, however, no biopsy was performed. In the United States, the National Prostatic Cancer Project began to develop new screening methods for prostatic cancer although they have not been achieved.

Rectal palpation of the prostate is an excellent procedure to get much diagnostic information. However, it has a serious weak point of objectivity

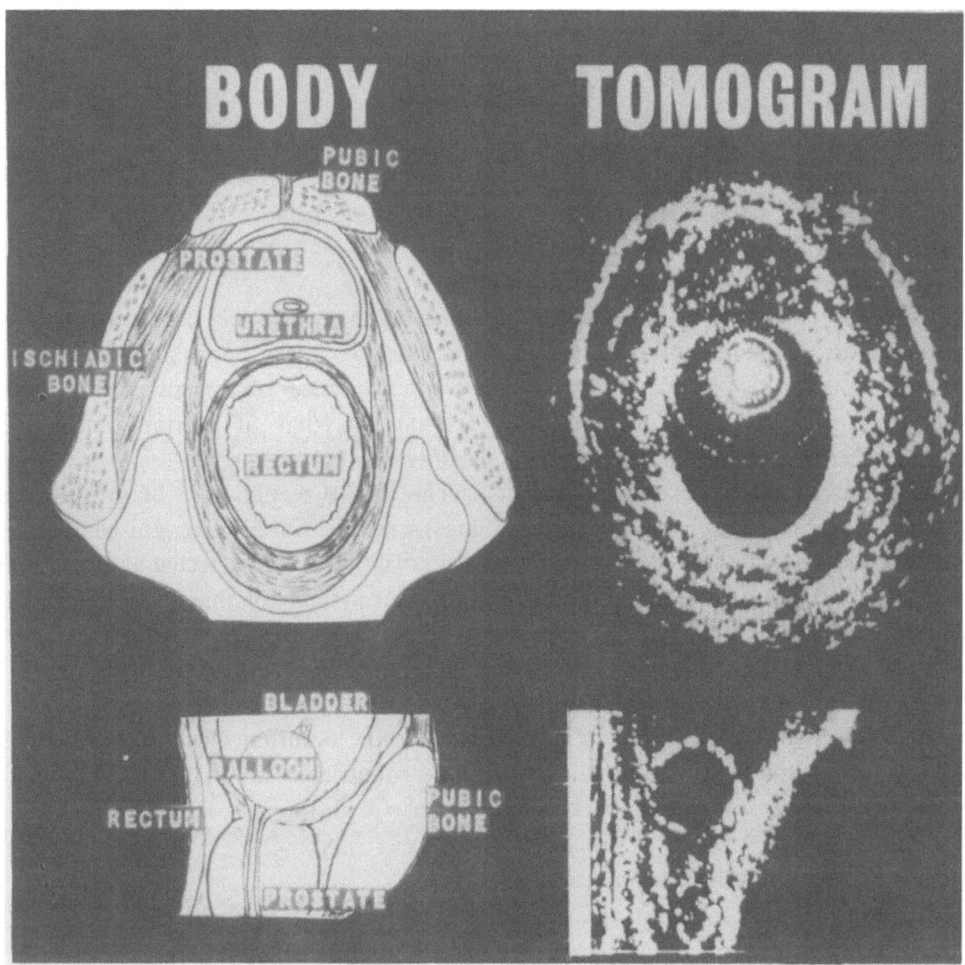

Figure 3. Horizontal structures of the intrapelvic organs around the rectum which are obtained by radial scanning.

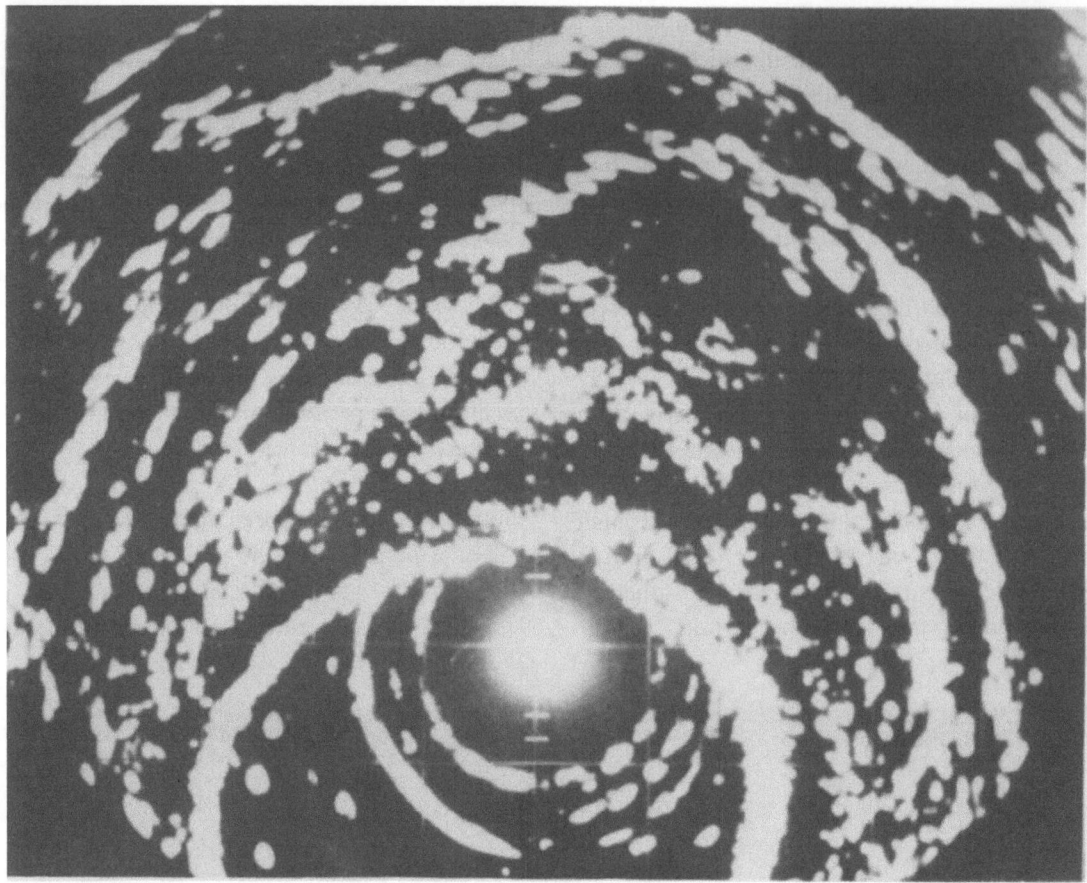

Figure 4. Ultrasonotomogram of prostatic cancer (case 1).

and reproductivity. In addition, rectal palpation gives some discomfort to both doctors and examinees.

We developed a mass screening program for prostatic cancer using transrectal ultrasonotomography, which was proved to be an excellent screening method for prostatic diseases. From the experiments described here, advantages of our mass screening system for prostatic diseases can be summarized as follows:

1) The primary study can be performed by technicians without urologist.
2) The primary study is non-invasive and painless.
3) The cost of the primary study is relatively less expensive.
4) The system is efficient from the viewpoint of the 4detection rate of diseases.

The detection rate of prostatic cancer in our experiments was much higher than mass screening for other organs, which had been performed in Japan. For example, it was reported that the detection rate of gastric cancer in mass screening was about 1/1,000 and that of uterine cancer was 1/600 (Hirayama 1978).

The high detection rate of prostatic cancer in mass screening was also recognized by Raasch et al. Moreover, BPH was detected at astonishingly high rate. Our system for mass screening program for prostatic diseases is now being considered to be generalized in Japan. The system might be even more useful in the United States and Europe because the occurrence rate of prostatic cancer in these countries is about ten times higher than in Japan.

VII. CONCLUDING REMARKS

A special chair-type apparatus for transrectal ultrasonotomography was developed in 1973. We per-

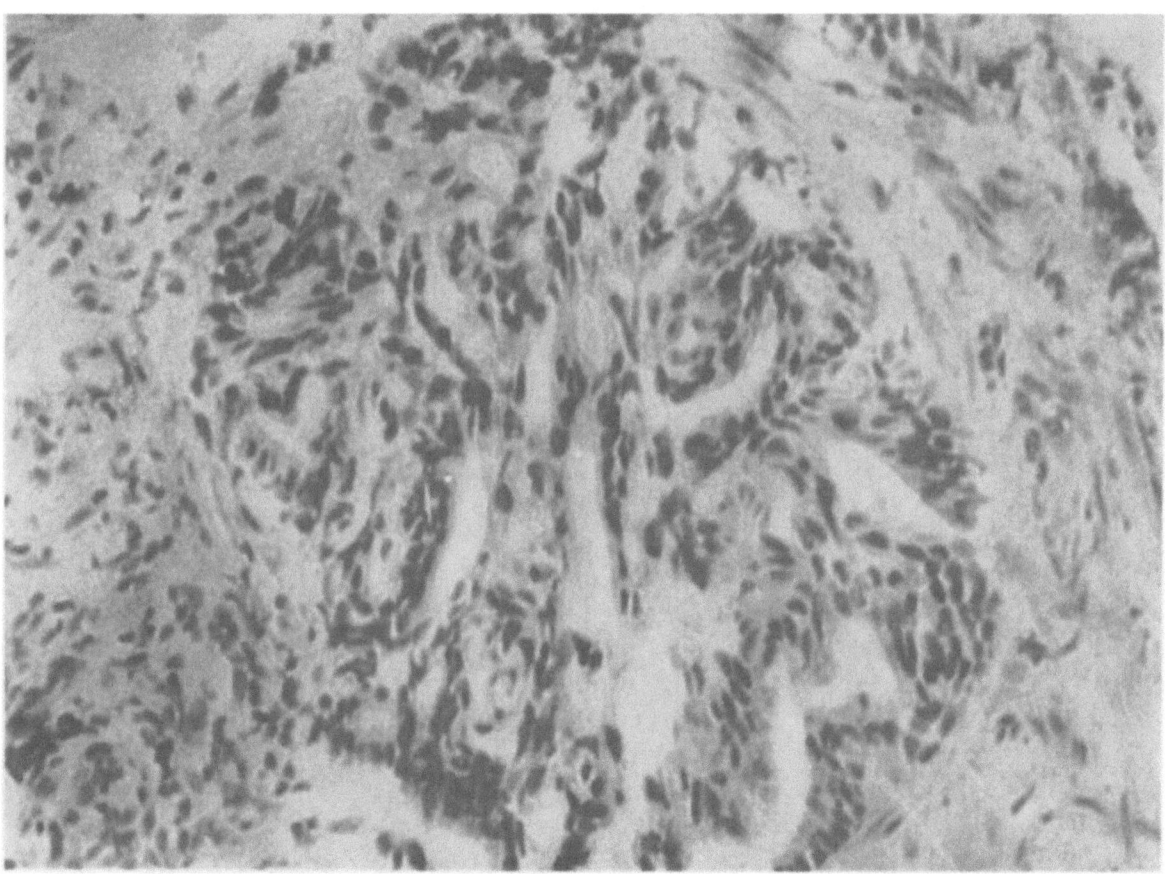

Figure 5. Histology (case 1).

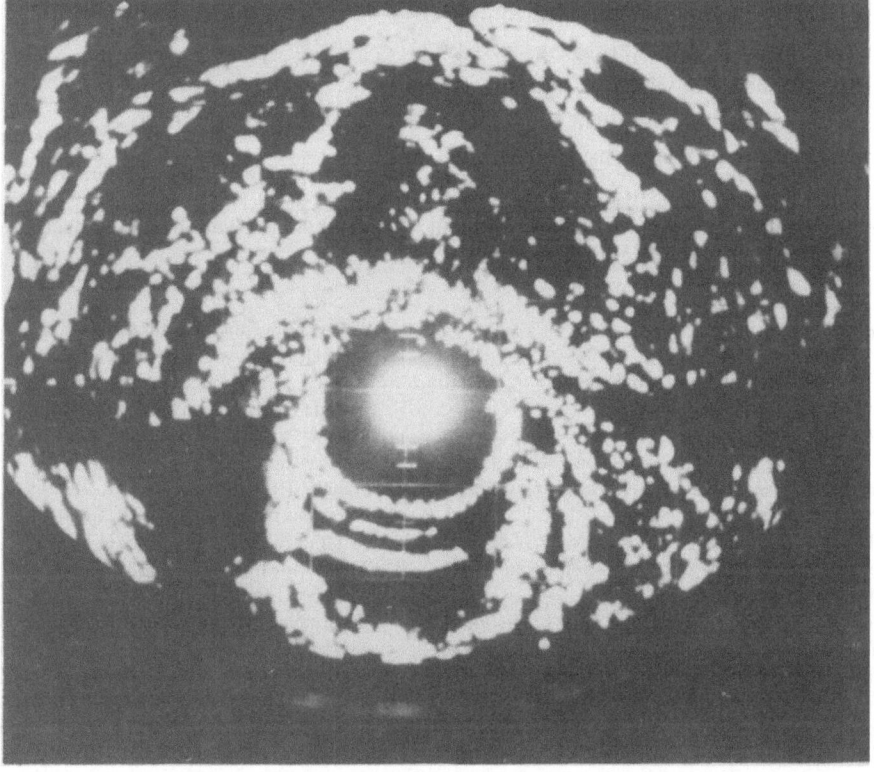

Figure 6. Ultrasonotomogram of prostatic cancer (case 2).

78

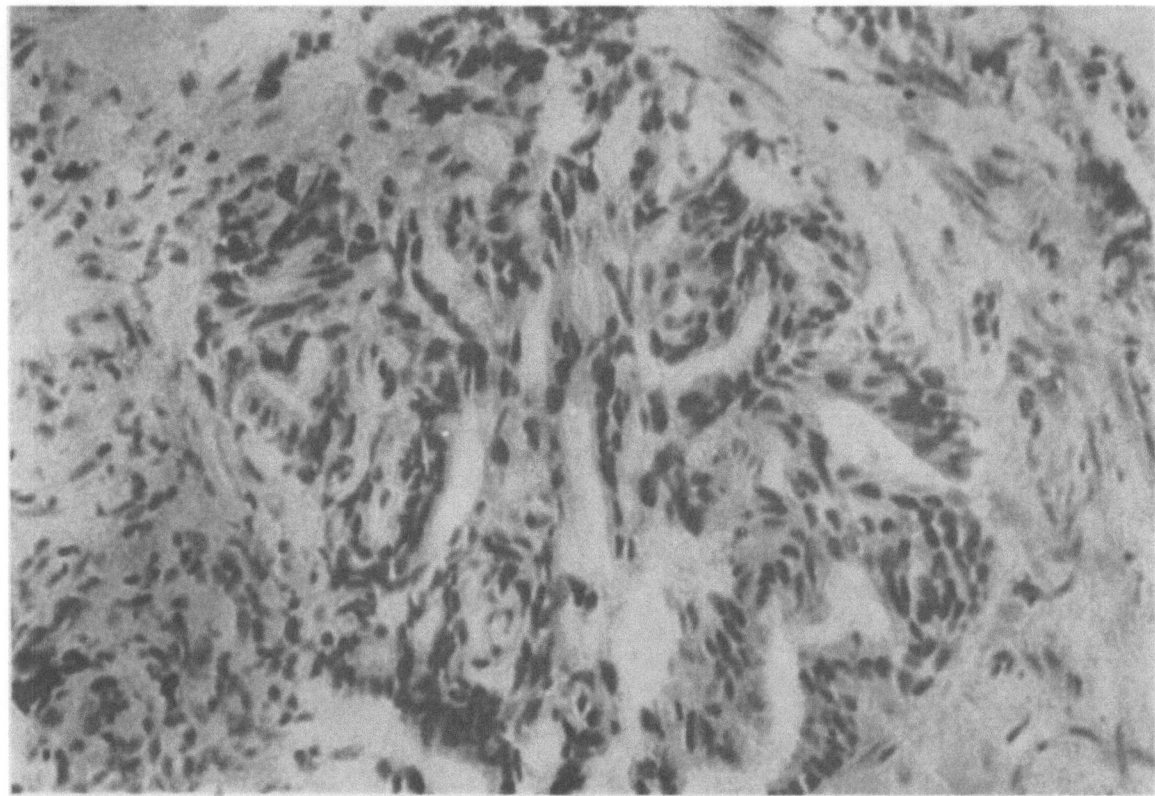

Figure 7. Histology (case 2).

formed a mass screening program for prostatic diseases, using this equipment as the primary study in the system. The 275 men evaluated ranged in age from 40 to 88 years, with an average age of 64.6. 108 subjects suspected of having prostatic diseases underwent secondary studies by usual urological examinations. Benign prostatic hyperplasia was detected in 56 cases (20.4 per cent), prostatic cancer in 2 (0.7 per cent), prostatitis in 7 (2.5 per cent) and other diseases in 4 (4.0 per cent). The system was reliable and efficient.

ACKNOWLEDGEMENT

This research was supported by grants for cancer research from the Ministry of Health and Welfare and for scientific research from the Ministry of Education, Japan.

REFERENCES

Hirayama T: Prostate in comparative epidemiology of cancer in the U.S. and Japan. Tokyo JSPS p 26, 1978.

Raasch G, Zakrzewski G, and Sonneborn D: Prostatakrebs-Vorsorgeuntersuchung im Kreis Worbis. Organisation, Durchführung und erste Ergebnisse. Deutsch Gesundh 30: 1116, 1975.

Watanabe H, Kaiho H, Tanaka M, Terasawa Y: Diagnostic application of ultrasonotomography to the prostate. Invest Urol 8: 548, 1971.

Watanabe H, Igari D, Tanahashi Y, Harada K, Saitoh M: Development and application of new equipment for transrectal ultrasonotomography. J Clin Ultrasound 2: 91, 1974.

Watanabe H, Igari D, Tanahashi Y, Harada K, Saitoh M: Transrectal ultrasonotomography of the prostate. J Urol 114: 734, 1975.

Watanabe H, Igari D, Tanahashi Y, Harada K, Saitoh M: A model experiment of mass screening program for prostatic cancer by means of transrectal ultrasonotomography. Jap J Med Ultrasonics 27: 177, 1975.

Watanabe H, Saitoh M, Mishina T, Igari D, Tanahashi Y, Harada K, Hisamichi S: Mass screening program for prostatic diseases with transrectal ultrasonotomography. J Urol 117: 746, 1977a.

Watanabe H, Saitoh M, Ohe H, Tanaka S, Itakura Y: A mass screening program for prostatic diseases by means of transrectal ultrasonotomography in two homes for the aged. Jap J Med Ultrasonics 32: 123, 1977b.

Watanabe H, Saitoh M, Ohe H, Tanaka S, Itakura Y: A first experiment of field mass screening program for prostatic diseases by means of transrectal ultrasonotomography. Jap J Med Ultrasonics 33: 151, 1978a

Watanabe H, Date S, Ohe H, Saitoh M, Tanaka S, Itakura K: A survey on 1,073 examinations by transrectal ultrasonotomography in our clinic during these 2 years. Jap J Med Ultrasonics 34: 203, 1978b.

7. CLINICAL MARKERS IN PROSTATIC CANCER

R.Y. KIRDANI, J.P. KARR, G.P. MURPHY and A.A. SANDBERG

I. INTRODUCTION

Attempts to correlate prostatic disease, particularly cancer of the prostate (CaP), with the levels of biochemical substances found in the serum, prostatic tissue and fluid and bone marrow of the involved patients have been a preoccupation of urologists, biochemists and immunologists. Even though a physician may suspect the presence of prostatic enlargement due to benign prostatic hyperplasia (BPH) or the presence of CaP, many cases of CaP cannot be confirmed by needle biopsy. One goal of the search for reliable prostatic markers for cancer of that organ is the development of biochemical assays for the early detection of CaP which may corroborate the need for further diagnostic tests such as biopsy of prostatic tissue. Another use for prostatic marker is to help determine whether a patient with CaP is responding to therapy. A further goal, still sought, is to identify a marker(s) for early detection of CaP.

In the present chapter, the various biochemical and other parameters which could be used as markers for CaP, particularly those which have been described since 1975 are reviewed and assessed. Most of the work has been directed towards finding prostatic markers in the blood. Recently, more emphasis has been given to determination of biochemical changes in prostatic tissue. Much work has been done on prostatic fluid, since conceivably malignant changes in the prostatic gland might first be reflected in its secretion. The markers are grouped by tissues or fluids in which they have been investigated, and some literature references prior to 1975 are cited where appropriate.

II. MARKERS IN BLOOD

A. Enzymatic markers

1. Acid phosphatase Since Gutman et al. (1936) reported elevated levels of serum acid phosphatase in CaP patients, especially those with metastases to the bone, measurement of serum prostatic acid phosphatase (PAP) has been a most useful marker for CaP. Acid phosphatases are a group of enzymes widely distributed in tissues; they are found in platelets, leukocytes, the liver, spleen and kidneys. These enzymes catalyze the hydrolysis of esters of orthophosphoric acid and are optimally active below pH 7. Acid phosphatases from various tissues are not identical and are distinguished by somewhat different substrate specificity and sensitivity to various inhibitors. The concentration of acid phosphatase in prostatic tissue is higher than in other tissues (Wajsman and Chu 1979; Chu 1980). Furthermore, acid phosphatases are known to be present as a group of molecular variants or isoenzymes (Murphy et al. 1978). PAP isoenzymes are a secretory product of prostatic glandular acini and are a natural component of semen.

Serum acid phosphatases, in general, become elevated in various diseases, such as those of bone, liver, kidney and in cases of cancer with liver or bony metastases (Batakis et al. 1970). Serum PAP becomes transiently elevated with prostatic massage, in prostatic infarction or BPH. PAP is, generally, highly elevated in CaP, particularly in advanced stages of the disease. Furthermore, the highest levels are generally with metastatic spread (Wajsman and Chu 1979). The question that remains to be answered is whether the concentration of PAP found in serum is a corollary to cancer of that organ in early stages of the disease.

Substrates that are believed to be specific for PAP have been developed and procedures refined. In one, for example, the hydrolysis of α-naphthyl phosphate is measured and the resulting α-naphthol is coupled to azo dyes which increase the sensitivity of the colorimetric determination (Babson and Philips 1966). In another procedure, L-tartrate is used as an inhibitor of PAP, and thus the inhibited activity represents that due to PAP (Bodansky 1975). This method may suffer from errors introduced because some acid phosphatases other than the prostatic enzymes may also be inhibited.

Even though the above enzymatic procedures are still widely used, they suffer from lack of sensitivity and rapid deterioration of acid phosphatases. Whereas measurement of the activity of serum PAP is used to ascertain the metastatic spread of CaP, more sensitive methods were needed if the plasma level of this enzyme is to be used as a marker for early stages of CaP. This required the development of immunological techniques particularly specific antisera to very highly purified PAP. Some of these purification procedures will be briefly described below. Three immunological techniques for measuring PAP have appeared to date: radioimmunoassay (RIA), counterimmunoelectrophoresis (CIEP) and, more recently, solid phase immunofluorescence (SPIF). While substantial progress has been made in the determination of PAP using these antisera, it is theoretically possible to develop antibodies against one or more of the PAP isoenzymes, and the use of such antisera would add considerably to the specificity of the immunological methods. However, at present this has not been accomplished, and PAP which is purified by conventional biochemical methods is still a mixture of its isoenzymes. It is hoped that more specific antisera can be obtained when PAP isoenzymes can

be individually prepared in quantities sufficient to inject into antibody-producing animals.

Initially, attempts at purification of PAP from prostatic fluid and development of a RIA was made by Cooper and Foti (1974, 1978a, b) and Foti et al. (1975, 1977a, c, 1978a, b, c, 1979). This group demonstrated the superiority of RIA over conventional methods in the detection of PAP at all stages of CaP as is shown in Table 1. However, Carroll (1978) stated that although the RIA is more sensitive than some of the spectrophotometric methods, it is not more specific or predictive of disease.

Choe et al. (1977, 1978) have purified human PAP obtained either from tissue homogenates or ejaculates by a modification of the procedure of Ostrowski et al. (1970). The method requires precipitation with ammonium sulfate, followed by chromatography of the crude preparation on Sephdex G-200. Subsequent DEAE-Cellulose chromatography yielded two crude PAP isoenzymes which were separately purified by affinity chromatography using Concanavalin A (Con A). The above yielded two purified isoenzymes. It has been established that differences in isoenzymes of PAP are due to differences in charge on the molecules due to variation in the number of neuraminic acid residues (Ostrowski et al. 1970). Choe et al. (1977) found that there were no immunological differences between the two isoenzymes. Antibodies to PAP were raised either in monkeys or rabbits and the antisera-PAP complexes were precipitated by the addition of goat anti-rabbit IgC, i.e., the double antibody technique (Choe et al. 1977).

Chu et al. (1976, 1978a) first proposed CIEP for PAP. This method entails the movement of antigen and antibody on agar slides in opposite directions in an electric field resulting in the formation of a precipitin line: human PAP moves towards the anode, whereas antibody moves towards the cath-

Table 1. A comparison of PAP values in sera of human subjects (ng/0.1 ml).

	RIA		CIEP	SPIF
	Cooper and Foti 1974	Choe et al. 1977	Choe et al. 1977	Lee et al. 1978
Normal men	1.5 → 6.5	1.6±0.8	<2.5	.14 → .98
BPH	3.1			
Non-prostatic carcinoma		1.8±0.6	<2.5	0.4 → 5.6
Prostatic carcinoma localized	10.6	0.5 → 2.1	5 → 100	0.63 → 430
Metastatic	13.3	5.5 → 100	5 → 100	2.0 → 570

ode. Plasma samples (or standards) are added to the cathodal wells of an immunoelectrophoresis apparatus, and the anti-PAP antiserum is added to the anodal wells. After electrophoresis, the antibody-PAP complexes in between the wells can be stained histochemically for visual comparison with standards. Alternatively, sensitivity can be increased by measuring PAP enzymatic activity of the complex in slices of the gel.

Other groups which have successfully used CIEP to measure PAP are Romas et al. (1978a, b), Rose et al. (1978) and Choe et al. (1978). CIEP as described above however, is at best a semi-quantitative procedure. Killian et al. (1980) have reported improvements on the CIEP; the method reported earlier had a sensitivity of 20ng PAP/ml serum (Chu et al. 1979). The improved colorimetric (CIEC) and densitometric (CIED) procedures resulted in greater sensitivity. Their results are depicted in Figures 1 and 2, which compare PAP levels in several cancers (including CaP) and in normal tissue. It should be noted that the normal range of PAP determined by CIEC is 0-2.13 ng PAP/ml and by CIED 0-1.4 ng PAP/ml.

Wajsman and Chu (1979), Gittes and Chu (1976), Chu (1977, 1978a, b), Lee et al. (1978) and Chu et al. (1977, 1978d) have introduced SPIF of PAP. Thus Lee et al. (1978) obtained crude PAP from human CaP tissue by extraction with Tween 80, followed by precipitation with 40 to 75% ammonium sulfate. A homogeneous PAP was obtained following a series of column chromatographies using affinity. DEAE- cellulose and Sephadex chromatography. An 85-fold purification with a recovery of 38% of initial enzyme activity was achieved.

The purified PAP was used to immunize rabbits (Lee et al. 1978). The antiserum formed was then isolated by ammonium sulfate precipitation followed by DEAE-cellulose column chromatography. The purified antibody (IgG) was coupled to a commercial preparation of cyanogen bromide (CNBr) activated sepharose 4B. This coupling does not interfere with the immunological reaction of the IgG. The IgG-sepharose was then reacted with either purified PAP or serum, in which case the PAP is bound to the IgG-sepharose. This antigen-antibody-sepharose complex retains its activity (the enzymatic and immunological sites are different)

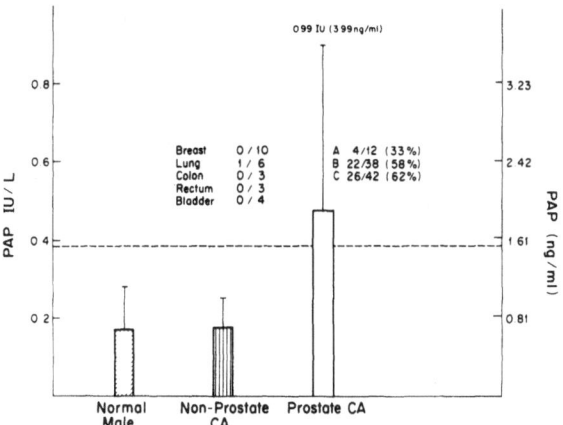

Figure 1. Results of determination of serum PAP by counter-immunoelectrophoresis using calcimetric determination in the final step (Killian 1980).

and is incubated with α-naphthyl phosphate, the liberated α-naphthol (a photonemitter) being measured spectrophotofluorometrically. In addition to the specificity of an immunological method, this assay offers solid phase support (sepharose) which has the advantage of decreased assay time (as compared to a double antibody technique) and the sensitivity of a fluorometric procedure. Furthermore, the antibody can be reused after PaP is dissociated from the IgG-sepharose 4B (Lee et al., 1978).

A variation of the SPIF method has been developed by Lee et al. (1979a). Lee et al. (1979a), who reported a SPIF which is very similar to the one reported earlier (Lee et al., 1978), except that the method of detection is colorimetric instead of spectrophotofluorometric. This results in not only a simplification of the procedure, savings in time and

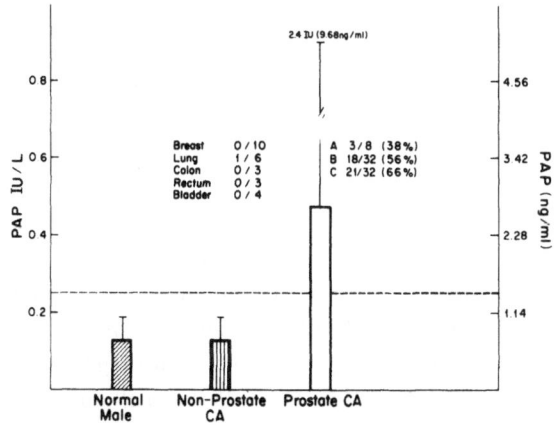

Figure 2. Results of determination of serum PAP by counter-immunoelectrophoresis using densitometry in the final step (Killian 1980).

the use of less expensive equipment, but also in a greatly reduced sensitivity.

The sensitivities of solid phase RIA and CIEP are (Chu 1980) 10ng/ml and 20ng/ml of plasma, respectively, whereas that of SPIF is 20pg/ml which is a thousand times more sensitive than the other two methods (Chu 1980). A comparison of sera PAP values using RIA and CIEP methods is given in Table 1. While values for normal subjects are comparable as determined by the three methods, PAP ranges in metastatic CaP are much higher with SPIF and CIEP than with RIA. The results have not always agreed with the diagnoses of the patients. For example, Foti et al. (1977a) stated that their RIA method correctly classified 33%, 79%, 71% and 92% of stage I, II, III and IV CaP patients, respectively, compared to 12%, 15%, 29% and 60%, respectively, found by enzymatic assay. Using CIEP, Wajsman and Chu (1979) reported positive results of 30%, 49% and 78% for stages II, III and IV, respectively. These authors emphasized that 19 BPH patients, 89 patients with other malignancies, 107 healthy volunteers and 50 normal men all gave negative results. Compared to the concurrent enzymatic determination of PAP, there were more positive correlations of CIEP data with the histological findings in all stages of the disease than was found by enzymatic assay (Wajsman et al. 1979). Even though 14% false CIEP positives in normal subjects were originally reported, upon follow-up by biopsy, early stages of CaP were present in some of these cases. It appears that presentation of assay results as percent positive or negative facilitates easy comparison and evaluation, but results should include a statement of the normal range of values used by authors to demark normal and cancer values.

From the above, it appears that work from several groups has been done towards the goal of establishing specific sensitive and reliable methods for determining PAP, and some researchers have been particularly encouraged by CIEP results (Wajsman et al. 1979). Work is underway to further develop SPIF and CIEP methods to simplify the procedures in the hope that they will be generally used in the future (Lee et al. 1979a, Killian et al. 1980).

2. Prostatic acid phosphatase isoenzymes Analysis of PAP from extracts of normal and malignant human prostates and/or sera of CaP patients shows PAP to be composed of several isoenzymes. Sur et al. (1962) separated 13 different isoenzymes of human PAP from extracts of the gland. Foti et al. (1977b) were able to isolate from a human prostatic tissue extract, analyzed on polyacrylamide gel electrophoresis, two bands of isoenzymes, the ratio of which differed between normal and cancerous tissue. One of the bands could be resolved by isoelectric focusing into at least five separate isoenzymes, however these bands did not differ between normal or cancerous tissues. Foti et al. (1977b) stated that normal prostatic tissue in addition to containing 5 to 15 times more PAP than cancer tissue also showed a quantitative difference of isoenzymes in normal versus cancerous tissue. Chu et al. (1978c) compared the isoenzymes of CaP extracts with the pattern in plasma. PAP extracts from human malignant tissue and sera of patients with CaP exhibited the same pattern of eight isoenzymes. Since these results (Sur et al. 1962, Foti et al. 1977b, Chu et al. 1978c) indicate a distinction between normal and CaP patients that could possibly be exploited as a prostatic marker, further work is in progress to extend this potentially important field.

3. Alkaline phosphatase (ALP) Serum contains isoenzymes of ALP orginating in several tissues, and as is the case of acid phosphatases, more than one isoenzyme of ALP may originate from the same tissue (Bodansky 1975). ALP isoenzymes originating in liver, kidney, intestine, placenta and bone were identified by Green (1972). In addition, there is a 'Regan' isoenzyme which is a placental-like isoenzyme of ALP present in sera of some cancer patients (Fishman 1968). Serum ALP (SALP) is elevated in metastases to the liver and/or the skeletal system (Woodard 1953, Bodansky 1975). SALP is markedly elevated in CaP metastatic to bone and measurements can monitor or may predict a patient's response to therapy (Wajsman et al. 1978).

Total SALP is measured by its activity in hydrolyzing p-nitrophenyl phosphate (pH $\simeq$ 9). The liberated p-nitrophenol is determined spectrophotometrically (Bowers and McComb 1975). ALP isoenzymes can be individually determined by inhibiting the activity of all isoenzymes except the one under consideration. This is achieved either by addition of chemical inhibitors or heat inactivation (Bodansky 1975). Thus, the addition of L-phenyl alanine inhibits intestinal, carcinoplacental (Regan) isoenzymes (77%, 79% and 79% inhibition, respectively), but not the liver or bone isoenzyme (7.7% and 10.3%, respectively) (Bodansky 1975). Heat inactivation for 16 minutes at 55°C reduces the activity of liver (50-70%), bone (90-100%) and intestinal (50-60%) isoenzymes, but has no effect on carcinoplacental (Regan) isoenzymes. More specificity is gained when measurements are carried out by using L-phenyl-alanine inhibition in addition to heating. Heating the serum for 5 minutes at 65°C totally inactivates liver, bone and intestinal isoenzymes but has no effect on either carcinoplacental (Regan) isoenzymes. Urea denaturation (Killian et al. 1976) separates bone and liver isoenzymes. Finally, cellulose acetate electrophoresis confirms the results of the inhibitions. Determination of SALP bone isoenzyme is a sensitive marker (Wajsman and Chu 1979).

Ishibe (1977) evaluated SALP determination in sera from 12 stage A-B patients, 54 stage C-D patients, 39 BPH patients, 21 patients without prostatic disease and 12 healthy women. Of the CaP patients, 28.8% had elevated SALP, with stage C-D having higher levels than the stage A-B group. Even though the SALP level was higher in patients with bony metastases (as opposed to patients without bone lesions), the difference was not statistically significant. Wajsman et al. (1978) determined SALP isoenzymes in 105 patients with metastatic CaP. Bone SALP isoenzyme was elevated in 91% of the patients with bony metastases, and subjects who had a higher pre-treatment level of SALP generally showed a poorer response to chemotherapy during the 18 months follow-up period. In another survey (Wajsman et al. 1978), the results of which are given in Table 2, of 357 patients with CaP metastases to the bone, 85% had elevated total SALP, mainly due to elevation of the bone isoenzyme fraction. An interesting result of the latter study was that 15% of the patients had normal total SALP but elevated bone isoenzyme, indicating that latter determination may be a more sensitive marker (Table 2).

It appears from the above, that the total and bone isoenzyme SALP is a very important marker for CaP. PAP and SALP should be determined (Wajsman et al. 1978), particularly since it was shown that PAP may be normal in some cases with elevated SALP (Goldberg and Ellis 1974). As a corollary, the liver SALP isoenzyme should also be quantitated in cases where prostatic metastases to that organ are suspected.

4. Serum ribonuclease activity (RNase) Serum ribonuclease activity was studied (Chu 1978a) as a marker for CaP, inasmuch as it was reported that higher levels are associated with CaP (Chu 1978a). Data listed in the report show that 71% of the CaP patients had elevated ribonuclease levels (i.e., greater than the normal range of 92-296 units), 78% of the same patients had elevated acid phosphatase and in 87% both ribonuclease and acid phosphatase were elevated. Lee et al. (1979b) have purified prostatic RNase for the development of a more specific and sensitive RIA using this marker. Three RNases were purified to homogeneity from human seminal plasma. The physico-chemical properties of these RNases were different. With the purified RNases, it may be possible to develop anti-sera to one or more of these ribonucleic acids for RIA use.

5. Serum amylase Ectopic (inappropriate) production of amylase has been identified for ovarian and pulmonary neoplasms (Lehner and Melman 1978), and the suggestion was made that CaP may also be a cause of hyperamylasemia. Hanafy et al. (1973) and Hafany (1979) reported that 19/20 BPH patients and 30/35 patients with CaP had elevated levels of plasma amylase. However, Lehner and Melman (1978) could not confirm these results, stating that analysis of serum amylase by two independent methods failed to establish an association with prostatic disease. In addition, there was no correlation of serum amylase with serum acid phosphatase and no amylase isozyme pattern unique for prostatic disease.

Further work needs to be performed to determine

Table 2. Bone alkaline phosphatase isoenzyme value (Wajsman et al. 1978).

	No.	(%)
No. pts. with bone metastases	357	(100)
Elevated total alkaline phosphatase	305	(85)
Normal total alkaline phosphatase	52	(15)
High bone alkaline phosphatase	22/52	(44)

the possibility of the use of serum amylase as a marker for CaP. Lehner and Melman (1978) did not perform serial assays over a period of time; these authors also found that patients with other cancers do not exhibit elevated serum amylase levels, and Hanafy (1979) has recently reviewed this previous data (Hanafy et al. 1973) and added new results which show elevated plasma amylase in prostatic disease.

6. Creatine phosphokinase This enzyme catalyzes the transfer of high energy phosphatases from creatine phosphate to adenosine diphosphate to produce adenosine triphosphate. Creatine kinase consists of three isoenzymes (MM, MB and BB). Whereas skeletal muscle contains relatively large quantities of MM, cardiac muscle contains MB and BB is found in several tissues, including the prostate. The high levels of the enzyme in blood of patients with myocardial infarction have been used in clinical biochemistry routinely to help diagnose the condition. Sjovall et al. (1975) histochemically showed a difference between epithelial cells of malignant and non-malignant human prostatic tissue in the uniformity of distribution of phosphokinase activity.

Feld and Witte (1977) found that even though the BB isoenzyme is rarely detectable in serum, of 19 patients with stage D CaP, 9 had high levels of the BB isoenzyme. The latter 9 subjects also had high serum ALP values. All 19 patients had high acid-phosphatase values (determined enzymatically), but the acid phosphatase values did not correlate with the presence of the BB isoenzyme. This may be due to the non-specificity of the method for determining PAP. Silverman et al. (1979) indicated a possible role for the BB isoenzyme as a tumor marker particularly for CaP. In 15/17 untreated CaP patients abnormal levels of the enzyme were found in prostatic fluid and peripheral serum using RIA and agarose electrophoresis. The isoenzyme was not found in serum of appropriate control patients (Silverman et al. 1979). The BB isoenzyme is a marker for malignancy and its detection in blood could possibly be used for diagnosis of CaP.

B. Hormonal markers

1. Serum steroids Hammond et al. (1978) deter-

mined the concentrations of several serum steroids (estradiol (E2), pregnenolone, progesterone, 17α-hydroxyprogesterone, androstenedione, testosterone (T), dihydrotestosterone (DHT) and androsterone) in 57 normal males (ages 30-80 years), 40 BPH patients (ages 50-80 years) and 11 untreated CaP patients (ages 59-79 years). When the control population was chosen from 25 normal males (ages 50-80 years), it was found that DHT and 17α-hydroxyprogesterone were significantly higher in BPH subjects. The average concentration of these two steroids in serum from cancer patients was slightly higher than those of the controls, but not statistically significant. No differences could be discerned in the concentration of the other steroids investigated.

Vermeulen et al. (1979) reported that in BPH and CaP patients mean androgen and estrogen plasma levels are slightly higher than in normals, and that more DHT is secreted which is of extraprostatic origin. While it is tempting to speculate that this increase in DHT plasma levels may be involved in the pathogenesis of BPH and/or CaP, the higher levels may be a result rather than a cause of the condition. Other studies on serum steroid concentration in CaP will be described below in the section on Sex Hormone Binding Globulin (Bartsch et al. 1979 and Leinonen et al. 1979).

2. Sex hormone or testosterone binding globulin (SHBG or TeBG) TeBG is a protein which upon electrophoresis migrates with the β-globulin fraction of plasma. It has its highest affinity for DHT, followed by T and then E2. The association constants of the reaction between the protein and these steroids are comparable to those of prostatic anfactors which influence the amount of TeBG present in blood, the most important of which is the sent in blood, the most important of which is the concentration of estrogens. Thyroid hormone and also liver diseases influence the concentration of TeBG.

The use of TeBG as a marker for CaP was first proposed by Houghton et al. (1977), whose results were given in moles 10^{-8} (values given in parentheses): BPH (5.1), untreated CaP (5.3), orchiectomized CaP (6.4), stilbestrol-treated CaP (25.4), and pregnant women (32.7). The authors found somewhat higher TeBG values in patients who had been treated with stilbestrol for longer than 3 years than in those treated for a lesser period of time (Houghton et al., 1977).

Bartsch et al. (1977) found no differences in the serum concentrations of TeBG, T, DHT, E_2 or estrone (E_1) between controls and newly diagnosed patients with CaP; their results were:

(1) Administration of cyproterone acetate, an anti-androgen, resulted in a significant decrease of T, E_2 and TeBG levels, with an increase in the DHT/T ratio.
(2) Orchiectomy caused a pronounced fall in steroid levels, but TeBG remained unchanged. The DHT/T ratio increased.
(3) Cyproterone acetate after orchiectomy caused elevated levels of prolactin.
(4) Estrogen treatment after orchiectomy increased both TeBG and prolactin.
(5) Treatment with corticosteroids after orchiectomy decreased T and TeBG levels, as compared to orchiectomy alone.

Karr et al. (1979a) determined serum T and TeBG in 133 subjects comprising two groups: controls and groups of CaP patients under various hormonal manipulations. T levels were higher in younger men and TeBG levels were higher in older men. Orchiectomy reduced T levels considerably, but did not affect TeBG. Estramustine phosphate or DES therapy in intact or orchiectomized subjects resulted in very low T and very high TeBG levels, particularly with the former drug.

Leinonen et al. (1979) measured TeBG binding capacity, the index of T binding of TeBG, and the levels of T, DHT and E_2 in sera of untreated CaP patients to assess the effectiveness of polyestradiol phosphate treatment, castration or the combination of both of these endocrine therapies in reducing biologically active plasma androgens. Orchiectomy was found to be the most effective treatment for lowering plasma androgens.

Murayama et al. (1977, 1978) have shown that TeBG levels in women may be used to predict the response of breast cancer to hormone therapy. In our opinion, it is too early to assign prognostic value to the measurement of TeBG, and the use of this parameter as a marker for CaP has to await further critical studies.

3. Serum prolactin The pituitary lactogenic hormone, prolactin, influences a number of physiological and biochemical changes in women. A complicated and not very conclusive picture emerges when plasma prolactin levels are correlated with health status of women (for example, breast cancer). A somewhat analogous situation exists for men, and attempts have been made to use serum prolactin as a marker for CaP. Bartsch et al. (1977) found serum prolactin levels higher in 15% of newly diagnosed CaP patients (see Sex Hormone Binding Globulin).

Saroff et al. (1977, 1979) have determined T, DHT and prolactin levels in sera from normal males and females, in patients with BPH and in clinically stable patients with CaP (intact and orchiectomized). The cancer patients were either untreated or on different modalities of therapy. The following is a summary of the results:
(1) Prolactin levels were higher in CaP, BPH and estrogenized patients.
(2) No significant difference was found between controls and patients treated with 5-fluorouracil (5-FU) plus cytoxan.
(3) T and DHT levels decreased in all non-control subjects.
(4) DHT levels in intact, untreated cancer patients or those receiving 5-FU plus cytoxan were significantly higher than in BPH patients.
Prolactin could possibly be used as a marker, however, from the results of Bartsch et al. (1977) and Saroff et al. (1977, 1979) it appears that prolactin determinations are potentially more useful as a marker for untreated, rather than treated, CaP patients.

C. Other markers

1. Carcinoembryonic antigen (CEA) There are certain proteins which are present in fetal and tumor tissue but are absent or found in small quantities in normal adult tissue. In malignant states, these proteins are often released in the circulation. One of these proteins, CEA, described by Gold and Freedman (1965), was originally thought to be elaborated by adenocarcinoma of the colon and fetal colon mucosa. It was found in patients with cancers other than those of the gastrointestinal tract (Reynoso et al. 1973). Chu et al.

(1975a) have measured CEA in patients with CaP and found elevated levels in 11 of 16 subjects. Williams et al. (1978) found elevated CEA in the media from 27 human BPH, CaP and normal primary prostatic cell cultures as compared to media from cultures of other tissues. Broder et al. (1977a) measured a number of parameters and found elevated CEA in 11/15 evaluable subjects with stage D CaP. Madduri et al. (1978) did not find elevated CEA in stage I and II CaP patients (only two subjects), whereas 10 of 11 subjects with stages III and IV had elevated CEA. Follow-up studies revealed that CEA does mirror the biologic behavior of the tumor.

The measurement of CEA as a marker for CaP has not been found to be as useful as it is in cancer of the colon.

2. Polyamines Interest in the determination of these polybasic compounds (putrescine, spermidine and spermine) as possible prostatic markers arose from reports that these compounds are found in high concentration in malignant tissue (Russell 1973). In rapidly metabolizing tissue, polyamines increase prior to stimulation of RNA and protein synthesis. These compounds exhibit high affinity for RNA. It has been shown (Dunzendorfer and Russell, 1978) that polyamine concentration is high in the normal prostate as compared to the normal kidney. Dunzendorfer and Russell (1978) reported high polyamine concentrations in BPH tissue.

A RIA procedure for measuring plasma spermine was developed by two groups of investigators. The assay of Bartos et al. (1975) had high cross-reactivity with spermidine. The procedure of Chaisiri et al. (1979) exhibited 12% cross-reactivity with spermidine and 0.18% with putrescine. The results were not encouraging: concentrations were only occasionally elevated in patients with CaP as compared to normals, and there was no difference between patients with CaP and those with BPH. It appears from the above that of RIA methods for measuring polyamines have not as yet been perfected. Other methods which depend on physical separation of polyamines, such as liquid chromatography, are of greater utility at present. Serial measurement of polyamines over a period of time may show greater promise as CaP markers.

3. Placental proteins Placental protein hormones are not detectable in adults except in pregnant women and in subjects with tumors which inappropriately produce these hormones. Prostate cancers are not known to be hormone secretors. As an exception, Broder et al. (1977b) measured human placental lactogen, placental ALP and human chorionic gonadotrophin and steroids in sera from 16 patients with stage-D CaP as well as in the NCI-Mayo Clinic Serum bank sera from 47 other patients with CaP. In all cases except one (of the sixteen subjects), there was no chorionic gonadotrophin production. Inappropriate hormone production of any nature by CaP remains an area to be further explored.

4. Neuraminic acid Serum glycoproteins are elevated in many diseases, including malignancy. The use of these compounds as markers for CaP would, ostensibly, be of little value, since they lack specificity. However, Moss et al. (1979) have determined the levels of N-acetyl neuraminic acid (NANA) in sera of normal subjects and patients with prostatic or bladder carcinoma. The results (μg/ml of plasma) were: normal (862), BPH (957), bladder cancer (1051), CaP (1000-1316, depending on stage). In patients with CaP, the NANA values correlated with both stage of disease and response to therapy. The authors state that the NANA test appears to be a more sensitive marker as to the stage of prostatic disease than is acid phosphatase. In view of the relatively small number of samples investigated in this work, compared to the number assayed for PAP, it would appear that NANA should be assayed more extensively to confirm these results.

5. Blood groups Wajsman et al. (1977) studied the relationship between blood groups and CaP in 264 patients. There was no statistical correlation with blood grouping as a marker. The reason for this study was based on several previous reports on a possible relationship between an increased susceptibility to carcinoma of the stomach, uterus, salivary glands, pancreas and prostate with blood group A.

III. MARKERS IN URINE

A. Polyamines

The polyamines, putrescine, spermidine and spermine have been determined in urine as possible markers for CaP. Fair et al. (1975) found polyamines in urine to be significantly higher in subjects with CaP, compared to controls 30 of 34 patients with grades II, III and IV had excessive urinary levels, with only one of 10 patients with grade I having high levels.

B. Urinary total and non-esterified cholesterol

Patients with cancer of the breast, testes, kidney and other sites have been reported to have high urinary cholesterol levels as compared to normals (Chu et al. 1975b, Acevedo et al. 1973, Chu et al. 1975b) and that the levels of non-esterified cholesterol in urine of patients with CaP were high and could possibly be used for evaluation of these patients. Juengst et al. (1979) have evaluated urinary cholesterol excretion in 79 men with BPH and in 48 patients with CaP. The authors compared their results with those of Acevedo et al. (1973) and Chu et al. (1975b), stating that the critical point is the cutoff used by investigators as the upper limit of the values for normal subjects. Juengst et al. (1979) used a value of 2.2 mg/24 hrs, which is very similar to that used by Chu et al. (1975b), but is about double that of Acevedo et al. (1973). Consequently, the two former workers report less abnormal results compared to the latter. Hypercholesteroluria is also a manifestation of other benign or malignant diseases, such as those of the testes and kidney. Juengst et al. (1979) concluded that if these diseases and BPH (with residual urine) can be excluded with reasonable certainty, then determinations of urinary non-esterified and total cholesterol may be of value in diagnosing CaP, even in early stages, especially in combination with serum acid phosphatase determinations.

C. Urinary hydroxyproline

Urinary hydroxyproline is found in a variety of bone disease and reflects bone matrix turnover. Bishops and Fellows (1977) determined 24 hr urinary hydroxyproline in 35 patients with CaP of whom 21 had bony metastases. Nine of the latter patients had had no treatment. These 9 subjects and most of the others with lung metastases had high levels of hydroxyproline. Patients who had no metastases had normal levels. These authors found that urinary hydroxyproline reflected bony metastases more accurately than serum acid or alkaline phosphatase and that hydroxyproline urinary levels fell in patients responding to treatment. In urine, hydroxyproline is found in both free and peptide-bound forms, which can be separated by dialysis against water. In a few cases, Bishop and Fellows (1977) separated bound and free and found the bound, non-dialyzable fraction to be below the limit of detection except in one patient with osteolytic lesions. In this patient's urine, the bound hydroxyproline levels did not change with treatment, though the amount of bound increased relative to the total excreted. Bishop and Fellows concluded that total urinary hydroxyproline measurements reflected the presence of bone metastases more accurately than plasma alkaline or acid phosphatase and found that serial measurements of hydroxyproline reflected progress in treatment. This work needs to be substantiated by other workers in view of the limited number of subjects used in the study.

IV. MARKERS IN PROSTATIC FLUID

Grayhack et al. (1977a, b, 1979) have concentrated their efforts on detecting differences in the composition of prostatic fluid that could serve as markers for CaP. Some of their work is based on an observation by Oliver et al. (1970) that changes in lactic dehydrogenase (LDH) isoenzymes may precede or be coincident with the development of recognizable malignancy. Grayhack et al. (1977a) measured this isoenzyme pattern in prostatic fluid, and, in addition, determined acid phosphatase and protein. The results indicate that a ratio of LDH V/LDH I in excess of 2 and in the absence of inflammation should be regarded as indicative of CaP. The authors also found results suggesting a decrease in the concentration of acid phosphatase and an increase in protein in prostatic fluid from subjects histologically diagnosed as having CaP. There was no indication as to the disease stages of the patients. The spectrum of prostatic fluid proteins analyzed by Grayhack et al. (1979) was expanded to encompass IgG, IgA, IgM, compliments C3 and C4 and transferrin. The LDH V/LDH I ratios were determined. The results of the study on 199 specimens from 99 patients indicated by both qualitative (immunoelectrophoresis) and quantitative (immunodiffusion) measurements that compliments C3 and C4 and transferrin were significantly elevated in prostatic fluid of cancer patients when compared to fluid from normals and subjects with prostatitis or BPH. Grayhack et al. (1979) suggested that the determination of these proteins together with LDH isoenzymes may assist in the identification of patients with a high risk of prostatic cancer.

V. MARKERS IN BONE MARROW

Prostatic acid phosphate found in bone marrow has been investigated as a marker for metastatic CaP. However, correlation with the disease has been controversial. Pontes et al. (1975) stated that bone marrow acid phosphatase might be a simple and quick method to be used in conjunction with established methods for accurate staging of CaP. However, other investigators (Veenema et al. 1977, Sadlowski 1978, Fossa et al. 1978, Cooper et al. 1978, Catane et al. 1978, Boehme et al. 1978) have been disappointed in the diagnostic value of bone marrow acid phosphatase. Pontes et al. (1978) and Belville et al. (1979) have compared enzymatic and immunological methods of determination of bone marrow acid phosphatase and found the latter yielded positive values, whereas the former did not show the presence of PAP, and caution must be exercised in interpreting the results depending on the method being utilized.

VI. MARKERS IN PROSTATIC TISSUE

A. Steroid oxido-reductase enzymes in prostatic tissue

The measurement of these enzymes by the determination of the amount of substrate and/or product transformed could provide an important prostatic marker, particularly since only a small amount of tissue is needed for the in vitro assay. Morfin et al. (1977) related the metabolism of labeled T and DHT in various types of human prostatic tissue to the histology and ultrastructure. Well differentiated cancer resembled the epithelium of BPH, and in both tissues T was metabolized mainly to DHT. Poorly differentiated adenocarcinomas and transitional-cell carcinomas lacked the cytoplasmic organelles responsible for the formation of DHT, with the concomitant predominance of metabolites involved in the 17-oxido-reductase pathway. The authors speculated that the findings may explain why poorly-differentiated prostatic neoplasms are frequently unresponsive to anti-androgen therapy. Kliman et al. (1978) confirmed the above results, i.e., major impairment in the formation of DHT by metastatic CaP tissue and a similar but less evident alteration of the metabolism of the primary tumor.

5α-reductase and the androgen receptor are critical with respect to biological activity of the prostate (Geller et al. 1978). Even though the in vitro measurement of this enzyme has been used to ascertain the effectiveness of potential anti-CaP drugs (Sandberg et al. 1977), there is a paucity of literature on endogenous 5α-reductase in the human prostate. Geller et al. (1978) measured prostatic 5α-reductase levels and DHT in four samples of carcinomatous tissue and compared the levels to those in BPH tissue. No differences were found in the levels of DHT, whereas 5α-reductase was reduced in three of the specimens. The patients from whom the 3 specimens were obtained were followed for six months and responded favorably to anti-androgen treatment. It should be noted that prostatic 5α-reductase activity and possibly its level depend on several factors in the cellular environment, such as the amount of zinc (Zn) and T (Habib 1977).

Bruchovsky and Lieskovsky (1979) have measured the ratio of 5α-reductase and $3\alpha(\beta)$-hydroxy dehydrogenase activities in prostatic homogenates (8 normal, 21 hyperplastic and four CaP). The normal tissue was obtained no later than 2-7 hours after death. According to Melanin (1975), the viability of prostatic tissue decreases after 15 hours post-mortem. The ratios of 5α-reductase/3α(β)-hydroxy dehydrogenase activities for normal, BPH and CA tissue were 0.42, 1.65 and 0.09, respectively; the higher ratio of the BPH tissue is due to higher levels of 5α-reduction.

Attempts at assigning specific receptor and 5-reductase functions to stromal and epithelial elements of the prostate have been reported. Wilkin et al. (1979) have indicated that the conversion of T to DHT in CaP is about 10% of normal and in BPH tissue, the level is about 300% of normal. Whole tissue concentration of DHT in CaP was within the normal range. Upon separation of the prostatic elements by simple mechanical means and measurements of enzymes activities, it was found that 70% of the 5α-reductase activity was in the stroma of both cancerous and normal tissues. The authors concluded that T is metabolized to DHT predominantly in the stroma, and that in cancer the concentrations of DHT and nuclear androgen receptors are regulated independently of 5α-reductase activity. It is possible, therefore, that anti-androgens would be more effective in therapy of cancer than 5α-reductase inhibitors.

B. β-Glucuronidase

Nilsson and Müntzing (1975) utilized histochemical methods for determining PAP and β-glucuronidase. No correlation was found between the numerical quotient of phosphatase/glucuronidase and therapeutic response to estramustine phosphate. However, in biopsy specimens, the quotient was lower in patients who had responded after two months of treatment.

C. Endogenous steroids

Hammond (1978) determined the levels (in ng/g wet weight) of steroids in prostatic tissue by RIA. The levels found in 18 (10 aged 20-49 years and 8 aged 50-75 years) normal adults (post-mortem) are given in Table 3. The steroid levels were compared to

those in prostates (normal, BPH and CaP) from males of all ages (ranging from 6 days to 75 years old). In newborns, steroid concentrations were high but decreased with age (with the exception of 3α-androstanediol which increased) until puberty when newborn levels were re-established.

In BPH (Hammond 1978), with the exception of the level of DHT, which was raised (5.33±0.12) and 3α-androstanediol and androsterone which were reduced (1.40±0.12 and 0.80±12 ng/g, respectively), there was no difference between BPH and normal tissue steroid content. This indicated a shift towards increased 5α-reduction and decreased 3α-hydroxysteroid dehydrogenase activity and corroborates the work of Bruchovsky and Lieskovsky (1979) in vitro with prostatic tissue.

In one sample of prostatic tissue from an untreated cancer patient, the concentrations of T, androstenedione, DHT and 3α-androstenediol were high, whereas those of 5β-androstanediol and androsterone were low (Hammond 1978). In cancer tissues from three patients treated with estrogen therapy, T and androstenedione virtually disappeared, but their reduced metabolites remained in concentrations similar to those observed in untreated cancer tissue.

The relationships described above are depicted in Figure 3. In normal tissue 3α-diol and androsterone were found in concentrations double that of DHT. There was a remarkable reversal in the concentration of DHT, 3α-diol and androsterone between normal and BPH tissue. The measurement of endogenous androgens as well as the determination of 5α-reductase and 3α-hydroxysteroid dehydrogenase activities appears to have potential for use as a marker, particularly since these determinations can be performed on a biopsy sample by using RIA for

Table 3. Endogenous steroid levels in human prostates (Hammond 1978).

Testosterone	0.25±0.04*
Androstenedione	0.13±0.03
5α-Androstane-3,17-dione	1.31±0.30
17β-Hydroxy-5α-androstane-3-one	1.22±0.14
5α-Androstane-3α, 17β-diol	4.32±0.49
Androsterone	4.15±1.07
Progesterone	0.39±0.07
17α-Hydroxyprogesterone	0.42±0.06

* ng/g wet weight tissue (mean ± standard error of the mean).

90

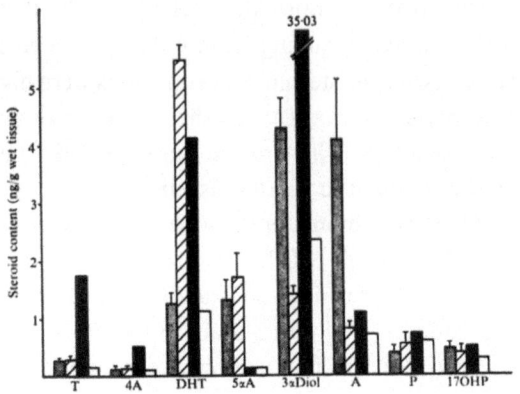

Figure 3. Comparison of the steroid contents of normal adult and diseased prostatic tissues. Stippled bars, normal tissue (n=18); hatched bars, tissues from patients with benign prostatic hypertrophy (n=10); solid bars, untreated carcinomatous tissue (n=1); open bars, oestrogen-treated carcinomatous tissue (n=3); T = testosteron; 4A = androstenedione; DHT = 17β-hydroxy-5α-androstan-3-one; 5αA = 5α-androstane-3,17-dione; 3αDiol = 5α-androstane-3α, 17β-diol; A =androsterone; P = progesterone; 17OHP = 17α-hydroxy-4-pregnene-3,20-dione. The S.E.M. is indicated for normal and benign prostatic hypertrophy samples (Hammond 1978).

the endogenous steroids and high specific activity androgen substrates for the measurement of enzyme activity.

Habib et al. (1979) have correlated the amount of endogenous Zn, T and DHT in prostatic tissue and observed that high Zn values are associated with DHT/T ratio of >1, whereas a value of <1 was found in CaP specimens and was usually associated with a low level of Zn (Table 4). It is interesting to note that both DHT and T accumulate in CaP tissue although there is greater conversion to DHT, as manifested by the change in the DHT/T ratio between normal and cancer prostatic tissue (Habib 1978, 1979, Hammond 1978). The increase in endogenous T may be ascribed to a change in the metabolic pattern of T, i.e. a decreased 5α-reductase activity as well as that of enzymes which metabolize T by pathways other than that involving DHT.

Krieg et al. (1979) have investigated androgen binding, in vitro metabolism and endogenous tissue concentration of androgens in CaP, BPH and normal human prostatic tissue. These authors (Krieg et al. 1979) stated that compared to CaP and BPH tissue, normal prostate seemed to be protected against excessive accumulation of T and DHT

because there was greater synthesis of 5α-andro-stanediols which in general did not bind with high affinity to the cytosolic androgen receptor. CaP and BPH tissues synthesized considerably more T and DHT which have high affinity for the receptor.

D. Receptors and binding proteins

1. Androgen receptors The use of steroid hormone receptor data in treatment related decisions in breast cancer has given impetus to such measurements as diagnostic and prognostic aids in CaP (Sandberg and Karr 1979). However, differences between breast and prostatic tissue have precluded direct application of available techniques and necessitated ongoing work to develop and/or to modify receptor assays for that purpose. Some of the factors that have complicated measurement of prostatic receptors include:

a) There are low levels of cytosolic androgen receptor sites which are 'unoccupied' by DHT molecules at the time of sampling due to the high levels of endogenous DHT. This androgen is formed by 5α-reduction of T and it accumulates against a blood gradient. The level of 'unoccupied' receptor sites has led some investigators to use exchange or nuclear receptor assays. For example, Hicks and Walsh (1979) and Sirett and Grant (1978) have found that about 70% of the labeled DHT in BPH tissue is in the nucleus.

b) There is a heterogeneous population of prostatic cells. Not only are there at least two different classes of cells in the normal prostate, viz., epithelial and stromal cells, but in CaP transformed tissue can adjoin normal tissue.

c) The amount of prostatic tissue available for receptor measurement is limited since open biopsies are infrequent. Transurethral resection (TUR) 'chips' are not suitable sometimes because of the possibility of heat inactivation of the receptor during resection (Snochowski et al., 1977). Needle biopsy specimens may contain other tissue and are frequently less than 100mg in weight. Therefore, prostate receptor methodology has to take into account the availability of prostatic tissue.

d) Even though the prostate is not as vascularized as other tissues, for example the liver, contamination from plasma during homogenization and the low levels of 'unoccupied' receptor molecules may cause TeBG concentration in the prostatic cytosol to be equal or greater than that of the receptor.

Recently there have appeared a number of publications on methodological and cancer correlative aspects of receptor data. These indicate that although much work remains to be done, oncologists can look forward to corroborative data on whether a newly diagnosed CaP patient will respond to hormonal therapy (20-30% do not) and if a patient is continuing to respond; all patients become refractory after a period of time. Studies which correlate receptor data with diagnosis will be described. A summary of the methods used is given in Table 5.

Lieskovsky and Bruchovsky (1979) reported that the mean concentration of nuclear androgen receptor molecules per nucleus was 1000 for tissue from normal subjects, 1,400 for BPH and 1,900 for well-differentiated carcinoma. Eckman et al. (1979) found that androgen and progestin and progestin cytosolic receptors were measurable in 4/5 and 2/5 of the cases, with no estrogen receptors being present, and in 3/5 of the cases glucocorticoid receptors were present.

Mobbs et al. (1978) assayed androgen receptors on 84 prostatic tissue specimens from 28 subjects with BPH and 54 patients with CaP. In untreated patients, receptor levels were low, but in estrogenized subjects in whom plasma T levels are low,

there was a range of receptor levels. Variability in number of sites was proportional to the extent of malignant involvement. Low androgen receptor levels in prostatic tissue from patients with low serum T were tentatively related by these authors to hormonal insensitivity of these tumors. They also pointed to the possibility of the androgen receptors consisting of more than one component, a fact that Liao et al. (1975) had pointed out previously as related possibly to the presence of a progesterone receptor. This may account for some of Mobbs et al.'s (1978) results of high prostatic cytosolic androgen receptors from patients who were not sensitive to treatment.

Krieg et al. (1978a) concluded that CaP cytosol samples as a whole had on the average a higher assayable DHT receptor concentration than the BPH cysotol. However, when the CaP samples were divided histologically, adenocarcinomatous tissue has lower DHT receptor concentration (N=7) than cribriform and/or undifferentiated cancer. Adenocarcinoma alone and BPH tissue did not differ. Wagner and Schulze (1978) using agar-gel electrophoresis could not correlate between the amount of androgen receptor and response to DES treatment in 11 patients from whom the tissues were obtained. Gustafsson et al. (1978b) correlated androgen receptor levels with clinical response to hormonal therapy in 16 patients: of 12 patients who had

Table 4. Zinc and androgen levels in normal and pathological prostates (Habib et al. 1979).

Type of specimen	No. of patients	Mean ± S.E.*	Range	DHT/T**
		Zn (μg/g dry wt)		
Normal	(8)	517± 51	121-1136	1.04
BPH	(20)	460± 53	131- 900	3.25
CaP	(10)	194± 19	112- 342	0.57
		Testosterone (ng/g dry wt)		
Normal	(8)	2.87±0.49	1.13-7.17	
BPH	(20)	3.23±0.47	1.14-12.7	
CaP	(10)	10.60±1.62	5.53-18.8	
		Dihydrotestosteron (ng/g dry wt)		
Normal	(8)	2.99±0.36	1.18- 5.35	
BPH	(20)	10.5±1.31	3.92-35.00	
CaP	(10)	6.06±0.74	2.30- 9.16	

* standard error of the mean
** Dihydrotestosterone/testosterone

measurable androgen receptor, one died; of the remaining eleven, 9 responded to treatment. The two subjects that did not respond had the lowest receptor level indicating a possible limit of androgen receptor below which no response can take place. Three of the four other subjects who had no measurable receptors did not respond; the remaining patient was 'false negative'.

2. Estrogen receptors Galli et al. (1977) determined receptor patterns in 3 BPH and 15 prostate cancers. No estrogen receptor was found in the BPH samples, whereas receptors were found in 40% of the prostatic cancers.

De Voogt and Dingjan (1978) determined steroid receptors in prostatic tissue from 68 BPH patients and 36 patients with different stages of CaP, 15 of whom had been treated with hormones. The receptors were separated by cold agar-gel electrophoresis. All BPH samples had E_2 receptors (800 femtomoles/mg tissue), 19/21 untreated cancers had 2,790 femtomoles/mg tissue and all hormonally treated cancers had 135 femtomoles/mg tissue. The authors

conclude that a relationship between response to endocrine therapy and E_2 receptor content does exist.

Sidh et al. (1979) determined androgen and estrogen receptors in 40 CaP patients. In subjects who were judged to be improving based on both subjective and objective observations, estrogen receptor concentrations were significantly higher than those of androgen receptors, whereas in subjects who were judged to be either stable or progressing, androgen receptor concentration was higher than that of estrogen receptor.

Karr et al. (1979b) analyzed the binding of labeled E_2 to cytosol from human prostatic tissue needle biopsy which were compared with DES and found in 11 prostate cancers a trend toward greater competition by DES for high affinity binding sites in differentiated tumors from men who were not receiving estrogen therapy. The assay values, expressed as the percentage reduction of $^3(H)$-estradiol binding in the presence of 100-fold molar excess of DES, were based on biopsies (average weight 16.8 mg) taken from CaP patients. The

Table 5. Estrogen receptors in prostate needle biopsies: bound estradiol displaced by diethylstilbestrol (%).

Age of patient	Endocrine therapy*	Wt. of tissue (mg)	Concentration ^3H-E_2-17β incubated (nM)**	% Competition	Histologic differentiation	Treatment	6 mos. follow-up
64	None	13.7	0.5	54	Well	Chemotherapy, diethylstilbestrol	Stable
59	None	15.8	0.5	47	Moderate	Orchiectomy recommended	—
62	Tace, Orchiectomy	27.7	0.5	43	Moderate	Chemotherapy, estramustine phosphate	Objective
58	Orchiectomy, 2 yrs.; estramustine phosphate. 2 mos.	19.9	0.5	28	Well	Chemotherapy, estramustine phosphate	Objective
64	None	19.4	0.5	22	Moderate	Diethylstilbestrol, radiation recommended	—
54	None	22.0	0.5	22	Moderate	Chemotherapy, estramustine phosphate	Stable
76	None	16.6	0.5	22	Poor	None	Stable
66	Diethylstilbestrol, orchiectomy Estramustine phosphate, 1 mo.	22.2 11.2	1.5 1.5	15 10	Poor	Chemotherapy, estramustine Progression phosphate	
62	Diethylstilbestrol	12.9	0.5	5	Moderate	Diethylstilbestrol recommended	—
71	Estramustine phosphate	7.0	1.5	0	Poor	Estramustine phosphate	Progression
67	Diethylstilbestrol, orchiectomy	13.1	1.5	0	Poor	Chemotherapy, estramustine phosphate	Progression

* At time of biopsy.
**20-hour incubations in presence of 0.5nM ^3H-E_2-17β. 2-hr incubations in presence of 1.5nM ^3H-E_2-17β.

striking feature of the data obtained is the difference in percentage competition in those patients who had not been on any hormonal therapy (54, 47 and 43%) and those who had been on estrogen therapy (5.0 and 0%). Ekman et al. (1979) found no estrogen receptors in five prostatic metastatic tissue specimens.

3. Progesterone receptors Cowan et al. (1977) in the course of determining the binding of R1881 to human prostatic tissue, reported the binding of R5020, the progesterone equivalent of R1881, in equal amounts. They found that the progesterone receptor-like binding sites are a feature of the prostatic stroma rather than the epithelium. A major contribution to defining progestin receptors in human prostatic BPH and cancer tissue came from Gustafsson et al. (1978a). Seventeen out of 21 patients with BPH and 3 patients with cancer had progestin receptors. A sample of normal tissue has no measurable receptor. This work had been undertaken since progestins had shown efficacy in treatment of CaP. More recently, Ekman et al. (1979) found progestin receptors in two out of five specimens of metastatic CaP.

Earlier contributions were by Hawkins et al. (1976), Cowan et al. (1977), Menon et al. (1977a, b), Ghanadian et al. (1978) and Geller et al. (1975). Reviews are given by Liao et al. (1975) and Karr and Sandberg (1979).

In summary, research on receptors in the prostate requires the solving of difficulties in methodology in order to evolve working methods for accurate assessment of the receptor levels.

4. Zinc binders The literature on the function and metabolism of zinc in the prostate and prostatic fluid is voluminous. Zinc is an important trace element, and prostatic tissue contains the second highest amount of zinc (about 7μmoles per gram dry weight), exceeded only by sperm, and is about ten times as high as that of soft tissues (Habib 1977). Animal work has suggested that the amount of zinc in the prostate is under hormonal control and that Zn plays an important role in hormonal effects; administration of estrogen and castration decrease prostatic Zn levels, whereas administration of androgens increases these levels (Habib 1977). Zinc is also important for the full function of 5α-reductase (Wallace and Grant 1975).

Willden and Robinson (1975) measured plasma zinc levels in 14 patients with CaP, 64 with BPH and in a large control group of men and women. It was found that plasma zinc levels rise in men over 55 years of age and fall in women of the same age group. The levels were higher in BPH patients though there was no correlation between plasma levels and prostate size. There was no significant difference between cancer patients (with or without metastases) and normal subjects. There was no correlation with serum acid or alkaline phosphatase, though as the latter levels increased, plasma zinc levels tended to decrease. It appears that plasma Zn levels may not be a reliable marker for CaP.

Reed and Stitch (1973) and Kirdani et al. (1979) have shown that labeled zinc binds to cytosolic protein in the prostate protein. Reed and Stitch (1973) showed that this protein does not bind T. Heathcode and Washington (1973) showed the protein to be an approximately 32,000 dalton molecule in which histidine comprised approximately 19% of the amino acids on a molar basis. Kirdani et al. (1979) have proposed the use of zinc binders in prostatic cytosol as marker for prostatic disease and in correlating the amount of labeled zinc bound to these peaks and their ratio with the state of the prostate. Using a dilute sucrose gradient ($1+1/2\%$ to 5%), Kirdani et al. (1979) have described two peaks which appear upon centrifugation of cytosol (human or rat) which has been pre-incubated with Zn. The peak with the higher molecular weight probably is identical to that identified previously by Reed and Stitch (1973).

ACKNOWLEDGEMENT

This work was supported in part by grants CA-20459 and CA-15436 from the National Prostatic Cancer Project. We are gratefully indebted to Dr. T Ming Chu for his interest and help. Mrs. Diane Smith and Miss Ann-Marie Conti provided clerical assistance.

94

REFERENCES

Acevedo HF, Campbell ER, Saier EL, Frich JC, Merkow LP, Hayslip DW, Bartok SP, Grauer RC, Hamilton JL: Urinary cholesterol. V. Its excretion in men with testicular and prostatic neoplasms. Cancer 32: 196, 1973.

Babson AL, Philips GE: An improved acid phosphatase procedure. Clin Chim Acta 13: 264, 1966.

Bartos D, Campbell RA, Bartos F, Grittie DP: Direct determination of polyamines in human serum by radioimmunoassay. Cancer Research 35: 2056, 1975.

Bartsch W, Horst, HJ, Becker H. Nehse G: Sex hormone binding globulin binding capacity testosterone 5α-dihydrotesterone, oestradiol and prolactin in plasma of patients with prostatic carcinoma under various types of hormonal treatment. Acta Endocrinol 85: 650, 1977.

Bashirelahi N, O'Toole JH. Young JD: A specific 17β-estradiol receptor in human benign hypertrophic prostate. Biochemical Medicine 15: 254, 1976.

Batsakis JG et al: Diagnostic enzymology. Chicago: Am Soc Clin Pathol, 1970.

Belville WD, Cox HD, Mahan DE. Stutzman RE. Bruce AW: Prostatic acid phosphatase by radioimmunoassay tumor marker in bone marrow. J Urol 121: 442, 1979.

Bishop MC, Fellows GH: Urine hydroxyproline excretion-A marker of bone metastases in prostatic carcinoma. Brit J Urol 49: 711, 1977.

Bodansky O: Biochemistry of human cancer. Academic Press, 1975.

Boehme WM, Augspurger RR, Wallner SF, Donohue RE: Lack of usefulness of bone marrow enzymes and calcium in staging patients with prostatic cancer. Cancer 41: 1433, 1978.

Bowers GN, McComb RB: Measurement of total alkaline phosphatase activity in human serum. Clin Chem 21: 1988, 1975.

Broder LE, Waalkes TP, Tajeda F, Weintraub BD. Cohen MH, Rosen SW: Biological markers in evaluating disease status in patients with stage D prostatic adenocarcinoma. Abstracts of the Am Assoc Can Res 18: 91. 1977a.

Broder LE, Weintraub BD. Rosen SW, Cohen MH, Tejada F: Placental proteins and their subunits as tumor markers in prostatic carcinoma. Cancer 40: 211, 1977b.

Bruchovsky N, Lieskovsky G: Increased ratio of 5α-reductase: 3α-hydroxysteroid dehydrogenase activities in the hyperplastic human prostate. J Endocrinol 80: 289, 1979.

Carroll BJ: Radioimmunoassay of prostatic acid phosphatase in carcinoma of the prostate. New England J Med 298: 912, 1978.

Catane R, Madajewicz S. Wajsman ZL, Chu TM, Mittelman A, Murphy GP: Immunochemical detection of prostatic acid phosphatase in serum and bone. New York State J of Med 78: 1060, 1978.

Chaisiri P, Harper ME, Griffiths K: Plasma spermine concentrations of patients with benign and malignant tumours of the breast or prostate. Clinica Chim Acta 92: 273, 1979.

Choe BK, Pontes EJ, McDonald I, Rose NR: Immunochemical studies of prostatic acid phosphatase. Cancer Treat Rep 61: 201, 1977.

Choe BK, Pontes EJ, Morrison MK et al: Human prostatic acid phosphatase. II. A double anti-body radioimmunoassay. Arch Androl 1: 227, 1978.

Chu TM: Serum acid phosphohydrolase (phosphatase) and ribonuclease in diagnosis of prostatic cancer. Antibiotics Chemotherapy 22: 98. 1978a.

Chu TM: Biochemical and immunologic techniques for acid phosphatase measurement in the diagnosis of prostate cancer. National Ca Inst Monograph 49: 239, 1978b.

Chu TM: Immunochemical assay for prostatic acid phosphatase and its application in diagnosis of prostate cancer. In: Biological markers for cancer, Chu TM, ed. Marcel Dekker, 1980.

Chu TM, Bhargava A, Barnard EA, Ostrowski W, Varkarakis MJ, Merrin C, Murphy GP: Tumor antigen and acid phosphatase isoenzyme in prostatic cancer. Can Chemother Rep 59: 97, 1975a.

Chu TM, Shukla SK, Mittelman A, Murphy GP: Comparative evaluation of serum acid phosphatase, urinary cholesterol and androgens in diagnosis of prostatic cancer. Urol 6: 291, 1975b.

Chu TM, Wang MC, Kajdasz R, Barnard EA, Kucil P, Murphy GP: Prostate-specific acid phosphohydrolase in the diagnosis of prostate cancer. Proceedings Am Assoc Can Res 17: 191, 1976.

Chu TM, Wang MC, Kuciel R, Valenzuela L, Murphy GP: Enzyme markers in human prostatic carcinoma. Cancer Treat Rep 61: 193, 1977.

Chu TM, Wang MC, Merrin C, Valenzuela L, Murphy GP: Isoenzymes of human prostate acid phosphatase. Oncology 35: 198, 1978c.

Chu TM, Wang MC, Scott WW, Gibbons RP, Johnson DE, Schmidt JD, Loening SA, Prout GR, Murphy GP: Immunochemical detection of serum prostatic acid phosphatase. Invest Urol 15: 319. 1978d.

Cooper JF, Foti AG: A radioimmunoassay for prostatic acid phosphatase. I. Methodology and range of normal male serum values. Invest Urol 12: 98, 1974.

Cooper JF, Foti AG: A radioimmunoassay for prostatic acid phosphatase. National Can Inst Monograph 49: 235, 1978a.

Cooper JF, Foti A, Herschman HH, Finkle W: A solid phase radioimmunoassay for prostatic acid phosphatase. J Urol 119: 388, 1978b.

Cooper JF, Foti AG, Shank PW: Radioimmunochemical measurement of bone marrow prostatic acid phosphatase. J Urol 119: 392, 1978c.

Cowan RA, Cowan SK, Grant JK: Binding of methyltrienolone (R1881) to a progesterone receptor-like component of human prostatic cytosol. J Endocrinol 74: 281, 1977.

Dunzendorfer U, Russell DH: Altered polyamine profiles in prostatic hyperplasia and in kidney tumors. Can Res 38: 2321, 1978.

Ekman P, Snochowski M, Dahlberg E, Gustafsson JA: Steroid receptors in metastatic carcinoma of the human prostate. Eur J Cancer 15: 257, 1979.

Fair WR, Wehner N, Brorsson U: Urinary polyamine levels in the diagnosis of carcinoma of the prostate. J Urol 114: 88, 1975.

Feld RD, Witte DL: Presence of creatine kinase BB isoenzyme in some patients with prostatic carcinoma. Clin Chem 23: 1930, 1977.

Fishman WH, Inglis NR, Stolbach LL, Krant MJ: A serum alkaline phosphate isoenzyme of human neoplastic cell origin. Cancer Res 28: 150, 1968.

Fossa SD, Sokolowski J, Theodorsen L: The significance of bone marrow acid phosphatase in patients with prostatic carcinoma. Brit J Urol 50: 185, 1978.

Foti AG, Cooper JF, Herschman H: Counterimmunoelectrophoresis in determination of prostatic acid phosphatase in human serum. Clin Chem 24: 140, 1978a.

Foti AG, Cooper JF, Herschman H, Malvaez RR: Detection of prostatic cancer by solid-phase radioimmunoassay of serum prostatic acid phosphatase. New England J Med 297: 1357, 1977a.

Foti AG, Cooper JF, Herschman H, Sapon SR: The detection of prostatic cancer by radioimmunoassay: a review. Human Pathol 9: 618, 1978b.

Foti AG, Cooper JF, Sapon SR, Herschman H: Radioimmunoassay for detection of prostatic cancer. Comp Ther 5: 24, 1979.

Foti AG, Herschman H, Cooper JF: A solid-phase radioimmunoassay for human prostatic acid phosphatase. Can Res 35: 2446, 1975.

Foti AG, Herschman H, Cooper JF: Isoenzymes of acid phosphatase in normal and cancerous human prostatic tissue. Can Res 37: 4120, 1977b.

Foti AG, Herschman H, Cooper JF: Comparison of human prostatic acid phosphatase by measurement of enzymatic activity and by radioimmunoassay. Clin Chem 23: 95, 1977c.

Foti AG, Herschman H, Cooper JF: Measurement of prostatic acid phosphatase in various cell lines. National Ca Inst Monograph 49: 55, 1978c.

Galli MC, De Giovanni C, Grilli S, Prodi G: Steroid receptors in human prostate and kidney. Eur Assoc Can Res, September 13-15, 1977.

Geller J, Cantor T, Albert J: Evidence for a specific dihydrotestosterone-binding cytosol receptor in the human prostate. J Clin Endo Meta 41: 854, 1975.

Geller J, Albert JA, de la Vega D, Loza D, Stoeltzing W: Dihydrotestosterone concentration in prostate cancer tissue as a predictor of tumor differentiation and hormonal dependency. Can Res 38: 4349, 1978.

Ghanadian R, Auf G, Chisholm GD, O'Donoghue EPN: Receptor proteins for androgens in prostatic disease. Brit J Urol 50: 567, 1978.

Gittes RF, Chu TM: Detection and diagnosis of prostate cancer. Seminars in Oncol 3: 123, 1976.

Gold P, Freedman SO: Demonstration of tumor-specific antigens in human colic carcinoma by immunological tolerance and absorption techniques. J Exp Med 121: 439, 1965.

Goldberg DM, Ellis G: An assessment of serum acid and alkaline phosphatase determination in prostatic cancer with a clinical validation of an acid phosphatase assay utilizing adenosine 3'-monophosphate as substrate. J Clin Pathol 27: 140, 1974.

Grayhack JT, Wendel EF, Lee C, Oliver L: Analysis of prostatic fluid in prostatic disease. Can Treat Rep 61: 205, 1977a.

Grayhack JT, Wendel EF, Lee C, Oliver L, Cohen E: Lactate dehydrogenase isoenzymes in human prostatic fluid: an aid in recognition of malignancy? J Urol 18: 204, 1977b.

Grayhack JT, Wendel EF, Oliver L, Lee C: Analysis of specific proteins in prostatic fluid for detecting prostatic malignancy. J Urol 121: 295, 1979.

Green S, Cantor F, Inglis NR, Fishman WH: Normal serum alkaline phosphatase isoenzymes examined by acrylamide and starch gel electrophoresis and by isoenzyme analysis using organ specific inhibitors. Am J Clin Pathol 57: 52, 1972.

Gustafsson JA, Ekman P, Pousette A, Snochowski M, Högberg B: Demonstration of a progestin receptor in human benign prostatic hyperplasia and prostatic carcinoma. Invest Urol 15: 361, 1979a.

Gustafsson JA, Ekman P, Snochowski M, Zetterberg A, Pousette A, Högberg B: Correlation between clinical response to hormone therapy and steroid receptor content in prostatic cancer. Can Res 38: 4345, 1978b.

Gutman EB, Sproul EE, Gutman AB: Increased phosphatase activity of bone at site of osteoplastic metastases secondary to carcinoma of prostate gland. Am J Cancer 28: 485, 1936.

Habib FK: Zinc and the steroid endocrinology of the human prostate. J Steroid Biochem 9: 403, 1977.

Habib FK, Mason MK, Smith PH, Stitch SR: Cancer of the prostate: early diagnosis by zinc and hormone analysis. Brit J Cancer 39: 700, 1979.

Hammond GL: Endogenous steroid levels in the human prostate from birth to old age: a comparison of normal and diseased tissues. J Endocrinol 78: 7, 1978.

Hammond GL, Kontturi M, Vihko P, Vihko R: Serum steroids in normal males and patients with prostatic diseases. Clin Endocrinol 9: 113, 1978.

Hanafy HM: Possible role of amylase enzyme in prostatic and seminal fluid. Urol Int 34: 11, 1979.

Hanafy HM, Gursel EO, Veenema RJ: Increased serum amylase levels in prostatic diseases. Urol 1: 37, 1973.

Hawkins EF, Nijs M, Brassinne C: Steroid receptors in the human prostate. Detection of tissue-specific androgen binding in prostate cancer. Clin Chimica Acta 75: 303, 1977.

Hawkins EF, Nijs M, Brassine C, Mattheiem WH: Enigmatic binding of corticosterone to protein in cytosols of human benign prostatic hypertrophy tissue. J Endocrinol 69: 17P, 1976.

Hawkins EF, Nijs M, Brassinne C, Tagnon HJ: Steroid receptors in the human prostate. 1. Estradiol-17β binding in benign prostatic hypertrophy. Steroids 26: 458, 1975.

Heathcote JG, Washington RJ: Analysis of the zinc-binding protein derived from the human benign hypertrophic prostate. J Endocrinol 58: 421, 1973.

Hicks LL, Walsh PC: A microassay for the measurement of androgen receptors in human prostatic tissue. Steroids 33: 389, 1979.

Houghton AL, Turner R, Cooper EH: Sex hormone binding globulin in carcinoma of the prostate. Brit J Urol 49: 227.

Ishibe T: Alkaline phosphatase in serum of patients with prostatic carcinoma. Urol 10: 227, 1977.

Juengst D, Pickel A, Elsaesser E, Marx FJ, Karl HJ: Urinary cholesterol excretion in men with benign prostatic hyperplasia and carcinoma of the prostate. Cancer 43: 353, 1979.

Karr JP, Sandberg AA: Steroid receptors in prostatic cancer. In: Prostatic Cancer, Murphy P, ed. Littleton, Mass: PSG Publishing Co, 1979.

Karr JP, Wajsman Z, Kirdani RY, Murphy GP, Sandberg AA: Effects of DES and Estracyt on serum sex hormone binding globulin and testosterone levels in prostate cancer patients. Submitted to J Urol, 1979. Abstract at the 1979 AUA Meeting, 1979a.

Karr JP, Wajsman Z, Madajewicz S, Kirdani RY, Murphy GP, Sandberg AA: Steroid hormone receptors in the prostate. J Urol 122: 170, 1979b.

Killian CS, Chu TM, Drzewiecki G, Schmidt K, Kajdasz R, Santalucia J, Saroff J, Murphy GP: A simple and reliable method for alkaline phosphatase isoenzyme in prostatic cancer. Clin Chem 22: 1174, 1976.

Killian CS, Wang MC, Lee CL, Chu TM, Murphy GP: Quantitative counter-immunoelectrophoresis assay of prostatic acid phosphatase. Submitted to investigative urology, 1980.

Kirdani RY, Müntzing J, Murphy GP, Sandberg AA: Specific zinc binding in the prostate and its application to clinical status. Abstract in the Endocrine Society Meeting, June 13-15, Anaheim, California, 1979.

Kliman B, Prout Jr Gr, MacLaughlin RA, Daly JJ, Griffin PP: Altered androgen metabolism in metastatic prostate cancer. J Urol 119: 623, 1978.

Krieg M, Bartsch W, Janssen W, Voigt KD: A comparative study of binding, metabolism and endogenous levels of androgens in normal, hyperplastic and carcinomatous human

96

prostate. In: UICC Workshop in Prostatic Cancer, Coffey D, Isaacs J, eds. Geneva, Switzerland, 1978a.

Krieg M, Grobe I, Voigt KD, Altenahr E, Klosterhalfen H: Human prostatic carcinoma: significant differences in its androgen binding and metabolism compared to the human benign prostatic hypertrophy. Acta Endocrinol 88: 397, 1978b.

Lee CL, Killian CS, Murphy GP, Chu TM: A solid-phase immunoadsorbant assay for serum prostatic acid phosphatase. Clin Chim Acta, 1979a.

Lee CL, Richards-Smith BA, Murphy GP, Chu TM: Purification and characterization of new human prostatic ribonuclease. XIth International Congress of Biochemistry, Ottawa, Canada, 1979b.

Lee CL, Wang MC, Murphy GP, Chu TM: A solid-phase fluorescent immunoassay for human prostatic acid phosphatase. Can Res 38: 2871, 1978.

Lehner LM, Melman A: Nonassociation of hyperamylasemia and prostatic disease. Urol 12: 461, 1978.

Leinonen P, Hammond GL, Lukkarinen O, Vihko R: Serum sex hormone binding globulin and testosterone binding after estradiol administration, castration, and their combination in men with prostatic carcinoma. Inves Urol 17: 24, 1979.

Liao S, Tymoczko JL, Castaneda E, Liang T: Androgen receptors and androgen-dependent initiation of protein synthesis in the prostate. Vit and Horm 33: 297, 1975.

Lieskovsky G, Bruchovsky N: Assay of nuclear androgen receptor in human prostate. J Urol 121: 54, 1979.

Madduri SD, Sporer A, Seabode JJ: Biologic and pathophysiologic prognosticating indices in prostatic cancer. Am Surg 44: 290, 1978.

Menon M, Tananis CE, McLoughlin MC, Lippman ME, Walsh PC: The measurement of androgen receptors in human prostatic tissue utilizing sucrose density centrifugation and a protamine precipitation assay. J Urol 11: 309, 1977b.

Menon M, Tananis CE, McLoughlin MG, Walsh PC: Androgen receptors in human prostatic tissue: a review. Can Treat Rep 61: 265, 1977a.

Mobbs BG, Johnson IE, Connolly JG, Clark AF: Androgen receptor assay in human benign and malignant prostatic tumour cytosol using protamine sulphate precipitation. J Steroid Biochem 9: 289, 1978.

Morfin RF, Leav I, Charles JF, Cavazos LF, Ofner P, Floch HH: Correlative study of the morphology and C_{19}-steroid metabolism of benign and cancerous human prostatic tissue. Cancer 39: 1517, 1977.

Moss Jr, AJ, Bissada NK, Boyd CM, Hunter WC: Significance of protein-bound neuraminic acid levels in patients with prostatic and bladder carcinoma. Urol 13: 182, 1979.

Murayama Y, Sakuma T, Udagawa H, Utsunomiya J, Okamoto R, Asano K: Sex hormone-binding globulin and estrogen receptor in breast cancer: technique and preliminary clinical results. J Clin Endo Meta 46: 998, 1978.

Murayama Y, Utsunomiya J, Asano K: Sex-hormone-binding globulin predicts response of breast cancer to hormone therapy. The Lancet, Dec. 24 and 31, p 1356, 1977.

Murphy GP, Karr J, Chu TM: Prostatic acid phosphatase: where are we? Ca-A Cancer Journal for Clinicians, 28 (no 5): 258, 1978.

Nilsson T, Müntzing J: the prognostic value of acid phosphatase and β-glucuronidase activity in biopsy specimens from patients with reactivated prostatic cancer. Scand J Urol Nephrol 9: 205, 1975.

Oliver JA, El Hilali MM, Belitsky P, et al: Lactic acid dehydrogenase (LDH) isoenzymes in benign and malignant prostate tissue. The LDH V/I ration as an index of malignancy. Cancer 25: 863, 1970.

Ostrowski W, Wasyl Z, Weber M et al: The role of neuraminic acid in the heterogeneity of acid phosphomonoesterase from the human prostate gland. Biochem Biophys Acta 221: 297, 1970.

Pertschuk LP, Zava DT, Gaetjens E, Macchia RJ, Brigati DJ, Kim DS: Detection of androgen and estrogen receptors in human prostatic carcinoma and hyperplasia by fluorescence microscopy. Res Commun Chem Pathol Pharmacol 22: 427, 1978.

Pontes JE, Alcorn SW, Thomas Jr, AJ, Pierce JM, Jr: Bone marrow acid phosphatase in staging prostatic carcinoma. J Urol 114: 422, 1975.

Pontes JE, Choe BK, Rose NR, Pierce JM, Jr: Bone marrow acid phosphatase in staging of prostatic cancer: how reliable is it? J Urol 119: 772, 1978.

Reed MJ, Stitch SR: The uptake of testosterone and zinc in vitro by the human benign hypertrophic prostate. J Endocrinol 58: 405, 1973.

Reynoso G, Chu TM, Guinan P, Murphy GP: Carcinoembryonic antigen in patients with tumors of the urogenital tract. Cancer 30: 1, 1972.

Romas NA, Hsu KC, Tomashefsky P, Tannenbaum M: Counter Immunoelectrophoresis for detection of human prostatic acid phosphatase. Urol 12: 79, 1978a.

Romas NA, Tannenbaum M: Immunologic detection of prostatic acid phosphatase: critique 1. Human Pathol 9: 620, 1978b.

Rose NR, Pontes JE, Choe BK: The use of antisera to prostatic acid phosphatase for the identification of cultured human cells. National Ca Inst Monograph 49: 29, 1978.

Russel DH: Polyamines in growth – normal and neoplastic. In: Polyamines in normal and neoplastic growth, Russel DH, ed. New York: Raven Press, 1973.

Sadlowski RW: Early stage prostatic cancer investigated by pelvic lymph node biopsy and bone marrow acid phosphatase. J Urol 119: 89, 1978.

Sandberg AA, Karr JP: Hormonal receptors in human neoplasia. Submitted to the 1980 International Advances of Surgical Oncology, 1980.

Sandberg A, Müntzing J, Kadohama N, Karr, JP, Sufrin G, Kirdani RY, Murphy GP: Some new approaches to potential test systems for drugs against prostatic cancer. Can Treat Rep 61: 289, 1977.

Saroff J, Kirdani RY, Chu TM, Wajsman Z, Murphy GP: Measurements of prolactin and androgens in patients with prostatic diseases. Surgical Forum 28: 568, 1977.

Saroff J, Kirdani RY, Chu TM, Wajsman Z, Murphy GP: Measurements of prolactin and androgens in patients with prostatic diseases. Oncology, 1979.

Shain SA, Boesel RW: Human prostate steroid hormone receptor quantitation. Current methodology and possible utility as a clinical discriminant in carcinoma. Invest Urol 16: 169, 1978.

Shain SA, Boesel RW, Lamm DL, Radwin HM: Characterization of unoccupied (R) and occupied (RA) androgen binding components of the hyperplastic human prostate. Steroids 31: 541, 1978.

Sidh SM, Young JD, Karmi SA, Powder JR, Bashirelahi N: Adenocarcinoma of prostate: role of 17β-estradiol and 5α-dihydrotestosterone binding proteins. Urology 13: 587, 1979.

Silverman LM, Dermer GB, Zweig MH, van Steirteghem AC, Tokes ZA: Creatine kinase BB: a new tumor-associated marker. Clin Chem 25: 1432, 1979.

Sirett DA, Grant JK: Androgen binding in cytosols and nuclei of human benign hyperplastic prostatic tissue. J Endocrinol 77: 101, 1978.

Sjovall K, Rubin S, Müntzing J: Creatine phosphokinase in prostatic tissue. Scand J Urol Nephrol 9: 181, 1975.

Slack NH, Chu TM, Wajsman ZL, Murphy GP: Carcino-placental isoenzyme (Regan) in carcinoma of the prostate. New England J Med, submitted, 1980.

Snochowski M, Pousette A, Ekman P, Bression D, Andersson L, Högberg B, Gustafsson JA: Characterization and measurement of the androgen receptor in human benign prostatic hyperplasia and prostatic carcinoma. J Clin Endo Metab 45: 920, 1977.

Sur BK, Moss DW, King EJ: Apparent heterogeneity of prostatic acid phosphatase. Biochem J 84: 55 P, 1962.

Veenema RJ, Gursel EO, Romas N, Wechsler M, Lattimer JK: Bone marrow acid phosphatase: prognostic value in patients undergoing radical prostatectomy. J Urol 112: 81, 1977.

Vermeulen A, Ven Camp A, Mattelaer J, De Sy W: Hormonal factors related to abnormal growth of the prostate. In: UICC Workshop in prostatic cancer. Coffey D, Isaacs J, eds. Geneva, Switzerland, 1978.

de Voogt HJ, Dingjan P: Steroid receptors in human prostatic cancer: a preliminary evaluation. Urol Res 6: 151, 1978.

Wagner RK, Schulze KH: Clinical relevance of androgen receptor content in human prostate carcinoma. Acta Endocrinol suppl 215 87: 139, 1978.

Wajsman Z, Chu TM: Detection and diagnosis of prostatic cancer. In: Prostatic cancer, Murphy P, ed. Littleton, Mass: PSG Publishing, 1979.

Wajsman Z, Chu TM, Bross D, Saroff J, Murphy GP, Johnson DE, Scott WW, Gibbons RP, Prout Gr, Schmidt JD: Clinical significance of serum alkaline phosphatase isoenzyme levels in advanced prostatic carcinoma. J Urol 119: 244, 1978.

Wajsman A, Chu TM, Saroff J, Slack N, Murphy GP: Two new, direct and specific methods of acid phosphatase determination. National field trial. Urology 13: 8, 1979.

Wajsman Z, Saroff J, Murphy GP: Blood group distribution in prostatic cancer patients. J Surg Oncol 9: 289, 1977.

Wallace AM, Grant JK: Effect of zinc on androgen metabolism in the human hyperplastic prostate. Biochemical Society Transactions 3: 540, 1975.

Wilkin RP, Bruchovsky N, Rennie PS, Comeau T: Stromal localization of testosterone 5α-reductase in normal, hyperplastic and carcinomatous prostates. ASCO Abstracts 20: 419, 1979.

Willden EG, Robinson MRG: Plasma zinc levels in prostatic disease. Brit J Urol 47: 295, 1975.

Woodard HQ: Changes in blood chemistry associated with carcinoma metastatic to bone. Cancer 6: 1219, 1953.

8. HORMONAL CONTROL OF PROSTATIC BIOCHEMICAL MARKERS: ACID PHOSPHATASE AS A MARKER OF ANDROGENIC CONTROL OF THE VENTRAL PROSTATE

A.F. Clark, M.P. Tenniswood, C.E. Bird, T.G. Flynn, F.A. Jacobs and P.A. Abrahams

I. INTRODUCTION

The hormonal dependence of the prostate glands of many species has been extensively studied since the prostate is an integral component of the male reproductive system and because there is a high incidence of pathological processes involving the gland in older men. While a great deal has been learned about the effects and actions of androgens in both prostatic carcinoma and benign prostatic hyperplasia (BPH), detailed studies of the biochemistry of these processes have been hampered by the lack of suitable animal model systems. The two most common animal models used have been the prostates of the dog and rat. In addition several prostatic tumour lines, derived from both rat and dog have been studied recently. However all these systems are morphologically and histologically distinct from the human gland and great care must be taken in extending the findings from these systems to humans.

The dog appears to be the only animal which develops BPH and this makes it a good model for studying BPH in humans. Work on the rate of appearance of the hyperplasia in castrated dogs with different hormone injection schedules has led to some interesting findings concerning the role of androgens in this system. 5α-Androstane-3α,17β-diol especially in combination with estradiol was more effective than either 5α-dihydrotestosterone or testosterone (Walsh and Wilson 1976).

Because of the availability and ease with which experiments can be performed, the rat has been the species used for many of the studies on prostatic biochemistry. As the rat prostate is the system used in our laboratory, the introduction will be concerned with a brief description of the various biochemical markers used in this organ to study the action of androgens.

A variety of approaches have been used in the study of the rat prostate. Experiments have been performed with a number of in vivo and in vitro preparations, which range from tissue homogenates and slices to organ and cell cultures. A number of hormones affect prostatic growth and function. Besides the well known androgen dependence of the prostate, other hormones including prolactin and estrogens have effects, most of which may be indirect. Studies on the ventral and the dorsolateral lobes which differ in their morphology and biochemical characteristics have shown that the hormonal effects on the two lobes are dissimilar in many instances. Some of those differences will be discussed briefly.

A. Mechanism of androgen action

Testosterone which is derived principally from the testes, is the most important androgen in the circulation. In the rat it circulates loosely bound to albumin. On entry into the prostate, testosterone is reduced by the enzyme, Δ^4-5α-reductase, to 5α-dihydrotestosterone which binds to the high affinity cytosolic androgen receptors. There appear to be two classes of such receptors in the prostate. One of them can be termed 'active' in that following combination with the steroid, it undergoes chemical and physical changes and the complex enters the nucleus (Fang and Liao 1971). In the nucleus the receptor 5α-dihydrotestosterone complex binds to chromatin and stimulates RNA synthesis which in turn will stimulate protein synthesis (Figure 1). There is a general stimulation of protein synthesis and of more specific proteins which can be used as biochemical markers of androgen effects. With time, there is a stimulation of DNA synthesis with the end result of increases in cell number and tissue weight. The second cytosolic androgen receptor can be termed 'passive' in that it does not appear to enter the nucleus after the binding of 5α-dihydrotestosterone and may simply act as a reservoir of this potent androgen and prevent its further metabolism (Hu and Wang 1978). There are several enzyme systems in the prostate which further metabolize 5α-dihydrotestosterone. As shown in Figure 2 these include 1) the interconversion of 5α-dihydrotestosterone (II) and 5α-androstane-3α,17β-diol (3α-androstanediol: III) which is catalyzed by 3α-hydroxysteroid dehydrogenase (Van Doorn et al. 1975); 2) the conversion 5α-dihydrotestosterone to 5α-androstane-3β,17β-diol (3β-androstanediol: IV) which is catalyzed by 3β-hydroxysteroid de-

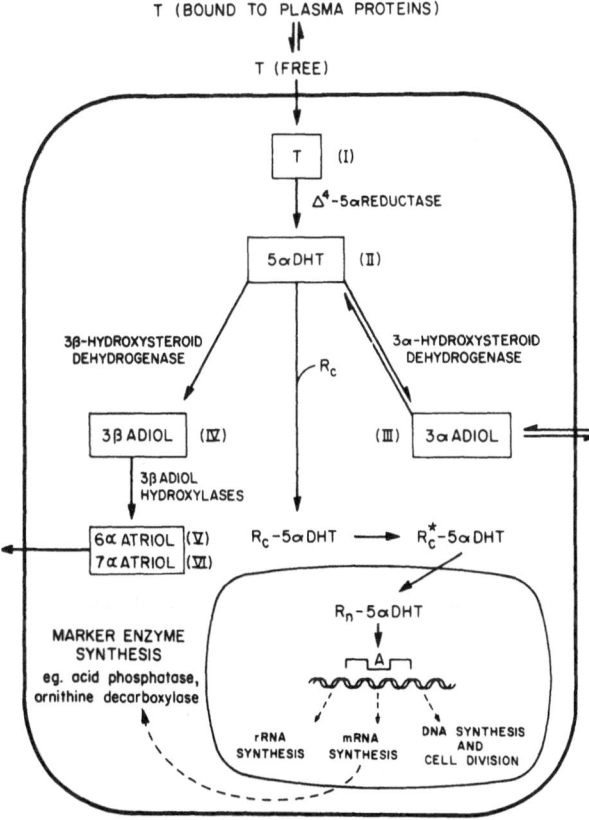

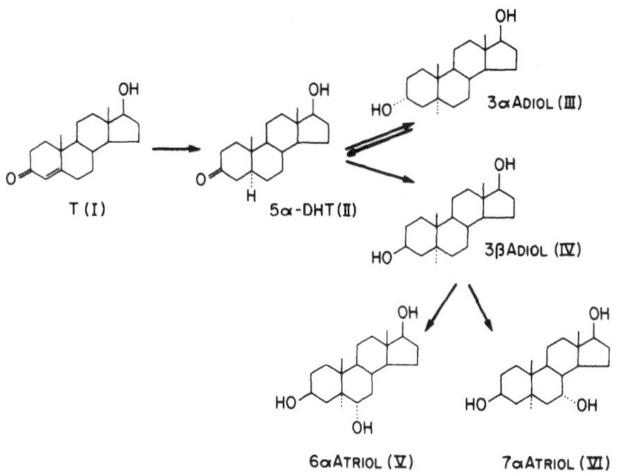

Figure 2. Steroid metabolism in the rat ventral prostate.
T = testosterone
5α-DHT = 5α-dihydrotestosterone
3α-ADIOL = 3α-androstanediol
3β-ADIOL = 3β-androstanediol
6α-ATRIOL = 5α-androstane-3β,6α,17β-triol
7α-ATRIOL = 5α-androstane-3β,7α,17β-triol

hydrogenase (Levy et al. 1974); and 3) the hydroxylation of 3β-androstanediol to form 5α-androstane-3β,6α,17β-triol (V) and 5α-androstane-3β,7α,17β-triol (VI) which are catalyzed by the 6α- and 7α-hydroxylases respectively (Isaacs et al. 1979). The enzymes catalyzing these reactions play an important role in modulating the intracellular levels of 5α-dihydrotestosterone and the other metabolites. One of the problems that has faced researchers in this field is the unravelling of the individual roles of each of these metabolites. A multimetabolite hypothesis of androgen action has been proposed which suggests that each metabolite exerts its own specific action on the prostate (Baulieu et al. 1968). In this scheme 5α-dihydrotestosterone specifically controls cell division, whereas 3β-androstanediol regulates the secretory processes, and it has been suggested that 3α-androstanediol may play a role in controlling some aspects of secretory activity. Their results leading to this hypothesis were obtained with an organ culture system.

B. *Markers of androgen actions*

A number of biochemical markers have been used to monitor androgen responsiveness of the rat prostate. Some examples are listed in Table 1. Several of these will be discussed briefly. In most instances,

Figure 1. Proposed mechanism of action of androgens in the rat ventral prostate as related to androgen metabolism.
T = testosterone
5α-DHT = 5α-dihydrotestosterone
3α-ADIOL = 3α-androstanediol
3β-ADIOL = 3β-androstanediol
6α-ATRIOL = 5α-androstane-3β,6α,17β-triol
7α-ATRIOL = 5α-androstane-3β,7α,17β-triol
RC = cytoplasmic receptor
RM = nuclear receptor
A = acceptor site

changes in these markers are monitored following castration and subsequent androgen replacement. A general indicator of androgen activity is prostate weight which can be followed as a ratio of prostate weight in milligrams to body weight in grams. Following castration this prostate weight/body weight ratio (PW/BW) decreases from 1.10 ± 0.04 to 0.15 ± 0.02. With this decrease there are corresponding decreases in cell and nuclei number and in the capacity of the organ to synthesize DNA, RNA and protein as measured by the incorporation of labelled precursors. Androgen injections to the castrated rat cause all the parameters to return to normal. More sensitive measurements of the changes in these macromolecules can be obtained by studying specific aspects of their assembly or function. For example, in DNA synthesis, DNA unwinding protein activity in the ventral prostate of castrated rats increases following the administration of androgens (Rennie et al. 1975) and RNA polymerase activities, both nucleolar and extra-nucleolar, are also increased (Mainwaring et al. 1971). Also RNA can be fractionated and the proportion of polysomal RNA estimated. This proportion is increased in the androgen stimulated state supporting the major role of androgens in controlling protein synthesis in the prostate (Mainwaring and Wilce 1973).

1. Steroid metabolizing enzymes The levels of some of the enzymes involved in the metabolism of androgens by the rat ventral prostate are at least in part controlled by androgens. The levels of Δ^4-5α-reductase (Shimazaki et al. 1969) and the 6α- and 7α-hydroxylases (Isaacs et al. 1979) decrease following castration and increase with androgen administration to castrated animals. Δ^4-5α-Reductase activity is found in both the outer nuclear membrane and the microsomes. It is in the latter fraction where the changes in activity occur following castration and with androgen replacement. Since the microsomal fraction is also the location of the

Table 1. Examples of useful biochemical markers for androgen actions in the rat prostate.

A. Steroid metabolizing enzymes (ventral prostate)

Δ^4-5α-reductase	Levels of microsomal enzyme decrease after castration and are restored to normal with administration of androgens (Moore and Wilson 1972).
3α-hydroxysteroid dehydrogenase	Some evidence suggests that the microsomal enzyme is under androgenic control (Massa et al. 1978).
6α- and 7α-hydroxylase	Levels of microsomal activity decrease after castration and are restored by androgens (Isaacs et al. 1979).

B. Chemical markers

Polyamines: Spermine	levels in the ventral prostate decrease after castration and are slowly restored on androgen administration.
Spermidine	levels in the ventral prostate decrease after castration and are restored more rapidly than spermine on androgen administration (Williams-Ashman et al. 1975).
Citrate	Concentration and content of citric acid in the dorsolateral prostate is decreased by castration.
Zinc	Uptake of zinc by the dorsolateral lobe of the prostate is greatly reduced by castration and can be restored to normal by androgen administration (Muntzing et al. 1977).

C. Protein markers

Ornithine decarboxylase	Very sensitive to castration, and rapidly restored by androgen administration (Williams-Ashman et al. 1972).
Aldolase	Levels decrease after castration and are restored by androgen administration. Changes correlate to alteration in aldolase mRNA (Mainwaring et al. 1974).
Spermine binding protein	Levels are decreased by castration and increase very rapidly on androgen stimulation (Liang et al. 1978).

hydroxylase activities it would appear that all the changes in enzymes involved in androgen metabolism occur at this subcellular site.

2. Polyamines Other biochemical indicators of androgen effects include the polyamines which are required for growth of prostate cells in culture. Spermine may have a role in the control of Mn^{++}-dependent RNA polymerase which is involved in mRNA synthesis (Moruzzi et al. 1971). Both the ventral and dorsolateral lobes of the rat prostate contain high levels of spermine and spermidine. Following castration the levels of both spermine and spermidine decrease to 20% of normal with the losses occurring both intracellularly and in the luminal secretions (Williams-Ashman et al. 1975). Androgen administration causes the levels to return to normal with that of spermidine being quite rapid and that of spermine requiring several days. The changes in the levels of spermidine and spermine are the result of changes in the activity of ornithine decarboxylase. This enzyme catalyzes the rate limiting step in polyamine biosynthesis and is extremely sensitive to androgen stimulation (Williams-Ashman et al. 1972). Spermine levels return completely to normal when prostatic secretory function returns with androgen administration to the castrated rat (Pegg et al. 1970). A specific spermine binding protein which has been recently identified in the cytosol of the ventral prostate is also under androgenic control and is probably involved in early or rapid responses to androgen stimulation. Increases in spermine binding protein levels can be seen within an hour of administration of androgens to a castrated rat (Liang et al. 1978).

3. Citrate Citrate is found in high concentrations in both lobes of the prostate but is under androgenic control in only the dorsolateral lobe, i.e. following castration the concentration and content of citrate in the dorsolateral lobe decrease. Testosterone administration increases both the content and concentration to normal (Slaunwhite and Sharma 1977). The high citrate levels in the ventral prostate are explained by an aconitase which favours citrate formation as opposed to citrate oxidation (Franklin and Costello 1978); this contrasts with the kidney enzyme which directs the reaction based on the relative levels of citrate and isocitrate with citrate oxidation being favoured at the high concentrations found in the prostate. One can speculate that aconitase activity in the dorsolateral prostate is also involved in the high citrate concentrations in this lobe.

4. Zinc uptake Like citrate, zinc is concentrated in all lobes of the prostate; its concentration in the dorsolateral lobe is 8 times higher than that of the ventral lobe. In the dorsolateral lobe zinc is associated with both stromal and epithelial elements. In the epithelium it is found at a number of cellular sites – lysosomes, nucleoli, nuclear chromatin, secretory granules and luminal secretions. In the stroma it is loosely associated with collagen and elastin. In the ventral lobe it is found mostly in the nucleus bound to proteins. Zinc uptake is under androgenic control only for the dorsolateral lobe (Muntzing et al. 1977). Following castration the rate of zinc uptake by the dorsolateral prostate decreased greatly while that for the ventral prostate is not significantly affected although there may be a subcellular redistribution within this lobe (Chandler et al. 1977).

5. Other markers There appear to be many biochemical parameters whose levels or rates of formation are controlled by androgens in the rat prostate. In addition to the examples discussed above, a number of others could be described but will only be mentioned in order to show that androgenic effects are widespread. A steroid-binding protein which is secreted into the lumen by the rat ventral prostate is under androgenic control (Heyns et al. 1977). Adenyl cyclase activity and cyclic AMP levels in the ventral prostate decrease following castration and increase with androgen administration. The activities of several of the glycolytic enzymes change in concert with the changes in cyclic AMP concentration. Other metabolic activities of the prostate may also be affected by the changes in cyclic AMP (Singhal et al. 1971). Aldolase synthesis in the ventral prostate is under androgenic control and it can be correlated to changes in the mRNA coding for the enzyme (Mainwaring et al. 1974).

C. Other hormones

The effects of hormones other than androgens will

not be discussed in any detail. Estrogens and prolactin may interact with androgens in the control of prostatic growth and function. While receptors for both these hormones have been demonstrated in the ventral prostate it has been difficult to delineate a direct physiological role for either estradiol or prolactin. Many effects of estrogens on the rat prostate are probably indirect since their primary role is to limit the availability of testosterone for uptake into the prostate cells. There are several ways this is accomplished including 1) inhibition of gonadotropin, in particular, LH secretion by the adenohypophysis which results in a decreased testosterone secretion by the testes (Verjans et al. 1974); 2) direct effects on the testes to inhibit testosterone biosynthesis (Bartke et al. 1977); 3) increased liver testosterone Δ^4-5α-reductase levels which increases the rate of clearance of testosterone from the circulation and hence decreases the amount of available androgen (Lee et al. 1974).

There is some evidence that prolactin may play a role in controlling some prostatic functions by acting synergistically with androgens. Evidence for this is strongest with the dorsolateral prostate where prolactin acts synergistically to increase zinc uptake and citrate production. Some of the conclusions on zinc have come through the use of 2-bromo-α-ergocryptine, an inhibitor of prolactin secretion. Administration of this compound decreases zinc content and zinc uptake in the dorsolateral lobe but has no effect in the ventral lobe of the rat prostate (Harper et al. 1976).

II. ACID PHOSPHATASE AS A MARKER OF ANDROGENIC CONTROL OF THE PROSTATE

This section summarizes the results obtained in our laboratory on the androgenic control of acid phosphatase characteristics in the rat ventral prostate. We initially chose this system because acid phosphatase has long been associated with human prostatic cancer. Increased levels in serum are customarily associated with spread of the malignancy outside the glandular capsule. As well, early studies in animals indicated that the levels of acid phosphatase in the prostate were at least in part under androgenic control.

Initially, methods for examining the characteristics of acid phosphatase activity were investigated. Extracts of rat prostate tissue were prepared for polyacrylamide gel electrophoresis (PAGE) by homogenization followed by several freeze-thaw cycles and filtration through 0.45μ Millipore filters. When extracts of mature rat prostates were run on PAGE, followed by staining for acid phosphatase activity utilizing α-naphthylphosphatase as substrate, examination revealed the presence of two bands (see left gel on Figure 3). These two bands of activity have been identified as the lysosomal and secretory isoenzymes of acid phosphatase. The lysosomal isoenzyme which is less mobile is found in all rat tissues while the secretory isoenzyme is found only in the mature male prostate (Tenniswood 1976). No additional bands on the gels appear if staining is allowed to proceed for 24 h rather than the normal 1 h. When staining is performed in the presence of tartrate the lysosomal band is qualitatively more inhibited than is the secretory band (centre gel on Figure 3), i.e. the secretory isoenzyme is more tartrate resistant (tartrate inhibition will be discussed in more detail later). Following castration the secretory isoenzyme on PAGE disappears in 4 days (see Figure 4); again the lysosomal isoenzyme is partially inhibited by tartrate and no further bands appear with 24 h of staining. If one of the androgens, testosterone (I), 5α-dihydrotestosterone (II) or 3α-androstanediol (III) are administered daily, starting immediately after castration the secretory acid phosphatase band on PAGE is retained. If, however these steroids are administered daily starting 7 days after castration (a time when the prostate has atrophied to 15% of its normal size) the secretory enzyme returns (see Figure 5) in 10 to 12 days (17-19 days after castration) which is approximately the same time the prostate gland returns to normal size. This suggests that the secretory acid phosphatase is androgen dependent (Tenniswood et al. 1978b). This idea is supported by the finding that the secretory enzyme is absent in the prostate extracts of immature rats. The presence or absence of the secretory acid phosphatase on PAGE also corresponds to the presence or absence of secretory granules staining for acid phosphatase activity on histochemical examination of prostate slices from the similar experimental groups of animals.

Tartrate has in the past been as an inhibitor of acid phosphatase activity in human serum to assist in determining whether the enzyme present was of prostatic origin. The addition of tartrate to the acid phosphatase assay which utilizes p-nitrophenol phosphate as substrate shows that mature rat prostate activity is inhibited to the extent of $41.1 \pm 1.0\%$ (% inhibition =

$$\frac{(\text{uninhibited activity} - \text{inhibited activity})}{\text{uninhibited activity}} \times 100).$$

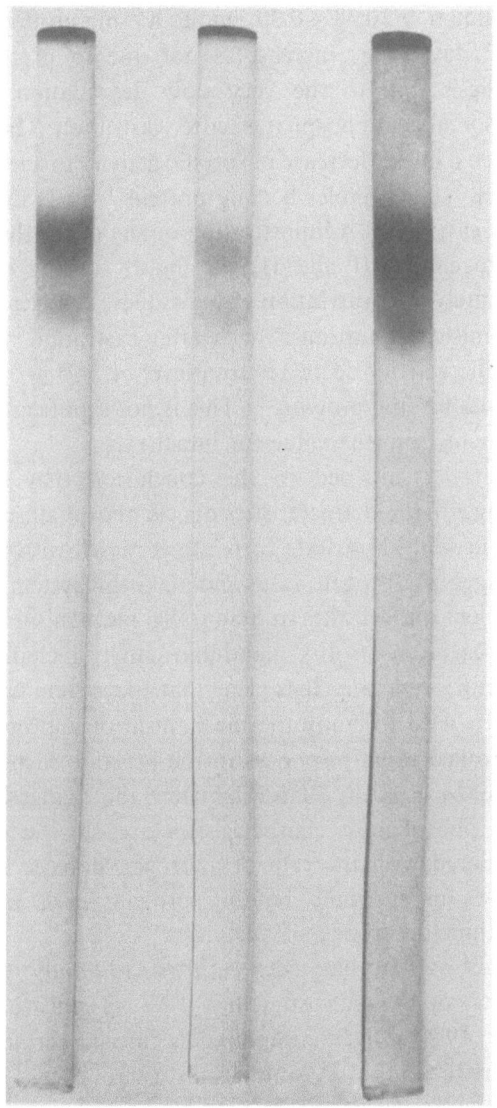

Figure 3. Polyacrylamide gel electrophoresis pattern of acid phosphatase from the prostate of an intact adult rat.

Acid phosphatase activity was localized on the gels using α-naphthylphosphate as the substrate and Fast Garnet GBC salt to couple the reaction product.

u = uninhibited stain
t = tartrate inhibited stain
24 = 24 hour stain

Following castration (see Figure 6) the extent of inhibition rises to $54.5 \pm 1.0\%$ within 7 days but then decreases to $31.0 \pm 2.0\%$ by 15 days. The initial increase is explained by the loss of the secretory isoenzyme of acid phosphatase as the studies with PAGE indicate it is more resistant to tartrate inhibition than the lysosomal enzyme. The drop in per cent inhibition from 55 to 30% is more difficult to explain. Based on available knowledge, it was first postulated that the relative amounts of the lysosomal forms are altered, resulting in a relatively more tartrate resistant mixture. While there are two isoenzymes of acid phosphatase in the prostate – lysosomal and secretory – neither of the isoenzymes is homogeneous and is apparently composed of a mixture of closely related glycoproteins differing slightly in the number or types of carbohydrate units attached to the polypeptide chain. If one of testosterone (I), 5α-dihydrotestosterone (II) or 3α-androstanediol (III) is administered (2 mg/day) starting immediately after castration, the % inhibition by tartrate remains within the normal range (Figure 6). When administration of any of these three androgens is initiated starting 7 days after castration, the % inhibition by tartrate first decreases from 55% to below normal but then increases to the normal range.

Further studies on the separation, partial purification and kinetic analysis of the prostatic acid phosphatases from normal and castrated rats have begun to clarify the problem. Both the lysosomal and secretory forms are associated with particles and hence with membranes. Release of the enzyme from these membranes requires sonication and/or several freeze-thaw cycles. Detergents such as Triton X-100 increase recovery of homogenate activity in soluble extracts. Removal of the enzyme from its natural state of membrane association leads to problems in purification. These include precipitation and aggregation which are often associated with loss of activity. However, separation and partial purification of several enzyme forms has been achieved and their kinetic constants measured (K_m for p-nitrophenol phosphate and K_i for tartrate). The values for a partially purified isoenzyme which, migrates as secretory acid phosphatase on PAGE are: $K_m = 0.24$ mM and $K_i = 104$ μM. Similarly those for a partially purified isoenzyme which migrates as the lysosomal isoenzyme are: $K_m = 3.2$ mM and $K_i = 43$ μM. The lower K_i for the lysosomal isoenzyme explains its greater sensitivity (or less resistance) to tartrate on PAGE. A third form which appears in significant amounts in extracts from 15 day castrated prostates has a K_m of 0.79 mM and a K_i of 1500 μM (Jacobs et al. submitted). This form was present in only very small amounts in extracts of prostates of rats castrated 7 days previously. The high K_i which indicates a relative insensitivity to tartrate when compared to K_i's of the other two isoenzymes explains why the per cent inhibition of total prostatic acid phosphatase activity has dropped from 55

Figure 4. Polyacrylamide gel electrophoresis pattern of acid phosphatase from the prostate of a rat castrated 7 Days previously. Other details as for Figure 3.

to 30 per cent between 7 and 15 days after castration. However it has been difficult to associate this with the lysosomal acid phosphatase as it tends to precipitate readily and it will not enter electrophoretic gels. This could be due to its being separated from other cellular components. Preliminary evidence for this has been found.

Following castration the specific activity of acid phosphatase increases from the level found for intact male rats (4.75 ± 0.30 μmoles p-nitrophenol phosphate hydrolyzed h^{-1} mg protein $^{-1}$) to a maximum of 10.38 ± 0.30 μmoles h^{-1} mg protein^{-1} by 7 days. This increase is not due to protein synthesis, but to the very slow degradation of lysosomal acid phosphatase after castration. There is then a linear decrease in specific activity to a level of 3.1 ± 0.60 μmoles h^{-1} mg protein^{-1} by 21 days after castration. Administration of any of the three androgens (I, II and III) (2 mg/d) starting immediately after castration prevents these changes. If administered starting 7 days after castration, the specific activity decreases to a level of 3.95 ± 0.40 μmoles h^{-1} mg protein $^{-1}$. This is not significantly different from the value for intact rats.

These results led to the conclusion that the changes in the characteristics of acid phosphatase in the rat ventral prostate correlate very well with the changes in androgen status and make this system an excellent model for studying the mechanism of androgenic control of glandular activity including secretory function. It is clear that the system cannot be used to study the mechanism of androgen controlled rapid responses in the prostate such as those discussed by Liao et al. since the changes in acid phosphatase characteristics are slow when compared with the rate of androgen induced increases in spermine binding protein levels and ornithine decarboxylase activity.

This system has been utilized to study the effects of 3β-androstanediol (IV) (Tenniswood et al. 1978b). This compound is formed through the reduction of 5α-dihydrotestosterone by 3β-hydroxysteroid dehydrogenase. As mentioned previously, this enzyme exists in the prostate gland, but the reduction is essentially irreversible because the product is efficiently hydroxylated and hence the 3β-androstanediol is not oxidized back to 5α-dihydrotestosterone to a significant extent. Originally it was suggested that different androgen metabolites controlled different functions in the prostate. It was postulated that 3β-androstanediol controlled prostate secretory function while 5α-dihydrotestosterone controlled cell growth and proliferation. In vivo 3β-androstanediol has little or no classical androgenic effects, i.e. it does not significantly stimulate growth of the gland in the castrated rat when compared to testosterone. In our system when 3β-androstanediol (2 mg/day, i.p.) is administered to castrated rats starting immediately after castration the PW/BW decreases but the secretory acid phosphatase does not disappear on PAGE or on histochemical examination of the tissue. However, the per cent inhibition by tartrate rises by day 5 to $51.5 \pm 0.7\%$ where it remains (Figure 6). The specific activity of acid phosphatase increases to a level of approximately 8.50 μmoles h^{-1} mg protein^{-1} and remains at this level. When administered daily starting 7 days after castration it causes a more rapid reappearance of the secretory acid phosphatase on PAGE than do those steroids which have classical androgenic activity since the secretory isoenzyme reappears after 6 days of 3β-androstanediol administration. In spite of a normal pattern of acid phosphatase isoenzymes on PAGE, the per cent inhibition by tartrate increases to $48.3 \pm 0.9\%$ indicating that the composition must be altered possibly through the production of forms with unusual patterns of glycosylation. We concluded from these experiments that 3β-androstanediol had unique effects on the ventral prostate in agreement with the previously discussed hypothesis.

However, we have subsequently shown that a very small dose of 5α-dihydrotestosterone (25 μg/day, i.p.) starting 7 days after castration will completely mimic the effects of 3β-androstanediol (2 mg/day, i.p.) (Tenniswood et al. submitted). This indicates that the effects of 3β-androstanediol may be asserted by a small amount of 5α-dihydrotestosterone produced peripherally. Such a postulate is supported by studies on the in vivo metabolism of 3β-androstanediol which have shown that small amounts of labelled 5α-dihydrotestosterone appear in the prostate after infusion of ^{3}H-3β-androstanediol (Tenniswood et al. submitted).

Thus very low doses of 5α-dihydrotestosterone (e.g. 25 μg/day) are capable of stimulating the synthesis of acid phosphatase even in the absence of prostate growth and the secretory acid phosphatase

reappears after only 6 days of androgen treatment. However as with 3β-androstanediol the % inhibition by tartrate is abnormally high, suggesting that the complement of enzyme forms synthesized is abnormal, probably in the pattern of its glycosylation. When the dosage of 5α-dihydrotestosterone is between 50 and 100 μg/day the growth of the prostate is still not enhanced, and the synthesis of acid phosphatase is also stimulated. However, the % inhibition by tartrate is within the normal range, being $38.5 \pm 1.5\%$ which suggests that the normal complement of enzyme forms is produced as the dose of 5α-dihydrotestosterone is increased. When

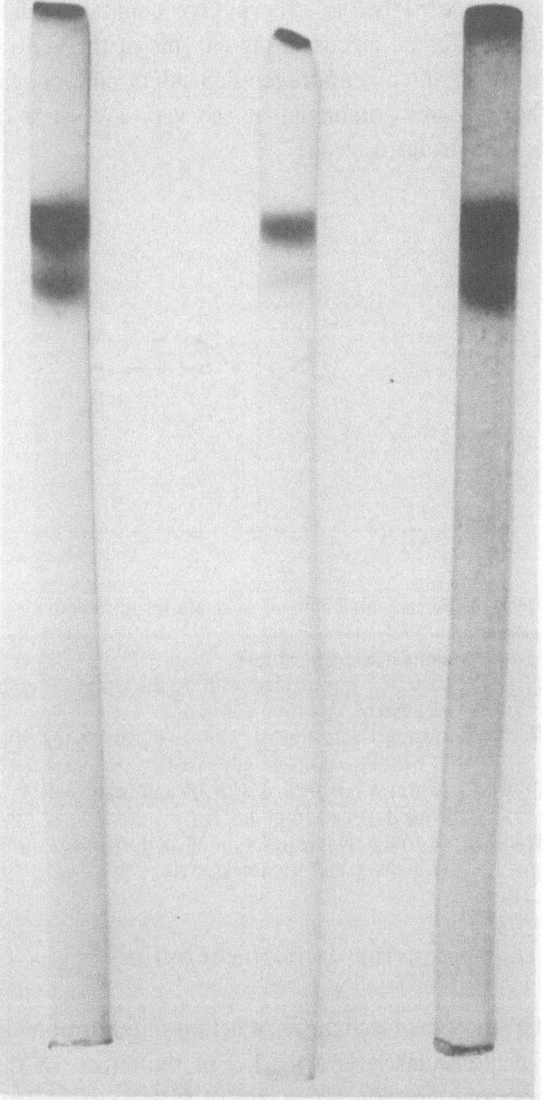

Figure 5. Polyacrylamide gel electrophoresis pattern of acid phosphatase from the prostate of a rat castrated 7 days prior to administration of 5α-dihydrotestosterone (2 mg/day, i.p.) for 10 days. Other details as for Figure 3.

the dose is higher still (e.g. 500 μg/day), prostate growth occurs and the secretory acid phosphatase does not appear until 10-12 days of treatment, at which point proliferation is complete.

This suggests that two mechanisms are involved in the control of secretory acid phosphatase. If there is sufficient androgen within the cell, proliferation occurs, and is followed later by the appearance of other androgen dependent responses including secretory function. However if the dose of androgen is below that required to produce growth then the androgen dependent responses appear much earlier. If the dose of androgen is lowered still further, some of the androgen stimulated responses are curtailed before others. One could speculate that there is a glycosylating enzyme in the ventral prostate which is androgen dependent and its synthesis is not stimulated at the very low dose of 5α-dihydrotestosterone.

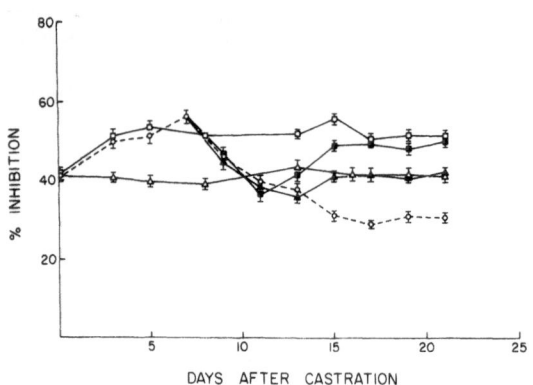

Figure 6. Percent inhibition of acid phosphatase activity by tartrate in:

○——○ untreated castrated rats.

△——△ castrated rats treated with 5α-dihydrotestosterone (2 mg/day, i.p.) from day zero.

▼——▼ castrated rats treated with 5α-dihydrotestosterone (2 mg/day, i.p.) from day seven.

□——□ castrated rats treated with 3β-androstanediol (2mg/day, i.p.) from day zero.

■——■ castrated rats treated with 3β-androstanediol (2 mg/day, i.p.) from day seven.

III. DISCUSSION AND CONCLUSIONS

To study the mechanism of action of a hormone at the molecular level a marker of the effects of the hormone in the target tissue is required. This marker should disappear or change significantly following removal of the hormone and return to normal with hormonal replacement.

The acid phosphatase characteristics described in this chapter appear to represent a complex system for the study of androgenic control. The secretory acid phosphatase is a good marker for androgen function in the rat ventral prostate in that it disappears following castration and returns with injections of the classical androgens – testosterone, 5α-dihydrotestosterone, 3α-androstanediol – when they are given at physiological or pharmacological doses. In addition, the changes in per cent inhibition of acid phosphatase activity by tartrate after the loss of the secretory isoenzyme following castration suggest that there are changes in the relative amounts of the lysosomal forms of acid phosphatase. The appearance of the form that is very tartrate resistant supports this hypothesis. We suggest that since acid phosphatase is a glycoprotein, there are androgen dependent changes in the degree or type of glycosylation leading to changes in the complement of lysosomal forms.

While the androgen dependent characteristics of acid phosphatase are complex, it does represent a system for studying a number of biochemical processes in the rat ventral prostate. The biochemical markers, citrate and zinc, which are also components of prostatic secretions are indicators of androgen effects on the dorsolateral prostate as opposed to secretory acid phosphatase and prostate binding protein which are indicators of ventral prostate function. That the hormonal control of the secretory functions of the ventral and dorsolateral lobes is probably different comes from an examination of the effects of prolactin. As mentioned in the Introduction, prolactin probably acts synergistically with testosterone in the control of zinc uptake and cellular redistribution by the dorsolateral prostate. We have found that testosterone injections will change the ventral prostate acid phosphatase characteristics from those of an immature rat to those of a mature rat more rapidly than will occur naturally; simultaneous prolactin administration does not alter the effects of testosterone (Tenniswood et al. unpublished results). Hence it appears that evidence to date indicates that prolactin affects the biochemistry of the dorsolateral but not the ventral prostate. The changes in acid phosphatase characteristics are not rapid as occurs for the spermine binding protein levels and hence cannot be utilized for the study of initial effects or actions of androgens.

Androgens in contrast to the other classes of steroid hormones are actively metabolized in some of their target tissues including the ventral prostate. The effects of testosterone and 3α-androstanediol are easily explained through their known conversions to 5α-dihydrotestosterone. The two required enzymes – Δ^4-5α-reductase and 3α-hydroxysteroid dehydrogenase – are both present in the ventral prostate. The cytosol androgen receptor which when bound to steroid translocates to the nucleus, is quite specific for 5α-dihydrotestosterone.

The studies with 3β-androstanediol are very interesting. It had been concluded from studies with a prostate organ culture system that while 5α-dihydrotestosterone controlled prostate growth, 3β-androstanediol controlled prostatic secretion. Using our acid phosphatase marker system, we have obtained strong evidence which indicates this conclusion is incorrect if applied to the in vivo situation. Microsomal receptors for 3β-androstanediol were reported (Robel et al. 1974) and it was suggested that they might be involved in androgen post-translational control of secretory processes. However, on examination of the data in that report it can be seen that these receptors have as high an affinity for 5α-dihydrotestosterone as for 3β-androstanediol. We conclude from our studies that there is no evidence that 3β-androstanediol has unique effects. All our results obtained with 3β-androstanediol can be explained by a low peripheral conversion to 5α-dihydrotestosterone which is then taken up by the ventral prostate. The same conclusion was not reached by Rennie et al. (1978) who also studied the effects of 3β-androstanediol on acid phosphatase in the ventral prostate utilizing PAGE; they did not examine the extent of inhibition by tartrate and hence did not note that the enzyme characteristics were still abnormal. The other marker systems described in the Introduction have not been studied with the detail required to arrive at such a conclusion.

It is hoped that further investigations will lead to a better understanding of androgen controlled processes in the rat ventral prostate including the control of secretory function. Despite the obvious species differences, studies with this system may contribute to knowledge on the production of acid phosphatase by human prostatic carcinomas.

ACKNOWLEDGEMENTS

The research described in this chapter was supported in part by grants from the National Cancer Institute of Canada and the Medical Research Council of Canada (MT-2338).

REFERENCES

Bartke A, Williams KIH, Dalterio S: Effects of estrogens on testicular production in vitro. Biol Reprod 17: 645-649, 1977.

Baulieu EE, Lasnitzki I, Robel P: Metabolism of testosterone and action of metabolites on prostate glands grown in organ culture. Nature 219: 115-1156, 1968.

Chandler JA, Timms BG, Morton MS: Subcellular distribution of zinc in the rat prostate studied by x-ray microanalysis. 1. Normal prostate. Histochem J 9: 103-120, 1977.

Fang S, and Liao S. Androgen Receptors. Steroid and tissue specific retention of a 17-hydroxyl-5α-androstane-3-one protein complex by the cell nuclei of ventral prostate. J Biol Chem 246: 16-24, 1971.

Franklin RB, Costello LC: Isocitrate uptake and citrate production by rat ventral prostate fragments. Invest Urol 16: 44-47, 1978.

Heyns W, Peeters B, Mous J: Influence of androgens on the concentration of prostatic binding protein (PBP) and its mRNA in rat prostate. Biochem and Biophys Res Comm 77: 1492-1499, 1977.

Hu A-L, Wang TY: Interaction of androgen binding cytosol proteins of rat prostate. J Steroid Biochem 9: 53-58, 1978.

Issacs JT, McDermott IR, Coffey DS: Characterization of two new enzymatic activities of the rat ventral prostate: 5α-androstane-3β,17β-diol 6α-hydroxylase and 5α-androstane-3β,17β-diol 7α-hydroxylase. Steroids 33: 675-692, 1979.

Jacobs FA, Flynn TG, Clark AF: Separation and kinetic characterization of acid phosphatase from the prostates of normal and castrated adult rats. Submitted to Mol Cell Endocrinol.

Lee DKH, Bird CE, Clark AF: Studies on the in vivo hormonal control of rat prostatic testosterone Δ^4-ene-5α-reductase activity. J Steroid Biochem 5: 609-617, 1974.

Levy C, Marchut M, Baulieu E-E, Robel P: Studies of the 3β-hydroxysteroid oxidoreductase activity in rat ventral prostate. Steroids 23: 291-300, 1974.

Liang T, Mezzetti G, Chen C, Liao S: Selective polyamine-binding proteins. Spermine binding by an androgen-sensitive phosphoprotein. Biochem Biophys Acta 542: 430-441, 1978.

Mainwaring WIP, Mangan FR, Peterken BM: Studies on the solubilized ribonucleic acid polymerase from rat ventral prostate gland. Biochem J 123: 619, 1971.

Mainwaring WIP, Wilce PA: The control of the form and function of the ribosomes in androgen dependent tissues by testosterone. Biochem J 134: 795-805, 1973.

Mainwaring WIP, Mangan, FR, Irving RA, Jones DA: Specific changes in the messenger ribonucleic acid content of the rat ventral prostate gland after androgenic stimulation: evidence from the synthesis of aldolase messenger ribonucleic acid.

108

Biochem J 144: 413-426, 1974.

Moore RJ, Wilson JD: Localization of the reduced nicotinamide adenine dinucleotide phosphate: Δ^4-3-ketosteroid 5α-oxido-reductase in the nuclear membrane of the rat ventral prostate. J Biol Chem 247: 958-967.

Moruzzi G, Barbiroli B, Corti A, Caldarera CM: Polyamines and testosterone on nucleic acid biosynthesis in the prostate gland of the rat. Ital J Biochem 20: 6, 1971.

Muntzing J, Kirdani R, Murphy JP, Sandberg AA: Hormonal control of zinc uptake and binding in the rat dorsolateral prostate. Invest Urol 14: 492-495, 1977.

Pegg AE, Williams-Ashman HG: Enzymic synthesis of spermine in rat prostate. Arch Biochem Biophys 137: 156, 1970.

Pegg AE, Lockwood DH, Williams-Ashman, HG: Concentrations of putrescine and polyamines and their enzymic synthesis during androgen-induced prostatic growth. Biochem J 117: 17-31, 1970.

Rennie RS, Symes EK, Mainwaring WIP: The androgenic regulation of the activities of enzymes engaged in the synthesis of deoxyribonucleic acid in rat ventral prostate gland. Biochem J 152: 1-16, 1975.

Rennie PS, Bruchovsky N, Hook SL: Androgenic regulation of a tissue specific isoenzyme of acid phosphatase in rat ventral prostate. J Steroid Biochem 9: 585-593, 1978.

Robel P, Blondeau JP, Baulieu E-E: Androgen receptors in rat ventral prostate microsomes. Biochim Biophys Acta 373: 1-9, 1974.

Shimazaki J, Matsushita I, Furuya N, Yamanaka H, Shida K: Reduction of 5α-position of testosterone in the rat ventral prostate. Endocr Jap 16: 453-458, 1969.

Shimazaki J, Kato N, Nagai H, Yamanaka H, Shida K. 3α-Reduction of 5α-dihydrotestosterone in the rat ventral prostate. Endocr Jap 19: 97-106, 1972.

Singhal RL, Parvlekar MR, Vijayvargiya R, Robinson GA: Metabolic control mechanisms in mammalian systems. Biochem J 125: 329-342, 1971.

Slaunwhite WR, Sharma M: Effects of hypophysectomy and prolactin replacement on prostatic response to androgen in orchiectomized rats. Biol Reprod 17: 489-492, 1977.

Tenniswood M, Bird CE, Clark AF: Acid phosphatases: androgen dependent markers of rat prostate. Can J Biochem 54: 350-357, 1976.

Tenniswood M, Abrahams P, Bird CE, Clark AF: Effects of castration and androgen replacement on acid phosphatase activity in the adult rat prostate gland. J Endocrinol 77: 301-308, 1978a.

Tenniswood M, Abrahams P, Bird CE Clark AF: Effects of 3β-androstanediol and 5β-dihydrotestosterone on acid phosphatase activity in the adult rat prostate gland. J Endo 79: 9-16, 1978b.

Tenniswood M, Bird CE, Clark AF: Kinetics of in vivo 5α-androstane-3β,17β-diol metabolism in adult normal and castrated male rats. Submitted to J Steroid Biochem.

Tenniswood M, Abrahams P, Bird CE, Clark AF: 5α-androstane-3β,17β-diol exerts its effects on acid phosphatase activity in the adult rat prostate gland through prior conversion to 5α-dihydrotestosterone. Submitted to J Endocrinol.

Van Doorn EJ, Bird CE, Clark AF: Nuclear 3α-hydroxysteroid dehydrogenase (3α-OHD) activity for 5α-dihydrotestosterone in the rat prostate. Endo Res Commun 2: 471-487, 1975.

Verjans HL, Eik-Nes KB, Aafjes JH, Vels FJ, van der Molen HJ: Effects of testosterone propionate, 5α-dihydrotestosterone propionate and estradiol benzoate on serum levels of LH and FSH in the castrated adult rat. Acta Endocrinol 77: 643-654, 1974.

Walsh PC, Wilson JD: The induction of prostatic hypertrophy in the dog. J Clin Invest 57: 1093-1097, 1976.

Williams-Ashman HG, Coppoc GL, Weber G: Imbalance in ornithine metabolism in hepatomas of different growth rates as expressed in formation of putrescine, spermidine and spermine. Can Res 32: 1924-1932, 1972.

Williams-Ashman HG, Corti A, Sheth AR: Formation and functions of aliphatic polyamines in the prostate gland and its secretions. In: normal and abnormal growth of the prostate, Goland M, ed. Springfield: Charles C Thomas, p 231, 1975.

9. PROSTATIC BIOPSY

N.K. Bissada and A.E. Finkbeiner

Prostatic carcinoma is the second most common malignancy in American men and the most common cause of cancer death in men over 55 years old (Catalona and Scott 1978). Although rectal examination is essential for early detection, the diagnosis of prostatic malignancy rests on microscopic examination of biopsy material from the suspicious area(s). Several methods of histologic and cytologic diagnosis of prostatic carcinoma have been advocated. Among these the needle biopsy is the most popular (Catalona and Scott 1978). In this chapter, the indications, advantages and techniques of the different methods of prostatic biopsy are described.

I. ASPIRATION BIOPSY AND CYTOLOGIC EXAMINATION

A. Perineal aspiration biopsy of the prostate

Cytological study of prostatic specimens obtained by perineal aspiration biopsy was introduced in 1930 (Ferguson 1930). In a subsequent evaluation of the method, Ferguson concluded that positive diagnosis of cancer from an aspiration biopsy by an experienced pathologist is reliable and that diagnosable tissue is obtained in 77 per cent of the cases (Ferguson 1937). However, others were less successful in their attempts to diagnose early prostatic carcinoma by perineal aspiration biopsy of the prostate (Franzen et al. 1960).

B. Transrectal aspiration biopsy

Transrectal aspiration biopsy using a specially designed syringe and needle holder seemed to yield better results than transperineal aspiration biopsy (Franzen et al. 1960, Linsk et al. 1972, Kurth et al. 1972, Bishop and Oliver 1977).

Technique The patient may be placed in the lithotomy or knee-chest position. The needle guide is drawn over the gloved finger. A finger cot is placed over the finger and the attached needle guide. The finger is then introduced into the rectum and the nodule is palpated. The long aspiration needle is threaded through the needle guide and passed through the tip of the guide into the prostatic nodule. The plunger of the syringe is drawn back as far as possible, creating a vacuum in the system. The needle is moved back and forth several millimeters within the mass with negative pressure applied. The plunger is then released to equalize the pressure within the syringe. The needle is withdrawn and is briefly separated from the syringe. Air is drawn into the syringe, the needle is reattached, and the aspirate is expressed onto a glass slide, after which it is evenly distributed and handed to the pathology technician.

In an extensive review of 1110 cases from Scandinavia, prostatic carcinoma was diagnosed cytologically in 336 cases (30 per cent) and none was considered falsely positive (Eposti 1966). However, histological diagnosis was obtained in only 162 patients. Of this group 55 were cytologically cancer of which 52 were confirmed histologically. Falsely negative results occurred in about 10 per cent of cases.

Advantages of transrectal aspiration biopsy are its being rapid and relatively atraumatic, almost without complications and, therefore, can be repeated as required to improve accuracy or to follow the results of treatment, especially after radiation therapy (Linsk et al. 1972, Bishop and Oliver 1977, Kurth et al. 1977). However, it is more difficult to perform than the conventional wide bore (needle) transrectal prostatic biopsy technique (Bishop and Oliver 1977). This fact is reflected in the fact that highly unsatisfactory results are seen initially. How much lower the unsatisfactory rate can be with experience is questionable (Williams et al. 1967). Also the recognition of prostatic carcinoma cells in the material obtained by this method requires experience in correlative study of cytology and histology of prostatic carcinoma. Cytologic grading has been attempted and seems to be promising as a possible prognostic indicator (Eposti 1971, Bishop and Oliver 1977). However, although close relationship between cytologic and histologic grading may be achieved by investigators with considerable experience (Eposti 1971), this has not been reproduced by less experienced investigators (Ekman 1967, Bishop and Oliver 1977).

In spite of the attractiveness of this method in diagnosing prostatic carcinoma, it is obvious that it requires considerable experience by both the urologist and pathologist. It is best to combine aspiration (cytological) biopsy with histological biopsy initially, until enough experience and confidence in the former is obtained, before relying solely on cytological diagnosis and grading.

C. Cytologic diagnosis of prostatic secretions

Cytologic examination of smears of expressed prostatic secretions was attempted by many investigators (Herbut and Lubin 1947, Albers et al. 1949, Gunn et al. 1954, Boyer 1950, Frank 1955, Mulholland 1931, Peters and Young 1951, Kaufman et al. 1954, Silberblatt 1956). However, the method proved to be generally unsatisfactory for diagnosing early prostatic carcinoma.

II. OPEN BIOPSY OF THE PROSTATE

A. Open retropubic biopsy

Open retropubic biopsy described by Culp (1958) has been used less frequently than open perineal biopsy.

Technique The prostate is exposed retropubically. The prostate is then mobilized and rotated laterally. Biopsy material is then obtained as described in open perineal biopsy.

B. Open perineal biopsy

Historically, open perineal prostatic biopsy was introduced by Young about 70 years ago (Kircheim 1975).

Technique In open perineal biopsy, the patient is placed in the exaggerated lithotomy position and the posterior aspect of the prostate is approached and exposed as for perineal prostatectomy. A generous wedge, including the nodule, on both sides of the posterior and posterolateral portions of the prostate, is removed with the scalpel. The defect is closed with catgut. If the frozen section is unequivocally positive the surgeon may proceed with the radical procedure at this time. If the frozen section is questionable or negative, or radical perineal prostatectomy is not planned, the biopsy area should be fulgurated, and the wound irrigated and closed. Further management is based on the results of the permanent section studies.

Among the different methods of diagnosing prostatic carcinoma, open perineal biopsy has been considered the most accurate (Hudson et al. 1955). Indeed, open perineal biopsy was found more accurate when compared to transperineal needle biopsy (Kaufman and Schultz 1962). However, no accurate comparison of needle transrectal biopsy with open perineal biopsy is available.

In a series of random open perineal biopsy (Hudson et al. 1954, 1955, Hudson 1957), the incidence, extent and behavior of prostatic cancer was studied in 686 men. Of the patients studied, 141 had minimal prostatic obstruction while the others had no evidence of prostatism. Open perineal prostatic biopsy resulted in the diagnosis of prostatic cancer in 11.1 per cent. Of those with cancer, 88 per cent were judged operable.

There was a recognized failure to detect cancer in 2 of 39 patients during initial hospitalization. In these 2 patients, cancer was discovered in tissue removed by enucleation prostatectomy. Further, in 30 to 50 months following negative random biopsy, 3 of 295 patients were found to have prostatic carcinoma (Hudson 1957). In another series, open perineal biopsy was accurate in 92 per cent (Colby 1953).

Since open perineal biopsy with frozen section studies is often attempted at the time of planned radical prostatectomy, the pitfalls of the frozen section study must be considered. A diagnosis of carcinoma was made by frozen section in 25 of 37 patients in whom complete histologic study of the specimen indicated carcinoma (Hudson 1954).

Open perineal biopsy obviously carried higher morbidity than needle biopsy. In addition to those complications inherent in an open surgical procedure under general or spinal anesthesia, rectal injury and impotence are recognized complications of this procedure. At present the postulated slightly increased accuracy of open perineal biopsy over transrectal needle biopsy does not justify the increased morbidity of the former procedure. Open perineal biopsy should be reserved for the rare patient with a potentially curable lesion in whom strong clinical suspicion of carcinoma remains after repeated negative transrectal biopsy.

III. TRANSURETHRAL BIOPSY OF THE PROSTATE AND TRANSURETHRAL PROSTATECTOMY

Transurethral biopsy of the prostate is not accurate in the diagnosis of early prostatic carcinoma (Hudson et al. 1954, Emmett et al. 1962, Fortunof 1962). On the other hand complete transurethral resection of the prostate for relief of obstructive uropathy can yield malignant tissue in the majority of patients with advanced carcinoma (Thompson 1942, Emmett et al. 1962) and even in a significant number of patients with clinically unsuspected carcinoma, especially when the tissue is step-sectioned and examined histologically (Denton 1965).

In a comparison of perineal needle prostatic biopsy with transurethral prostatectomy in the diagnosis of prostatic carcinoma, perineal needle biopsy was performed prior to or at the time of transurethral prostatectomy on 300 unselected men (Denton et al. 1967). In all cases in which the needle biopsy was positive for carcinoma, the surgical specimen of the transurethral prostatectomy was also positive.

The diagnostic accuracy of transurethral prostatectomy was compared to transrectal biopsy in 139 patients with obstructive uropathy and clinically suspected prostatic carcinoma in whom both techniques were carried out in each patient (Bissada 1977). Eighty-five patients had carcinoma detected in the tissues obtained by transurethral resection,

transrectal biopsy or both. The diagnosis was missed on transurethral resection in 11 patients and on transrectal biopsy in 12 cases. It was concluded that transurethral resection of the prostate performed to relieve obstructive uropathy was as accurate as standard transrectal prostatic biopsy in diagnosing prostatic carcinoma.

Often the urologist is faced with a patient who has obstructive urinary symptoms and suspected prostatic carcinoma. Some of these patients are candidates for radical treatment and diagnosis is preferably confirmed by needle biopsy. However, many of these patients are not candidates for radical treatment. In such instances the urologist may proceed directly to transurethral resection to relieve the obstruction and to obtain tissue diagnosis at the same time.

IV. NEEDLE BIOPSY OF THE PROSTATE

Two approaches have been utilized for needle biopsy of the prostate, the transperineal and transrectal.

Prostatic needle biopsy may be performed using the Vim-Silverman needle, the Franklin modification of the Vim-Silverman needle (Figure 1) or with the Travenol disposable biopsy needle (Figure 2). The

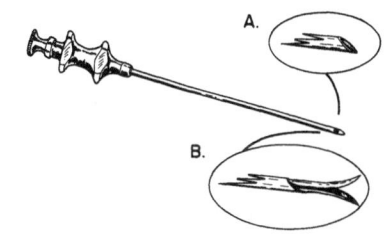

Figure 1. Franklin modification of Vim-Silverman Biopsy needle. Inset: close up of the needle tip. A) with obturator, B) with biopsy blades.

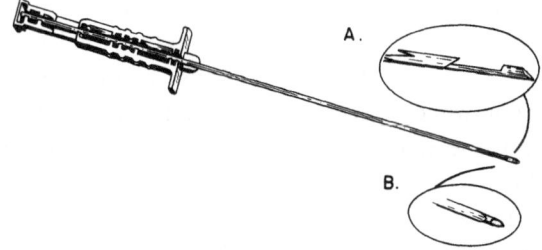

Figure 2. Travenol disposable biopsy needle. Inset: close up of needle tip. A) open, B) closed.

Franklin modification differs from the Vim-Silverman needle in that it has à metal block built into the hollow grooves of the biopsy blades at the tip. This prevents biopsied tissue from pulling out of the blades as they are retracted into the sheath. We have utilized the Franklin modification in our series (of 306 patients) and were satisfied with it although recently we have shifted to the disposable Travenol biopsy needle and feel that we can get better tissue cylinders with it.

A. Transperineal needle biopsy

Technique With the patient in the lithotomy position, the perineum is prepped and draped. A finger is then inserted into the rectum, the prostate is palpated and the site(s) for biopsy is (are) selected. The site of puncture in the perineum is infiltrated with a local anesthetic as are the deeper tissues down to the prostatic capsule. If the Franklin modification of the Vim-Silverman needle is used, it is introduced, with the stylet in place, through the perineal skin and advanced to the prostatic capsule at the site to be biopsied (directed by the rectal finger). The stylet is removed and the biopsy blades are gently inserted until they meet resistance at the prostatic capsule. They are then advanced into the nodule. The sheath is then advanced over the blades. The blades are then withdrawn and the tissues are placed in formalin. The sheath is withdrawn to the capsule again and the procedure is repeated in an adjacent area. Usually two and sometimes three specimens are obtained before removing the sheath. Pressure is applied for several minutes on the prostate by the rectal finger and over the site of puncture in the perineum to stop any transient bleeding. A small dressing is then applied.

If the Travenol needle is used, it is advanced to the capsule. The outer sheath is steadied in place while the trocar is pushed into the nodule. The trocar is then steadied and the outer cutting sheath is pushed into the lesion trapping a cylinder of prostatic tissue. The closed biopsy needle is then withdrawn, care being taken to keep it closed until the tissue sample is removed on the instrument table.

Transperineal needle biopsy is generally felt to be less accurate than transrectal biopsy (Barnes et al. 1972, Bissada 1977, Davison and Malament 1971,

Emmett and Barber 1962, von Buedingen 1976, Zincke et al. 1973). In early prostatic carcinoma, the incidence of false negative transperineal needle biopsy was reported from 24 to 40 per cent (Colby 1953, Kaufman 1954, Goodwin 1957). In one series transperineal needle biopsy detected carcinoma of the prostate in 85 of 105 patients ultimately proven to have adenocarcinoma of the prostate (Fortunof 1962). In the series reported by Kaufman (1962) a false negative punch biopsy was present in 27 per cent of the patients. In patients with isolated nodules in the prostate and those with lesions limited to the prostate, the incidence of false negative transperineal biopsy was 33 and 27 per cent respectively (Kaufman 1962).

B. Transrectal needle biopsy

Transrectal biopsy of the prostate was introduced in 1937 (Astraldi). The simplicity and efficacy of the procedure was reaffirmed in 1953 (Grabstald and Elliott). Thereafter, several series were published in the English literature indicating the popularity of the procedure (Barnes et al. 1972, Bissada et al. 1977, Daves et al. 1961, Emmett et al. 1962, Wendel and Evans 1967, Zincke et al. 1973).

Technique Transrectal biopsy using any of the previously described needles is similar to transperineal needle biopsy but more simple. The left index finger palpates the nodule while the right hand holds the biopsy needle, which is advanced into the rectum over the left index finger and is inserted through the rectal wall directly overlying the prostatic nodule. Two or three cylinders of tissue are obtained as described above and pressure is applied to the prostate for several minutes.

C. Accuracy of transrectal needle biopsy

The only method to determine absolutely the accuracy of biopsy would be the removal and examination of the entire prostate by step sections. However, this is unpractical in a patient with negative biopsy of the prostate. Other less reliable methods are comparisons with results of repeated biopsy by the same or other routes, examination of sections of prostatic tissue obtained during prostatectomy, or of autopsy findings. Since different authors use different criteria to estimate the accuracy of biopsy, comparison of different biopsy routes is difficult. However, careful analysis of the results of transrectal and transperineal biopsy routes seems to indicate markedly improved accuracy with the transrectal route. The accuracy of transrectal needle biopsy of the prostate was evaluated in 306 consecutive patients suspected to have prostatic carcinoma (Bissada et al. 1977). Of 155 patients who initially had negative biopsy, 20 were ultimately proven to have carcinoma. Of these 14 were detected in specimens obtained by repeated transrectal biopsy that was performed in 33 patients in whom clinical suspicion persisted in spite of negative first biopsy. The yield of positive biopsy in the second and third attempts in this particular group was 42.2 per cent. Twelve more patients were found to have carcinoma in tissues obtained during transurethral resection of the prostate that was performed for obstructive uropathy. Carcinoma was found at autopsy in three patients who had initial negative prostatic biopsy. Thus, the overall accuracy of a single and multiple transrectal biopsy was 81.3 and 90.4 per cent respectively. Using somewhat similar criteria to evaluate accuracy of transrectal biopsy of the prostate, others reported false negative results in 12 per cent of the first biopsy and 6 per cent after repeated biopsy (Zincke et al. 1973).

D. Complications of transrectal needle biopsy

Complications of needle biopsy of the prostate are reported variably from uncommon to rather frequent (Bissada et al. 1977, Daves et al. 1961, Emmett et al. 1962, Fawcett et al. 1975, Fortunof 1962, Grabstald and Elliott 1953, von Buedingen 1976, Wendel and Evans 1967). Complications are generally due to trauma or infection and include bladder, urethral and ureteral injuries; gross hematuria, hematospermia; perineal and retropubic hematoma; acute urinary retention; seeding of the needle tract with malignant tissue; fever; urinary tract infection; prostatitis, epididymitis; pyelonephritis; prostate, perineal or retroperitoneal abscess; bacteriuria, osteomyelitis of the vertebrae and disc space infection; and death (Desai and Woodruff 1974, Dowlen 1974, Fortunof 1962, Grabstald and Elliott 1953, Hogan and Johnson 1972, Mobley

et al. 1971, Stuppler et al. 1974, Wendel and Evans 1967). There is no correlation between the type of instrument used and the incidence of complications (Wendel and Evans 1967). Similarly, except for increased incidence of infectious complications with the transrectal route (Dowlen et al. 1974, Fawcett et al. 1975, Fortunof 1962, von Buedingen 1976) there is no correlation between the needle route of approach to the prostate and the incidence of other complications (Wendel and Evans 1967). In one series 121 of 306 patients (39 per cent) developed 158 complications (Bissada et al. 1977). Infection developed in 35 per cent of the cases. Preoperative antimicrobial therapy significantly reduced the incidence of infection in the patients who had biopsy alone from 38 per cent to 6 per cent. There was no advantage to antibiotics if they were used postoperatively. Other investigators (Davison and Malament 1971, Fawcett et al. 1975) also indicated that pre-biopsy antimicrobials would be effective in reducing the incidence of infectious complications. It is, therefore, recommended that antimicrobials should be started prior to undergoing transrectal needle biopsy of the prostate (Bissada et al. 1977).

V. CONCLUDING REMARKS

The indications and merits of different prostatic biopsy techniques have been discussed. At present, transrectal needle biopsy seems to offer the best compromise of high accuracy with acceptable morbidity. Patients with obstructive prostates and suspected prostatic carcinoma, who are not candidates for curative treatment may have transurethral prostatectomy to relieve the obstruction and confirm the diagnosis of prostatic carcinoma simultaneously. While transrectal needle aspiration biopsy is attractive because of its low morbidity, considerable experience must be gained with this technique before it can replace conventional histological biopsy techniques.

REFERENCES

Albers DD, McDonald JR, Thompson GJ: Carcinoma cells in prostatic secretions. J Am Med Ass 139: 299, 1949.
Astraldi A: Diagnosis of cancer of the prostate: biopsy by rectal route. Urol and Cutan Review 41: 421, 1973.

Barnes RW, Ninan CA: Carcinoma of the prostate: biopsy and conservative therapy. J Urol 108: 897, 1972.

Bishop D, Oliver JA: A study of transrectal aspiration biopsies of the prostate, with particular regard to prognostic evaluation. J Urol 117: 313, 1977.

Bissada NK: Accuracy of transurethral resection of the prostate versus transrectal needle biopsy in the diagnosis of prostatic carcinoma. J Urol 118: 61, 1977.

Bissada NK, Rountree, GA and Sulieman JS: Factors affecting accuracy and morbidity in transrectal biopsy of the prostate. Surg Gynec and Obstet 145: 869, 1977.

Boyer WF: Carcinoma of the prostate: A cytological study. J Urol 63: 334 1950.

Catalona WJ, Scott WW: Carcinoma of the prostate: A review. J Urol 119: 1, 1978.

Colby FH: Carcinoma of the prostate: Results of total prostatectomy. J Urol 69: 797, 1953.

Culp OS: Significance and treatment of prostatic nodules. Journal of Mich Med Soc 58: 585, 1959.

Culp DA, Flocks RH, Porto JR: Retropubic biopsy of the prostate. J Urol 79: 873, 1958.

Daves JA, Tomskey GC, Cohen AE: Transrectal needle biopsy of the prostate. J Urol 85: 180, 1961.

Davison P, Malament M: Urinary contamination as a result of transrectal biopsy of the prostate. J Urol 105: 545, 1971.

Day E: Early case finding. In: Proc Third Nat Cancer Conf Philadelphia: JB Lippincott, 1957, p 196.

Denton SE, Choy SH, Valk WL: Occult prostatic carcinoma diagnosed by the step-section technique of the surgical specimen. J Urol 93: 296, 1965.

Denton SE, Valk WL, Jacobson JM, Kettunen RC: Comparison of perineal needle biopsy and the transurethral prostatectomy in the diagnosis of prostatic carcinoma: an analysis of 300 cases. J Urol 97: 127, 1967.

Desai SG, Woodruff LM: Carcinoma of the prostate: Local extension following perineal needle biopsy. Urology 3: 87, 1974.

Dowlen DW Jr, Block NL, Politano VA: Complications of transrectal biopsy examination of the prostate. South Med J 67: 1453, 1974.

Ekman H, Hedberg K, Persson PS: Cytologic versus histological examination of needle biopsy specimens in the diagnosis of prostatic cancer. Br J Urol 39: 544, 1967.

Emmett JL, Barber KW Jr. Jackman RJ: Transrectal biopsy to detect prostatic carcinoma: A review and report of 203 cases. J Urol 87: 460, 1962.

Eposti PL: Cytologic diagnosis of prostatic tumors with the aid of transrectal aspiration biopsy. A critical review of 1,110 cases and a report of a morphologic and cytochemical studies. Acta Cytol 10: 182, 1966.

Eposti PL: Cytologic malignancy grading of prostatic carcinoma by transrectal aspiration biopsy: A five year followup study of 469 hormonetreated patients. Scand J Urol Nephrol 5: 199, 1971.

Fawcett DP, Eykyn S, Bultitude MI: Urinary tract infection following trans-rectal biopsy of the prostate. Br J Urol 47: 679, 1975.

Fortunof S: Needle biopsy of the prostate: A review of 346 biopsies. J Urol 87: 159, 1962.

Frank IN: A cytologic evaluation of the prostatic smear in carcinoma of the prostate. J Urol 73: 128, 1955.

Franzen S, Giertz G, Zajieck J: Cytological diagnosis of prostatic tumours by transrectal aspiration biopsy: A preliminary report. Br J Urol 32: 193, 1960.

Ferguson RS: Prostatic neoplasms: Their diagnosis by needle puncture and aspiration. Am J Surg 9: 507, 1930.

Ferguson RS: Diagnosis and treatment of early carcinoma of the prostate. J Urol 37: 774, 1937.

Goodwin WE: Early case finding. In: Proc Third Nat Cancer Conf Philadelphia: JB Lippincott, 1975, p 196.

Grabstald H, Elliott JL: Transrectal biopsy of the prostate. JAMA 153: 563, 1953.

Gunn SA, Ayre JE, Coplan MM, Woods FM, Melvin PD: Clinical application of cytology of prostatic cancer. J Urol 72: 722, 1954.

Herbut PA, Lubin EN: Cancer cells in prostatic secretions. J Urol 57: 542, 1947.

Hogan JM, Johnson DE: Ureteral perforation. A complication of transrectal needle biopsy of the prostate. J Urol 108: 297, 1972.

Hudson PB: Prostatic cancer: XIV. Its incidence, extent and behavior in 686 men studied by prostatic biopsy. J Am Geriatr Soc 5: 338, 1957.

Hudson PB, Finkle AL, Hopkins JA, Sproul EE, Stout AP: Prostatic cancer: XI. Early prostatic cancer diagnosed by arbitrary open perineal biopsy among 300 unselected patients. Cancer 7: 690, 1954.

Hudson PB, Finkle AL, Jost HM, Trifilio A, Stout AP: Prostatic cancer: X. Comparison of open and 'punch' biopsy techniques. Arch Surg 70: 508, 1955.

Hudson PB, Finkle AL, Trifilio A, Wolan CT: Prostatic cancer: IX. Value of transurethral biopsy in search of early prostatic carcinoma. Surg. 35: 897, 1954.

Kaufman JJ, Rosenthal M, Goodwin WE: Methods of diagnosis of carcinoma of the prostate: A comparison of clinical impression, prostatic smear, needle biopsy, open perineal biopsy and transurethral biopsy. J Urol 72: 450, 1954.

Kaufman JJ, Schultz JI: Needle biopsy of the prostate: A re-evaluation. J Urol 87: 164, 1962.

Kirchheim D: Prostatic biopsy. In: Glenn JF, ed. Urologic surgery, second edition. Hagerstown: Harper and Row, 1975, chap 39, pp 539-545.

Kurth KH, Althwein JE, Skoluda D, Hohenfellner R: Follow-up of irradiated prostatic carcinoma by aspiration biopsy. J Urol 117: 615, 1977.

Linsk JA, Axilrod HD, Solyn R, Delaverd C: Transrectal cytologic aspiration in diagnosis of prostatic carcinoma. J Urol 108: 455, 1972.

Mobley JE, Redman JF, Black RM, Sellars JR: Hemorrhage from transrectal needle biopsy of prostate. JAMA 216: 1867, 1971.

Moore RA: The morphology of small prostatic carcinoma. J Urol 33: 224, 1935.

Mulholland, SW: A study of prostatic secretion and its relation to malignancy. Proc Staff Meet Clin 6: 733, 1931.

Parry WL, Finelli JF: Biopsy of prostate. J Urol 84: 643, 1960.

Peters H, Young JD: Prostatic smear in cancer diagnosis. JAMA 145: 556, 1951.

Silberblatt JM, Solomon C, Hyman RM: Exfoliative cytology as screening method of prostatic carcinoma. J Urol 75: 734, 1956.

Stuppler SA, Kandzari SJ, Milam DF: Transrectal needle biopsy of prostate. Complications. Urology 3: 82, 1974.

Thompson GJ: Transurethral resection of malignant lesions of the prostate gland. JAMA 120: 1105, 1942.

von Buedingen RP: Prevention of infection during transrectal biopsy of prostate through double-glove technique. Urology 7: 296, 1976.

Wendel RG, Evans AT: Complications of punch biopsy of the prostate gland. J Urol 97: 122, 1967.

Williams JP, Still BM, Push RCB: The diagnosis of prostatic cancer: Cytological and biochemical studies using the Franzen biopsy needle. Br J Urol 39: 549, 1967.

Zincke H, Campbell J, Utz DC, Farrow GM, Anderson MJ Jr: Confidence in the negative transrectal needle biopsy. Surg Gynec Obstet 136: 78, 1973.

10. SERIAL PROSTATIC BIOPSIES: APPLICATION IN CONTROL AND MANAGEMENT OF BENIGN AND MALIGNANT PROSTATIC DISEASE

H. WOLF

The advent of prostatic biopsy – whether performed as needle biopsy or needle aspiration biopsy – has made it possible preoperatively to diagnose prostatic diseases with acceptable accuracy. It has also made it possible, at least theoretically, to follow histologically the effect of a specific treatment by performing serial prostatic biopsies. The diagnosis of benign prostatic hypertrophy is largely a clinical one, whereas the final diagnosis of prostatic cancer is a microscopic one. The diagnostic value of needle biopsy for the diagnosis of cancer of the prostate has been discussed in the preceding chapter.

The need for histological follow-up by serial prostatic biopsies is primarily present when non-surgical modalities of treatment with curative intention are used both for benign prostatic hypertrophy and cancer of the prostate. This chapter is a review of the value of serial prostatic needle biopsies used for that purpose.

I. BENIGN PROSTATIC HYPERTROPHY

A. Hormonal treatment

Treatment of benign prostatic hypertrophy is at present surgical, but during the past, several attempts have been made to treat this disease with hormones either singly or in combination (Wolf and Madsen 1968). Trials of hormone treatment have been based on the assumption that this disease is hormone dependent and/or induced by the changing hormone ratios in elderly men. Generally such trials have not been successful, and hormonal manipulation in the treatment of benign prostatic hypertrophy seems at present not to be indicated.

However, with increasing knowledge of the etiology of benign prostatic hypertrophy the possibility still exists that hormonal management of this disease some day may become the treatment of choice.

One way of evaluating a therapeutic effect would be to follow the histological changes induced by such treatment in serial prostatic biopsy specimens. This has also been done in some of the studies performed.

B. The significance of histological changes in serial prostatic biopsy specimens

Castration induces atrophy of the prostate and changes in the histological appearance of benign prostatic hypertrophy in man (Huggins and Stevens 1940). These changes include microscopic signs of atrophy such as: 1) increased number of acini per microscopic field, 2) smaller lumina of the acini, 3) less papillary infoldings of the epithelium into the acini, and 4) decreased cell height of the epithelium. Hormonal treatment of benign prostatic hypertrophy with intended cure would be believed to result in similar changes in order to be effective.

The histological appearance of benign prostatic hypertrophy is, however, known to be very variable. Therefore, it is questionable whether a single biopsy specimen can give a representative picture of the entire gland and whether minor changes of the histological appearance observed in biopsy specimens such as those mentioned above are of any significance in judging a possible effect of treatment.

This question has been systematically evaluated in a study of the appearance of preoperative needle biopsy specimens compared with the appearance of 20 randomly chosen areas from the same prostates removed at operation, the size of these areas being comparable to the size of a needle biopsy specimen (Wolf 1975).

116

In this study a quantitative evaluation of the prostatic tissue was made as described by Huggins and Stevens (1940) recording the number of acini, the average maximal epithelial height of the acini and the average maximal diameter of the acini for the biopsy specimen and for each randomly chosen area.

This study reemphasized the great variability of the histological appearance of benign prostatic hypertrophy. A few examples will illustrate this. A preoperative biopsy specimen from a benign hypertrophied prostatic gland consisted of fibromuscular tissue with rather uniformly looking acini (Figure 1A). Such areas were also found in the removed prostate. However, other areas showed a greater number of acini, whereas still other areas showed highly dilated acini. Thus, in some areas the average maximal diameter of the acini was large and there were few acini and vice versa. Some of the randomly chosen areas had both types of acini (Figure 1B). The average epithelial height of the acini was rather uniform in dilated as well as non-dilated acini in all 20 randomly chosen areas from this particular prostate (Figure 1C, D).

Two areas from another prostate showed completely different types of acini (Figure 1E, F). The number of acini per area and the average diameter of the acini from these 2 areas were again different. However, in this prostate there was also a great variation in the average maximal height of the acinar epithelium (Figure 2A, B). Such variation was found in about 75 per cent of the prostates studied and was also found in adjacent acini with equal diameters (Figure 2C).

Figure 2D shows a preoperative biopsy with rather uniformly looking acini. This area shows signs of atrophy according to the criteria of Huggins and Stevens (1940). Such areas were also found in the removed prostate (Figure 2E). However, the appearance of other areas of the same prostate was quite different. Some areas showed acini with cylindrical epithelium and numerous infoldings into the acini (Figure 2F), whereas other areas showed dilated acini lined with cuboidal epithelium without infoldings (Figure 3A).

Thus, it appears that hyperplastic prostatic tissue has a multiplicity of changes, that is varying proportions of acinar, and fibrous and muscular tissue together with cystic changes throughout the same prostate. The epithelium may be flat and atrophic or tall and secretory with numerous epithelial infoldings. Any area of the size comparable to biopsy specimens does not give a representative picture of the entire gland and it will not be possible from the appearance of single, serial biopsy specimens to draw any conclusions on the effect of a given treatment. Such conclusions will invariably lead to misinterpretations, at least if they are based on the criteria of Huggins and Stevens (1940).

II. CANCER OF THE PROSTATE

A. Histology

1. Grading of cancer of the prostate The histological criteria for the diagnosis of cancer of the prostate need not be reviewed here, since they are generally well established and noncontroversial. Most carcinomas of the prostate are adenocarcinomas.

Grading of adenocarcinomas of the prostate is carried out on basis of cellular differentiation and histological pattern. Generally adenocarcinomas of the prostate are not anaplastic. Thus, Pool and Thompson (1956) found only 3 percent grade IV tumors. Grading of cancer of the prostate is essential, because there seems to be a correlation between tumor differentiation and development of metastases and survival (Boxer et al. 1977, Culp 1968, Gleason et al. 1974, Pool and Thompson 1956, Vickery and Kerr 1963) both in patients treated with radical prostatectomy or more conservative measures. Others were, however, not able to demonstrate such correlation (Franks et al. 1958).

2. Variability of histology in operative specimens The great variety of cellular and glandular appearance of the cancerous tissue found within the same tumor makes it extremely difficult to categorize these tumors. This fact has recently been reemphasized (Byar and Mostofi 1972), but has previously been demonstrated by several investigators (Starklint 1950, Utz and Farrow 1969). Within the same tumor there may be a wide variety of tumor differentiation. Well differentiated glan-

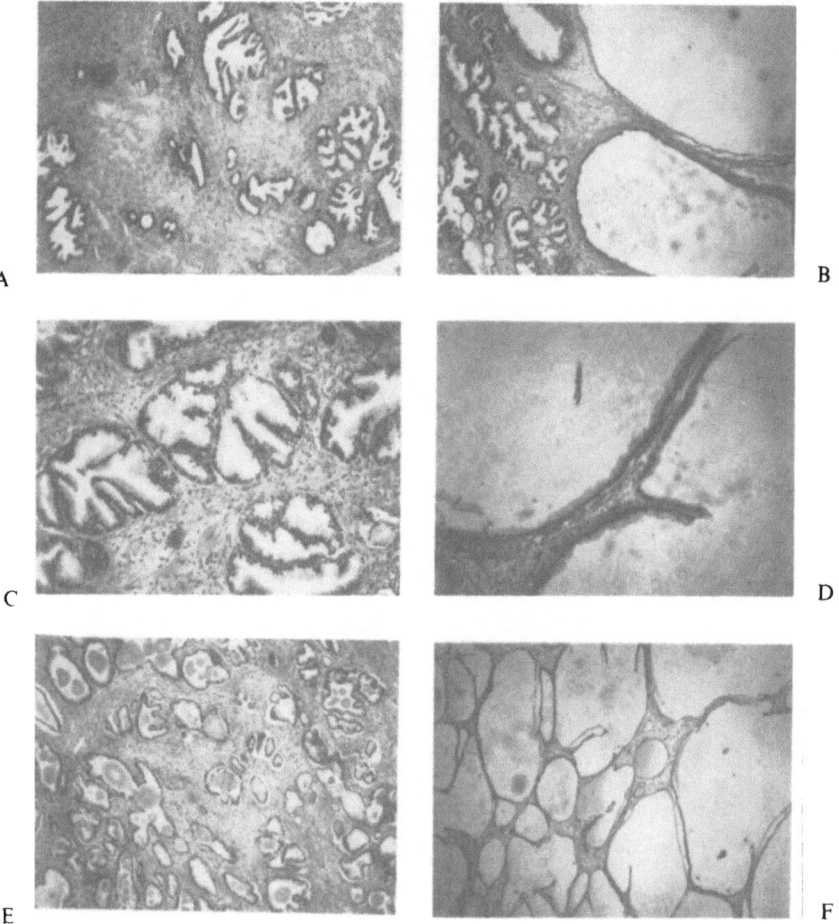

Figure 1. A. Preoperative biopsy from a hypertrophied prostatic gland, consisting of fibromuscular tissue with rather uniformly looking acini. Reduced from ×80.

B. Randomly selected area from the same hypertrophied prostatic gland removed at operation as in A, showing in addition to acini of the same appearance as in the preoperative biopsy highly dilated acini, in this particular area adjacent to each other. Numerous papillary infoldings of the epithelium into the acini are seen in the acini of small diameter. Such infoldings are not seen in the highly dilated acini. Reduced from ×80.

C. Micrograph demonstrating the epithelial height of the small acini of the same hypertrophied prostatic gland as in A and B. Reduced from ×200.

D. Micrograph demonstrating the epithelial height of the dilated acini of the same hypertrophied prostatic gland as in A and B, the epithelial height being of the same size as in non-dilated small acini as shown in C. Reduced from ×200.

E. Randomly selected area from a second hypertrofied prostatic gland showing numerous small acini in fibromuscular tissue. Reduced from ×80.

F. Another randomly selected area from the same hypertrophied prostatic gland as in E, showing fewer acini per microscopic field, the acini being highly dilated and the fibromuscular tissue more sparse. Reduced from ×80.

dular areas of prostatic adenocarcinoma (Figure 3B), solid areas of poorly differentiated adenocarcinoma (Figure 3C), or even fields of anaplastic carcinoma (Figure 3D). Most tumors may thus be placed in one or several categories depending on the field studied, and even the same examiner has difficulties in repeating himself unless exactly the same microscopic field is examined (Byar and Mostofi 1972).

3. The significance of grading based on biopsies To overcome these difficulties of grading, it has been

118

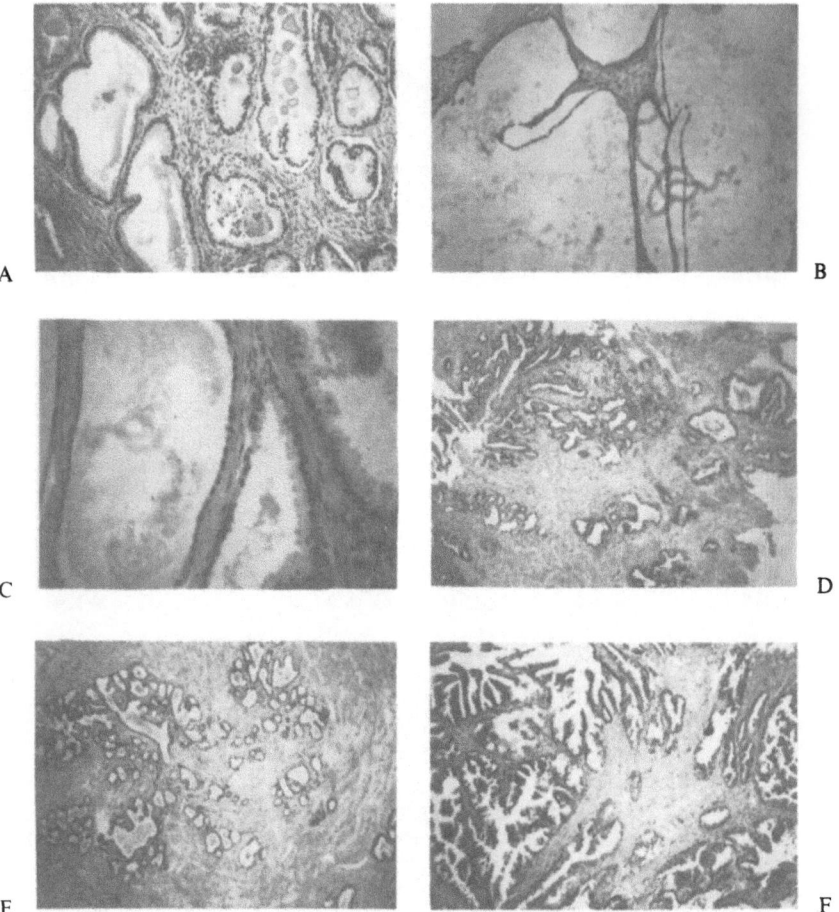

Figure 2. A. Micrograph demonstrating the high epithelium of the non-dilated acini of the same randomly selected area as shown in Figure 1E. Reduced from ×200.
B. Micrograph demonstrating the flat, atrophic epithelium of the dilated acini of the same randomly selected area as shown in Figure 1F. Reduced from ×200.
C. Micrograph demonstrating flat cuboidal epithelium and high cylindrical epithelium in adjacent acini of similar diameter. Randomly selected area from the same hypertrophied prostatic gland as in Figure 1E and F. Reduced from ×320.
D. Preoperative biopsy from a third hypertrophied prostatic gland consisting of fibromuscular tissue with uniformly looking acini. Reduced from ×80.
E. Randomly selected area from the same hypertrophied prostatic gland removed at operation as in D, showing a similar proportion of fibromuscular tissue and acini of similar size as in the biopsy specimen. Reduced from ×80.
F. Randomly selected area from the same hypertrophied prostatic gland as in D and E, showing acini with cylindrical epithelium and numerous infoldings into the acini. Reduced from ×80.

proposed to classify the tumor by its most malignant area (Shelley et al. 1958) and to use only two grades of differentiation, either well differentiated or poorly differentiated (Vickery and Kerr 1963). This may easily be done with radical prostatectomy or transurethral resection specimens, where several areas are available for study.

However, this considerable variation in histology certainly invalidates any attempts of grading cancer of the prostate on basis of a single needle biopsy specimen, so that the prognostic guide of such grading may be limited and attempts to evaluate various modalities of treatment in relation to the degree of differentiation of a needle biopsy may be uncertain (Cantril et al. 1974).

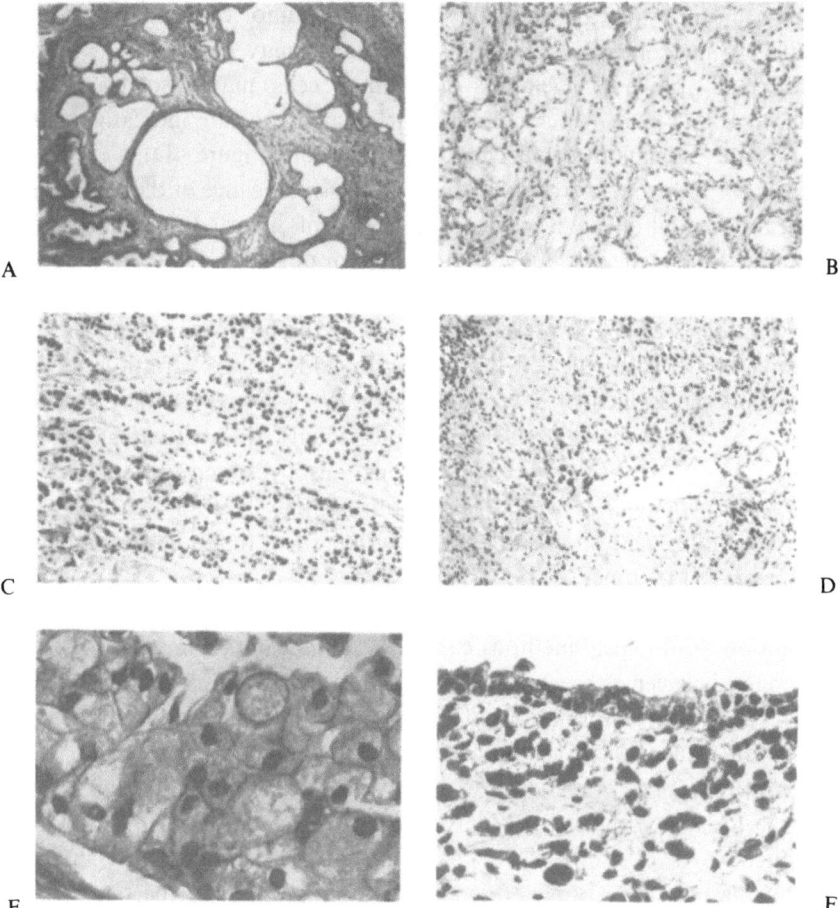

Figure 3. A. Another randomly selected area from the same hypertrophied prostatic gland as in Figure 2E and F, showing dilated acini without any infoldings and lined with cuboidal epithelium. Reduced from ×80.

B. Randomly selected area from a prostatic adenocarcinoma, showing well differentiated glandular tissue. Reduced from ×80.

C. Randomly selected area from the same prostatic adenocarcinoma as in B, showing less well differentiated glandular tissue. Reduced from ×80.

D. Randomly selected area from the same prostatic adenocarcinoma as in B and C, showing a field of poorly differentiated carcinoma. Reduced from ×80.

E. Micrograph of prostatic carcinoma showing signs of influence by estrogens. Intracytoplasmatic basal vacuoles and large swollen cells (balloon cells) with the nucleus pushed aside are seen. Reduced from ×480.

F. Micrograph of prostatic carcinoma showing late signs of influence by estrogens. Strands of distorted or ruptured cells are seen in fibrous tissue and seen beneath the epithelium of a prostatic duct. Reduced from ×400.

B. Treatment with estrogens

1. Histological changes The changes that occur in most prostatic cancer cells after treatment with estrogens have been described by several authors (Franks 1960, Schenken et al. 1942). These changes may appear within a very short time after start of treatment. They include (Figure 3E) the appearance of intracytoplasmatic basal vacuoles that coalesce and form large swollen cells (balloon cells) with the nucleus pushed aside. The nuclei become condensed, hyperchromatic and later pyknotic and the swollen cells may rupture with dissolution of the normally sharp epithelial-stromal margins and diffusion of cells and alveolar contents into the stroma. Dense knots or strands of distorted cells in fibrous tissue may then be seen (Figure 3F). In some cases squamous metaplasia after estrogen treatment may be seen. These changes are also seen in metastatic lesions.

Many tumor cells seem to disappear completely, but even in tumors showing pronounced degenerative changes as described above small clumps of apparently undamaged cells (Figure 4A) can almost always be found. In some patients these degenerative changes do not occur following estrogen medication. The biological potential of the degenerated tumor cells is unknown, but generally judged inactive, although we do not know whether these shrunken and distorted cells are capable of renewed tumor growth activity or whether renewed tumor growth always arises in the islands of surviving, undamaged cells.

2. Variation of response and significance of serial biopsies Thus, the morphological response of prostatic cancer cells to estrogen treatment varies from tumor to tumor, but also from part to part of the same tumor. In addition, histological methods can not reveal any difference between estrogen resistant and sensitive cells. Therefore, information of a correlation between differences in morphological changes and the clinical course of patients with cancer of the prostate treated with estrogens have until now been limited.

The significance of demonstration of the presence or absence of morphological changes in serial prostatic biopsy specimens is therefore extremely doubtful. Variation in structure or response to treatment throughout the tumor may give a quite erroneous impression if only one or two areas are fortuitously selected for biopsy in analogy with benign prostatic hypertrophy.

C. Radiotherapy

1. Histological changes Together with radical perineal prostatectomy external beam irradiation and/or interstitial radiotherapy has been advocated as a modality of definitive curative treatment for localized cancer of the prostate.

The histological appearance of the irradiated cancer of the prostate – after the acute irradiation changes including bizarre tumor cell morphology, balloon cells, vacuolation of the cytoplasm, irregular nuclei of individual tumor cells, and abnormal mitotic figures – is characterized by intense fibrosis (Figure 4B). In the fibrotic areas small nests of tumor cells mainly in the form of clumps of nuclei may be present (Figure 4C). Abundant tumor cells may also be present in the post-irradiated prostate indicating minimal response to irradiation (Figure 4D).

The significance of the presence of single or small groups of distorted tumor cells is unknown. It is at present not known whether these cells are viable or may be able to develop regrowth of the cancer during the lifetime of the patient.

In addition to variation in response to radiotherapy of cancer of the prostate among different individuals, different areas of the same prostate may also respond differently. Areas of intense fibrosis may be found together with fibrotic areas with nests of tumor cells or areas with intact tumor tissue.

2. Serial biopsies in follow-up Determination of the size or consistency of a carcinoma of the prostate and its clinical response to irradiation by rectal palpation is imprecise (Byar and Mostofi 1972, Carlton et al. 1976, Cox and Stoffel 1977). The frequent finding of residual tumor tissue at autopsy even though the palpable prostatic tumor has disappeared further stresses that rectal palpation is of little use. On the other hand radiation fibrosis occasionally results in a hard prostate that on histological examination is benign.

Therefore, serial prostatic biopsies have been advocated to judge the effect of external beam irradiation and/or interstitial radiotherapy. These serial biopsies are usually designated as either histologically positive or histologically negative for malignancy.

The frequency of positive biopsies following irradiation has been communicated by several authors. Many of these studies include only a few patients, and the biopsy follow-up has in many cases not been systematic. A review of the published series will appear from Table 1.

The over-all fall in percentage of positive biopsies during an observation period of several years has been demonstrated by several authors and will also appear from Table 1. This may indicate a very slow regression rate of cancer of the prostate after irradiation, which also has been observed clinically (Hill et al. 1974). The latter authors are of the opinion that although the tumor cells are lethally

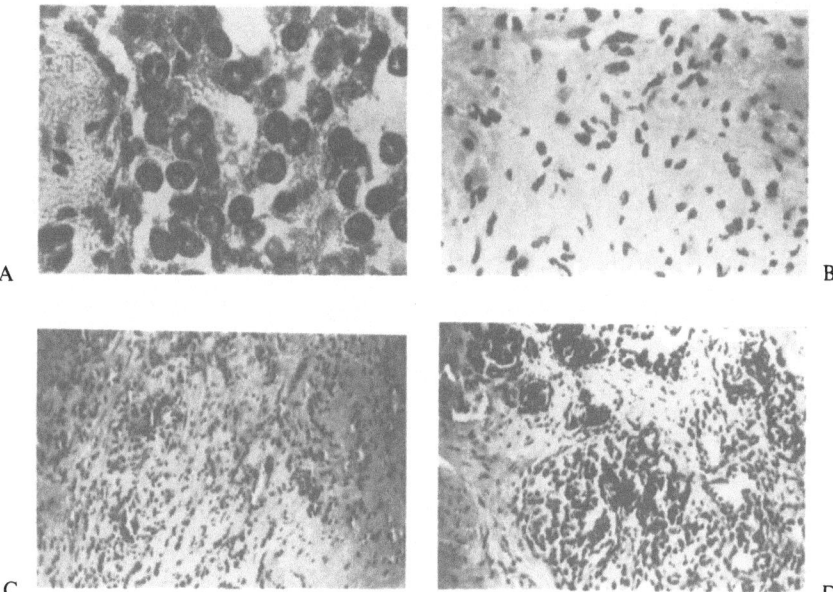

Figure 4. A. Micrograph of prostatic carcinoma treated by estrogens for several years showing clumps of apparently undamaged cancer cells. To the left inactive cells in fibrous tissue. Reduced from ×800.

B. Micrograph of prostatic carcinoma treated by external irradiation (6000 R) showing intense fibrosis apparently without any viable tumor cells. Reduced from ×400.

C. Micrograph of prostatic carcinoma treated with external irradiation (6000 R) showing intense fibrosis, but apparently small nests of tumor cells that may be viable. Reduced from ×80.

D. Micrograph of prostatic carcinoma treated with external irradiation (6000 R) showing abundant apparently viable tumor cells. Reduced from ×80.

damaged by irradiation and incapable of mitosis, they may still be present microscopically for a prolonged period. The regression rate does not seem to be influenced by the degree of differentiation of the cancer (Cantril et al. 1974, de Muelenaere et al. 1974).

3. Significance of changes in serial prostatic biopsies
There are many problems with the interpretation of the clinical and histological features of cancer of the prostate following irradiation. Unfortunately biopsies at present represent the only objective means of following the local response to treatment.

Several authors have reported on the post-irradiation biopsy as a means of predicting further evolution of the disease (Hill et al. 1974, Mollenkamp et al. 1975). A critical look at these reports indicates that any predictive value of such biopsies is uncertain. Most series are small and the cases not well staged, so that an interrelationship between local response to treatment and patient survival is indeed difficult to establish. In addition, the histo-

logical pattern of cancer of the prostate is not always geometrically uniform within the tumor (Franks et al. 1958, Starklint 1950), the response of the tumor to irradiation is variable within various parts of the tumor, the interpretation of the presence of residual nests of tumor cells is uncertain and so is the finding of changes in differentiation to a more anaplastic type, which some authors (Rhamy et al. 1972) have found alarming.

Recent studies (Cox and Stoffel 1977, Harisiadis et al. 1978, Kagan et al. 1977) have not shown any prognostic significance of a positive or negative biopsy even if taken a year or more following irradiation.

The 'reappearance' of tumor in a needle biopsy is a frequent finding (Kagan et al. 1977). Similarly, Cox and Stoffel (1977) found that 9 out of 38 patients had a positive biopsy after two or more negative biopsies, 7 of these being clinically free of disease. Does such 'reappearance' of tumor represent a new growth or a previous sampling error? It does indeed represent a clinical problem! These authors con-

Table 1. Biopsy following radiotherapy for carcinoma of the prostate.

Authors	Dose	Pos. Biopsy ≦ 1 year	Pos. Biopsy > 1 year
Grout et al. (1971)	5300-7200	9/9	16/28
Loh et al. (1971)	6500	—	4/14
Carlton et al (1972)	6000-7500	3/11	8/26
Rhamy et al. (1972)	6000-7000	9/11	13/17
Rodriguez-Antunez et al. (1973)	6000-7000	6/7	2/3
Cantril et al. (1974)	7000-7500	5/9	5/9
Hill et al. (1974)	6000	—	5/21
de Muelenaere et al. (1974)	5400-6000	—	17/38
Praetorius et al. (1974)	6000	7/9	3/8
Mollenkamp et al. (1975)	5500-7500	45/77	—
Cosgrove and Kaempt (1976)	5500-7500	—	5/10
Cox and Stoffel (1977)	7000	12/31	7/37
Kagan et al. (1977)	7000-7500	9/18	3/6
Harisiadis et al. (1978)	5000-7000	3/5	0/3
		108/187 (58%)	88/220 (40%)

cluded that for a given patient a negative random biopsy at any time means nothing.

With these uncertainties in mind it is indeed doubtful whether we gain any information from post-irradiation biopsies. Similarly, the significance of a positive or negative post-irradiation biopsy for the individual patient with cancer of the prostate or the prognostic value for a population of such patients is uncertain.

III. CONCLUSIONS

Random prostatic biopsies give a limited and often erroneous picture of the histology of the entire prostatic gland, since both benign prostatic hypertrophy and cancer of the prostate show a multiplicity of histological changes distributed unevenly throughout the prostate. Response to treatment varies in different parts of the prostate. Therefore, random prostatic biopsies in the follow-up of any specific treatment of these diseases are invalidated by sampling error. In addition, the significance of changes in serial biopsies for the individual patient and for a population of patients is uncertain. Justification at present of performing serial prostatic biopsies in the follow-up of treatment of benign or malignant prostatic diseases seems doubtful.

REFERENCES

Boxer RJ, Kaufman JJ, Goodwin WE: Radical prostatectomy for carcinoma of the prostate: 1951-1976. A review of 329 cases. J Urol 117: 208, 1977.

Byar DP, Mostofi FK: Carcinoma of the prostate: prognostic evaluation of certain pathological features in 208 radical prostatectomies. Examined by the stepsection technique. Cancer 30: 5, 1972.

Cantril ST, Vaeth JM, Green JP, Schroeder AF: Radiation therapy for localized carcinoma of the prostate. Correlation with histopathological grading. Front Radiation Ther Oncol 9: 274, 1974.

Carlton CE Jr, Hudgins PT, Guerriero WG, Scott R Jr: Radiotherapy in the management of stage C carcinoma of the prostate. J Urol 116: 206, 1976.

Cosgrove MD, Kaempf MJ: Prostatic cancer revisited. J Urol 115: 79, 1976.

Cox JD, Stoffel TJ: The significance of needle biopsy after irradiation for stage C adenocarcinoma of the prostate. Cancer 40: 156, 1977.

Culp OS: Radical perineal prostatectomy: its past, present and possible future. J Urol 98: 618, 1968.

Franks LM: Estrogen-treated prostatic cancer. The variation in responsiveness of tumor cells. Cancer 13: 490, 1960.

Franks LM, Ferguson JD, Murnaghan GF: An assessment of factors influencing survival in prostatic cancer – the absence of reliable prognostic features. Brit J Cancer 12: 321, 1958.

Gleason DF, Mellinger GT: The Veterans Administration Co-operative Urological Research Group: Prediction of prognosis for prostatic adenocarcinoma by combined histological grading and clinical staging. J Urol 111: 58, 1974.

Grout DC, Grayhack JT, Moss W Holland JM: Radiation therapy in the treatment of carcinoma of the prostate. J Urol 105: 411, 1971.

Harisiadis L, Veenema RJ, Senyszyn JJ, Puchner PJ, Tretter P,

Romas NA, Chang CH, Lattimer JK, Tannenbaum M: Carcinoma of the prostate. Treatment with external radiotherapy. Cancer 41: 2131, 1978.

Hill DR, Crews QE Jr, Walsh PC: Prostate carcinoma: Radiation treatment of the primary and regional lymphatics. Cancer 34: 156, 1974.

Huggins C, Stevens RA: The effect of castration on benign hypertrophy of the prostate in man. J Urol 43: 705, 1940.

Kagan AR, Gordon J, Cooper JF, Gilbert H, Nussbaum H, Chan P: A clinical appraisal of post-irradiation biopsy in prostatic cancer. Cancer 39: 637, 1977.

Loh ES, Brown HE, Beiler DD: Radiotherapy of carcinoma of the prostate. J Urol 106: 906, 1971.

Mollenkamp JS, Cooper JF, Kagan AR: Clinical experience with supervoltage radiotherapy in carcinoma of the prostate. A preliminary report. J Urol 113: 374, 1975.

de Muelenaere GFGO, Sandison AG, Coetzee FD: Radiotherapy in Prostaatkarsinoom. S Afr Med J 48: 321, 1974.

Perez CA, Bauer W, Garza P, Royce RK: Radiation therapy in the definitive treatment of localized carcinoma of the prostate. Cancer 40: 1425, 1977.

Pool TL, Thompson GJ: Conservative treatment of carcinoma of the prostate. JAMA 160: 833, 1956.

Praetorius M, Faul P, v Lieven H, Buttler R: Zur Strahlenbehandlung niederdifferenzierter Prostatakarzinome. Ein vorläufiger Bericht. Münch Med Wochenschr 116: 27, 1974.

Ray GR, Cassidy JR, Bagshaw MA: Definitive radiation therapy of carcinoma of the prostate. A report on 15 years of experience. Radiology 106: 407, 1973.

Rhamy RK, Wilson SK, Caldwell WL: Biopsyproved tumor following definitive irradiation of resectable carcinoma of the prostate. J Urol 107: 627, 1972.

Rodriguez-Antunez A, Cook SA, Jelden GL, Hunter TW, Straffon RA, Stewart BH: Management of primary and metastatic carcinoma of the prostate by the radiotherapist. Am J Roentgenol Radium Ther Nucl Med 111: 876, 1973.

Shelley HS, Auerbach SH, Classen KL, Marks CH, Wiederanders RE. Carcinoma of the prostate. A new system of classification. Arch Surg 77: 751, 1958.

Schenken JR, Burns EL, Kahle PJ: Effect of diethylstilbestrol and diethylstilbestrol dipropionate on carcinoma of prostate gland; II. cytologic changes following treatment. J Urol 48: 99, 1942.

Starklint H: Studies on latent and manifest cancer of the prostate (thesis). Copenhagen: E. Munksgaards Forlag, 1950.

Utz DC, Farrow GM: Pathological differentiation and prognosis of prostatic carcinoma. JAMA 209: 1701, 1969.

Vickery AL Jr, Kerr WS Jr: Cancer of the prostate treated by radical prostatectomy. A clinicopathological survey of 187 cases followed for 5 years and 148 cases followed for 10 years. Cancer 16: 1598, 1963.

Wolf H: The significance of histological changes in serial prostatic biopsy specimens. J Urol 113: 75, 1975.

Wolf H, Madsen PO: Treatment of benign prostatic hypertrophy with progestational agents. J Urol 99: 780, 1968.

11. BONE MARROW ACID PHOSPHATASE IN PROSTATE CANCER

N.A. ROMAS, R.J. VEENEMA and M. TANNENBAUM

Carcinoma of the prostate remains the most common malignancy of the genitourinary tract and constitutes the second leading cause of death from cancer in men fifty years old or more (Cancer statistics 1975). Earlier recognition of metastasis, with more accurate means of staging should improve the length and quality of survival. Therefore, the search by investigators for earlier staging in prostate carcinoma has led to the identification of tumor cells and recently, acid phosphatase determinations in bone marrow.

In 1935, Kutscher and Wolbergs reported elevated levels of acid phosphatase in the prostate. In 1938, Gutman and Gutman determined that elevated serum levels of this enzyme reflected metastatic prostate carcinoma. However, it is now known that up to 40% of patients with known metastasis may have normal serum acid phosphatase (London et al. 1954). The Gutmans also demonstrated increased acid phosphatse activity at the site of metastasis and believed that tumor cells produced acid phosphatase at the metastatic site similar to that of normal prostatic tissue. Based on this observation, much effort was placed on the direct identification of tumor cells in bone marrow aspirates and subsequently, the measurement of acid phosphatase.

Alyea and Rundles (1949) studied 32 cases of carcinoma of the prostate and found bone marrow metastasis in 18 cases. The sternum was the sight of metastasis in 15 cases, the ilium in 2, and the vertebral body in 1. Most of their patients demonstrated evidence of wide spread metastases. In 1952, Clifton and associates demonstrated that in random biopsies, carcinoma cells from the prostate could be found with equal frequency in the sternum and ilium. In 1963, Flocks found approximately 10% positive bone marrow cytology in prostatic carcinoma patients. Welch and McKenny (1964) studied 18 patients and found 38% with positive cytology of the bone marrow aspirates from the iliac crest. In 1966, Mehan and associates studied 49 patients with carcinoma of the prostate and found 22% with positive bone marrow cytology. In 1969, Chua and associates studied 70 patients who had documented cancer of the prostate by means of random bone marrow biopsies of the posterior iliac spine or selective biopsies of suspicious areas in the skeletal survey. Of these patients, 32 had radiographic findings diagnostic of bone metastasis. Nineteen of 32 patients had selective marrow biopsies of the involved bone and 13 patients had random biopsies of the posterior iliac spine. Eighteen of 19 selective biopsies confirmed the presence of bone marrow metastasis and one biopsy showed non-neoplastic osteosclerosis. Thirteen random biopsies in these 32 patients showed carcinoma cells in the bone marrow from 8 patients but 5 had falsely negative biopsy results. In selective bone marrow biopsies from 11 patients who had suspected metastatic areas in the bone, only two patients had documented metastasis. In 3 out of 27 patients, the only evidence of the extension of disease was by means of random vertebral bone marrow biopsy.

In reviewing 556 bone marrow aspirations performed on 449 patients within a ten year period, Nelson and associates (1973) found an overall 7.6% positive cytology. The authors concluded that the low yield of routine positive cytology made this technnique of questionable value in assessing patients with carcinoma of the prostate.

In 1970, Chua and associates were the first to indicate the potential value of measuring acid phosphatase in bone marrow. Since that initial report, there have been various methodologies employed to measure acid phosphatase in bone marrow. A controversy has arisen as to methodology and the meaning of acid phosphatase elevations in bone marrow.

Discussion of bone marrow acid phosphatase determinations will be subdivided into biochemical and immunological assays.

I. BIOCHEMICAL

While the activity of acid phosphatase has been described in high concentrations in the cells and the secretions of the prostate gland, acid phosphatase activity has a rather wide tissue distribution (Sodeman and Batsakis 1977). Activity is present in erythrocytes, platelets, leukocytes, liver, spleen, kidney and other tissues. Most of these tissues including the prostate gland contain two or more molecular variants. Bone marrow has many cells such as megakaryocytes and osteoclasts which are potential sources of acid phosphatase.

The biochemical methods do not measure acid phosphatase directly, but use substrates for the measurement. The substrates that have been used for the measurement of serum acid phosphatase activity have been beta-glycerophosphate or various phenolic or naphtholic phosphates. Methods using the former substrates measure the released inorganic phosphate. If aromatic substrates are used, the organic moiety is usually measured. Many substrates and various inhibitors have been utilized in order to achieve specificity for prostatic acid phosphatase but no know biochemical test has been universally accepted as measuring only acid phosphatase of prostatic origin (Yam 1974).

Chua and his associates reported the first measurements of bone marrow acid phosphatase using a modification of the Bodansky method with sodium betaglycerophosphate as a substrate. This substrate was chosen because Woodard (1959) felt that the acid phosphatase elaborated by bone was relatively inactive to this particular substrate. She had studied extracts of normal and abnormal bones and found that there was a minimal amount of acid phosphatase activity present when this substrate was utilized. She also reported that serum acid phosphatase activity was not elevated in patients with primary bone disease.

In the initial study, by Chua (1970), 12 patients

with benign prostatic hypertrophy were found to have levels that were normal in the serum and bone marrow fluid. Eight of 12 patients with clinically localized stages I and II carcinoma of the prostate also had normal serum and bone marrow acid phosphatase. In their group, four patients had elevated bone marrow acid phosphatase with normal serum acid phosphatase levels and their skeletal series were negative for metastasis. Three of these four patients had negative random biopsies but one patient had a positive biopsy. In patients with extensive disease, there was a high correlation of serum and bone marrow acid phosphatase. They concluded that the determination of bone marrow acid phosphatase is a simple and safe procedure which could be done in conjunction with bone marrow biopsy. It appears to be a better index of early bone metastasis than the serum acid phosphatase or routine skeletal survey since 40% of the bone must be involved before metastasis is visible radiographically (Bachman and Sproul 1955).

In 1974, Gursel and associates reported their comparative evaluation of bone marrow acid phosphatase and bone scanning in the staging of prostate cancer. They found 16 of 39 patients with carcinoma of the prostate who had negative bone scans and skeletal surveys but elevated bone marrow acid phosphatase. Nine of these 16 patients had normal serum acid phosphatase but, subsequently, two of these patients had high serum acid phosphatase values and died of metastasis. In the remaining seven patients who had elevated bone marrow acid phosphatase levels alone, repeated skeletal surveys were negative and the serum acid phosphatase remained normal. The possible reasons for the high bone marrow acid phosphatase levels in these patients were not discussed.

The prognostic value of bone marrow acid phosphatase in patients undergoing radical prostatectomies was reported by Veenema and associates in 1977. In all 31 patients studied, the modified Bodansky method utilizing beta-glycerophosphate as substrate was utilized. Eighteen of the 31 patients had pre-operatively elevated bone marrow acid phosphatase levels and 13 were normal. The serum acid phosphatase levels were normal in all 31 patients. Only one of 13 patients who had normal bone marrow acid phosphatase levels developed metastasis and may be considered a 'false negative'.

The microscopic sections of the prostate from this patient showed extra-prostatic extension and metastasis occurred within the first year. Six of the 18 patients who had elevated bone marrow acid phosphatase levels developed radiological evidence of metastasis within one to four years. In 3 of 7 patients in whom the histology sections did not detect microscopic extra-prostatic carcinoma invasion, metastasis appeared 3 to 4 years later and 1 of 3 patients died at 4 years. Thus only 4 of 7 patients can still be considered to have 'false positive' elevation of bone marrow acid phosphatase levels and will continue to be followed. Three of the 11 patients who had elevated bone marrow acid phosphatase and also microscopic findings of extra-prostatic extension of carcinoma had developed radiological evidence of metastasis in 1 to 4 years. In summary this clinical study indicated that there was a higher incidence of metastasis in patients who had elevated bone marrow acid phosphatase.

Bruce et al. in 1977 made a comprehensive study utilizing various methods in an attempt to stage 75 patients with histologically documented carcinoma of the prostate. They used serum and bone marrow acid phosphatase, bone scanning including bone tomography, lymphangiography, seminal vesiculography, pelvic lymphadenectomy and bone marrow cytology. They concluded that the estimation of bone marrow acid phosphatase appears to be the most sensitive test to detect blood-borne metastasis (Table 1). In their study of 75 patients, there were only seven who had elevated serum acid phosphatase as compared to 29 patients with an elevated bone marrow acid phosphatase and 17 patients with positive bone scans. They had 18 patients with elevated bone marrow acid phosphatase as the only

Table 1. Serum and bone marrow phosphatase estimations and technetium bone scans in 75 patients with primary prostatic adenocarcinoma.

	Normal	Abnormal
Serum acid phosphatase	68	7
Bone marrow acid phosphatase	46	29
^{99m}Tc Polyphosphate scan	58	17
Increase in bone marrow acid phosphatase, positive scan		11
Positive scan		6
Increase in bone marrow acid phosphatase		18

evidence of spread of disease and after one year, positive scans were obtained in 2 of these patients. In the early part of this study, they utilized alpha-naphthyl as the substrate for the measurement of serum and bone marrow acid phosphatase levels but in the later group of patients, they also used beta-glycerol in an effort to compare the accuracy of these two substrates. They reported close correlation between the two techniques.

In 30 patients who had undergone pelvic lymphadenectomies there were 11 patients with metastatic lymph nodes present. Eight patients had elevated bone marrow acid prosphatase. A close correlation was found between stage and grade of disease and the incidence of nodal pathology. There was some correlation between the degree of nodal involvement and evidence of blood spread as detected by bone marrow acid phosphatase levels.

Sadlowsky in 1978 studied early stage prostatic cancer by pelvic lymph node biopsy and bone marrow acid phosphatase. Patients with histologically proven stage B_1, B_2 or C adenocarcinoma of the prostate were entered into the study. Thymolphthalein (Roy method) as the substrate, was used to determine the bone marrow acid phosphatase. Thirteen patients (28%) had tumor in the pelvic lymph nodes. Using the Roy method, the bone marrow acid phosphatase was not elevated to more than the normal value for serum. Combined high grade and stage tumors seemed to demonstrate an increased incidence of pelvic lymph node metastasis. A surprisingly high incidence of B_1 lesions (5 of 21 patients or 24%) had positive lymph nodes. Generally, the nodes were moderately well- or well-differentiated lesions. The metastases were unilateral, frequently only microscopic and involved one or only a few nodes. He concluded that pelvic lymphadenectomy seems to have a well-defined role in the diagnostic study of early stage prostatic cancer, while bone marrow acid phosphatase determinations are of no value.

Klaber et al. in 1976 reported on the role of bone marrow acid phosphatase and lymphangiography in the evaluation of patients with carcinoma of the prostate. Thirty patients with carcinoma of the prostate underwent lymphangiography and bone marrow acid phosphatase as well as conventional staging studies prior to radical prostatectomy or radical irradiation. They concluded that bone marrow acid phosphatase may indicate regional extension not always demonstrated by lymphangiography.

Although the above reports have been favorable, some reservation about the value of this procedure has been expressed by various investigators who found a large number of falsely positive results in patients without prostatic disease. The main problem is that it is difficult to accept the value of a single chemical determination as evidence of metastatic disease with the absence of histological proof. This is compounded by the knowledge that the acid phosphatase determinations used in most hospitals are not specific for prostatic acid phosphatase.

Kahn and associates in 1977 reported the measurement of bone marrow acid phosphatase using a substrate of sodium alpha-naphthyl phosphate in 25 patients with biopsy-proven adenocarcinoma of the prostate and 90 patients without clinical evidence of prostatic malignancy who underwent marrow acid phosphatase as part of their bone marrow examination. Approximately 20% of the control patients were female subjects. Of the 90 control patients who had no clinical evidence of prostatic malignancy 22 (24%) had elevations of bone marrow acid phosphatase. Six of these patients also had elevated serum acid phosphatase. Commonly found conditions in these patients were acute and chronic leukemias, lymphomas and various anemias. Of the 25 patients in their study with histologically proven prostatic malignancy, 18 had elevations of bone marrow acid phosphatase, while only 11 patients had elevated serum acid phosphatase. Also falsely negative results were seen in three patients with clinical evidence of skeletal metastasis by means of positive bone scans. The control patients in this study with elevated bone marrow acid phosphatase and no clinical evidence of malignancy, suggest that falsely positive results may be common with primary hematological disease. Therefore, bone marrow acid phosphatase should never be performed without a complete microscopical analysis of the bone marrow in order to rule out hematological disorders.

In 1977, Diaz and Barnett studied bone marrow acid phosphatase values in 24 patients (12 men and 12 women) who were selected at random, including 6 at autopsy. The acid phosphatase level was determined using the Bessey-Lowry technique with p-nitrophenyl phosphate as a substrate. False positive results were noted in 8 of the 18 patients who were alive and all 6 patients studied at autopsy. They concluded that bone marrow acid phosphatase is a test of poor specificity and should not be used as the sole test on which vital decisions regarding management of patients are to be based.

In 1978 Boehm et al. measured bone marrow acid and alkaline phosphatase, lactic dehydrogenase, and calcium in a group of 84 patients with a variety of problems, including 18 with cancer of the prostate. The methods used for determining acid phosphatase included the alpha-naphthyl phosphate (Babson), p-nitrophenyl phosphate (Bessey-Lowry) and thymolphtalein monophosphate (Roy method). Bone marrow aspirates, were collected by one of two methods. For 'fast' aspiration the plunger of a 60 cc disposable syringe was rapidly withdrawn to the 55-60 cc mark and held there until about 10 cc of aspirate was obtained. For a 'slow' aspirate, the plunger was gently withdrawn so that at no time was there more than 5cc above the level of the aspirate entering the syringe. They found that the bone marrow acid and alkaline phosphatase and lactic dehydrogenase were elevated and calcium was depressed in most patients. Among patients with prostate cancer, bone marrow acid phosphatase was not significantly different between those with or without bone metastasis. In addition, the patients with metastatic cancer did not have higher levels of bone marrow acid phosphatase than the subjects with other malignant and non-malignant diseases.

In comparing results of 'fast versus 'slow' samples, a marked difference appeared. In 23 of 24 samples, the value for bone marrow acid phosphatase on the 'fast' sample was greater or equal to that of the 'slow' sample. In every case, the 'fast' value was greater than that of the simultaneous serum value. The levels of acid and alkaline phosphatase, lactic dehydrogenase, and calcium were independent of sex, disease state or method of chemical determination. Due to this variation, they concluded that bone marrow enzyme and calcium levels were of no value in the detection of metastasis in patients with prostate cancer.

II. IMMUNOLOGICAL DETECTION OF PROSTATIC ACID PHOSPHATASE

In 1960, prostate-specific antigens in dogs were suggested by the in vivo studies of Flocks et al. In 1964, Shulman et al. demonstrated antibodies which reacted with human prostatic acid phosphatase. Subsequent studies by Moncure and Prout (1970) and Ablin (1973) attested to the apparent antigenic specificity of prostatic acid phosphatase. The practical application of an immunological assay was first demonstrated by Milisauskas and Rose (1972). Subsequently a radioimmunoassay and a counterimmunoelectrophoretic method were developed for the specific determination of prostatic acid phosphatase (Choe et al. 1977, Foti et al. 1977, Chu et al. 1978, Romas et al. 1978). Romas et al. (1979) have recently reported on an extensive review on this subject. The determination of bone marrow acid phosphatase by the use of these methods has revived an interest for correlative staging of prostate cancer.

III. GEL IMMUNODIFFUSION

In 1972, Moncure et al. employed radial immunodiffusion to compare prostatic acid phosphatase levels in serum and bone marrow. In their experience, levels of prostatic acid phosphatase in a patient's marrow which were greater than concurrent serum levels, indicate stage IV disease and usually correlate with a demonstration of tumor cells in the marrow. In only one female patient with chronic myelogenous leukemia was there a questionable positive bone marrow reaction.

This same group of investigators in 1978 emphasized the importance of immunological testing (radial immunodiffusion) as a procedure for staging prostate carcinoma (Drucker et al. 1978). When the bone surveys were negative, the immunodiffusion was positive in 45% of the patients studied. In this same group of patients, the serum acid phosphatase was elevated in 18% and bone marrow aspirates were positive in 16%. In those patients with negative isotope scans, 16% were positive by the radial immunodiffusion method for detecting prostatic acid phosphatase. Thus, it would appear that immunodiffusion may be a more accurate means of identifying metastatic disease than bone surveys or isotope scans.

IV. RADIOIMMUNOASSAY (RIA) AND COUNTER-IMMUNOELECTROPHORESIS (CIEP)

Pontes et al. in 1978 analyzed 50 bone marrow samples collected at random from the hematology service at his hospital. The samples were measured for acid phosphatase content by a colorimetic method using sodium thymolphthalein monophosphate as a substrate and by two immunochemical assay methods developed at their laboratory (CIEP and RIA.) They found a high percentage (61%) of falsely positive results in patients with various hematological diseases without evidence of prostatic carcinoma by the colorimetric evaluation. All of these patients except one had negative immunochemical determinations. Until a specific prostatic acid phosphatase assay is developed for clinical use, caution should be excercised against the use of a single chemical determination of bone marrow acid phosphatase as a parameter of metastatic disease. This same group of investigators studied a small group of patients; 20 men with known carcinoma and 20 men of comparable age without clinical evidence of prostatic cancer with the three methods enumerated above. Again, the large percentage of falsely positive results obtained by the colorimetic determination invalidates this method as the sole parameter for metastatic prostate carcinoma.

Belville et al. (1978) utilized a double-antibody RIA to measure prostatic acid phosphatase in bone marrow aspirates. An upper limit of 12.0 ng/ml of prostatic acid phosphatase in the bone marrow of patients with benign prostatic hypertrophy was chosen. Eighty percent of the patients with proven stage D_2 disease had levels above 12.0 ng/ml. In stages C and D, the elevated values were 18% and 25% respectively. In stages A and B, only one value exceeded this upper limit. Their experience with use of an enzymatic method showed a poor correlation with the presence or absence of metastatic adenocarcinoma.

A limited clinical study by Cooper et al. (1978) on the use of RIA for bone marrow acid phosphatase indicated that it was technically superior to the p-nitrophenyl phosphate enzymatic method in bone marrow and serum samples.

Since 1975, our group has utilized a counter-immunoelectrophoretic assay for the specific determination of prostatic acid phosphatase (Romas et al. 1978). The measurement of simultaneously obtained bone marrow and serum acid phosphatase in 72 patients who had various stages of prostate cancer and 13 patients who did not have prostate cancer were compared by the CIEP assay and a standard biochemical method (sodium thymolphthalein) (Romas et al. 1980).

The biochemical test of the bone marrow gave 65% false positive results overall which makes it of no value in measuring bone marrow acid phosphatase. The CIEP used to detect bone marrow metastasis showed a 13% false positive rate overall, but only 4.4% false positive if the CIEP test was considered positive above 1 international unit per liter. The percentage accuracy (Stage C Neg.; Stage D pos.) was 62.5% for the Roy Method and 89.6% for the CIEP (Table 2).

The study also elaborated on other factors such as temperature and pH which could effect acid phosphatase determinations. It has been reported that there can be a 50% reduction in the enzyme level in 1 hour during warm weather (Woodard 1952). This finding has been confirmed with CIEP. Transportation of the specimen in an ice filled beaker, or any other temperature controlled device in warm weather should therefore reduce the number of false negatives.

When serum is separated from the clot and kept at room temperature (25°C), enzyme activity decreases considerably within one to two hours owing to the increase in pH as a result of the loss of carbon dioxide. This increase in pH, which may go from 7.6 to 8.5 in several hours, may be slowed by storing ther serum in tightly *stoppered containers*. Preliminary results with CIEP indicate that blood collected in a tightly stoppered container at room temperature will not show any appreciable change in acid phosphatase activity up to 4 hours (unpublished data).

The trauma that occurs incidental to bone aspiration carries with it the possibility for releasing many non-prostatic acid phosphatase enzymes present in bone marrow. In the literature, the lack of substrate specifity in measuring bone marrow acid phosphatase has led to conflicting reports regarding the value of bone marrow acid phosphatase determination for the detection of prostate acid phosphatase in bone metastases. Based on our early experience using beta-glycerophosphate and our present observations using thymolphthalein, we find the beta-glycerophosphate substrate method to be suited if bone marrow acid phosphatase is to be measured by biochemical tests, but immunological methods, such as CIEP are much perferred.

V. FUTURE DEVELOPMENTS

As noted in this review, the immunological methods were felt to be potentially the best methods suited for measuring bone marrow acid phosphatase. Such questions as what antigen should be employed for the production of prostatic acid phosphatase antibody has not been clearly defined. As the source of acid phosphatase investigators have used seminal fluid, benign prostatic hypertrophic tissue, and prostate cancer tissue. A standardized, simplified immunological method for routine hospital use has not been developed. Studies are also necessary on the diffusion of acid phosphatase between the bone marrow and the circulatory system.

Table 2. Bone marrow acid phosphatase (BMAP) in 24 stage C and in 24 stage D prostate cancers.

BMAP results	Roy method	CIEP
% error (stage C pos; stage D neg)	18/48 (37.5%)	5/48 (10.4%)
% detection of metas. (pos. in both stages C & D)	42/48 (87.5%)	27/48 (56.3%)
% accuracy (stage C neg; stage D pos)	30/48 (62.5%)	43/48 (89.6%)

REFERENCES

Albin RJ: Immunochemical identification of prostatic tissue-specific acid phosphatase. Clin Chem 19: 786, 1973.
Alyea EP, Rundles RW: Bone marrow studies in carcinoma of the prostate. J Urol 62: 332, 1949.

Bachman AL, Sproul EE: Correlation of radiographic and autopsy findings in suspected metastases in the spine. Bull NY Acad Med 31: 146, 1955.
Belville WD et al: Bone marrow acid phosphatase by radio-immunoassay. Cancer 41: 2286, 1978.
Boehme UM et al.: Lack of usefulness of bone marrow enzymes

130

and calcium in staging patients with prostatic cancer. Cancer 41: 1433, 1978.

Bruce AW et al: Carcinoma of the prostate: a critical look at staging. J Urol 117: 319, 1977.

Cancer Statistics, 1975. Ca 25: 2, 1975.

Choe BK et al: Immunochemical studies of prostatic acid phosphatase. Cancer Treat Rep 61: 2, 1977.

Chua DT et al: Bone marrow biopsy in patients with carcinoma of the prostate. J Urol 102: 602, 1969.

Chua DT et al: Acid phosphatase levels in bone marrow: value in detecting early bone metastasis from carcinoma of the prostate. J Urol 103: 462, 1970.

Chu TM et al: Immunochemical detection of serum prostatic acid phosphatase. Invest Urol 15: 319, 1978.

Clifton JA et al: Bone marrow and carcinoma of the prostate. Amer J Med Sci 224: 121, 1952.

Cooper JF et al: Radioimmunochemical measurement of bone marrow prostatic acid phosphatase. J Urol 119: 392, 1978.

Dias SM, Barnett RN: Elevated bone marrow acid phosphatase: problems of false positives. J Urol 117: 749, 1977.

Drucker JR et al: Immunologic staging of prostatic carcinoma: three years of experience. J Urol 119: 94, 1978.

Flocks RH et al: Studies on the antigenic properties of prostatic tissue. I. J Urol 84: 134, 1960.

Flocks RH: Combination therapy for localized prostatic cancer. J Urol 89: 889, 1963.

Foti AG et al: Detection of prostatic cancer by solidphase radioimmunoassay of serum prostatic acid phosphatase. N Engl J Med 297: 1357, 1977.

Gursel EO et al: Comparative evaluation of bone marrow acid phosphatase and bone scanning in staging of prostatic cancer. J Urol 111: 53, 1974.

Gutman EB, Sproul EE, Gutman AB: Significance of increased phosphatase activity of bone at the site of osteoblastic metastasis secondary to carcinoma of the prostate gland. Amer J Cancer 28: 485, 1936.

Gutman AB, Gutman EB: An 'acid' phosphatase occurring in the serum of patients with metastasizing carcinoma of the prostate gland. J Clin Invest 17: 473, 1938.

Kabler R et al: Bone marrow acid phosphatase and lymphangiography in the evaluation of patients with carcinoma of the prostate. Presented at annual meeting of American Urological Association, Las Vegas, Nevada. May 18, 1976.

Khan R et al: Bone marrow acid phosphatase: another look. J Urol 117: 79, 1977.

Kutscher W, Wolbergs H: Prostataphosphatase. Z Physiol Chem 236: 237, 1935.

London M, McHugh R, Hudson PB: On low acid phosphatase values of patients with known metastatic cancer of prostate. Cancer Res 14:718, 1954.

Mehan DJ et al: Bone marrow findings in carcinoma of the prostate. J Urol 95: 241, 1966.

Milisauskas V, Rose NR: Immunochemical quantitation of prostatic phosphatase. Clin Chem 18: 1529, 1972.

Moncure CW, Prout GR Jr: Antigenicity of human prostatic acid phosphatase. Cancer 25: 463, 1970.

Moncure CW et al: Immunological and histochemical evaluation of marrow aspirates in patients with prostatic carcinoma. J Urol 108: 609, 1972.

Nelson CMK et al: Bone marrow examination in carcinoma of the prostate. J Urol 109: 667, 1973.

Pontes JE et al: Bone marrow acid phosphatase in staging of prostatic cancer: how reliable is it? J Urol 119: 772, 1978.

Romas NA et al: Counterimmunoelectrophoresis for detection of human prostatic acid phosphatase. Urol 1279-83, 1978.

Romas NA, Rose NR, Tannenbaum M: Acid phosphatase: new Developments. Human Pathology 10: 501-512, 1979.

Romas NA et al: Bone marrow acid phosphatase in prostate cancer: an assessment by immunoassay and biochemical methods. J Urol 123: 392, 1980.

Sadlowski RW: Early stage prostatic cancer investigated by pelvic lymph node biopsy and bone marrow acid phosphatase. J Urol 119: 89, 1978.

Shulman S et al: The detection of prostatic acid phosphatase by antibody reactions in gel diffusion. J Immunol 93: 474, 1964.

Sodeman TM, Batsakis JG: Acid phosphatase. In: Urologic pathology: the prostate, Tannenbaum M ed. Philadelphia: Lea and Febiger, 1977, p 129.

Veenema RJ et al: Bone marrow acid phosphatase: Prognostic value in patients undergoing radical prostatectomy. J Urol 117: 81, 1977.

Woodard HQ: Factors leading to elevation of serum acid glycerphosphatase. Cancer 5: 236, 1952.

Woodard HQ: The clinical significance of serum acid phosphatase. Amer J Med 27: 902, 1959.

Welsh JF, Mackinney CC: Experiences with aspiration biopsies of the bone marrow in the diagnosis and prognosis of carcinoma of the prostate gland. Amer J Clin Path 41: 509, 1964.

Yam LT: Clinical significance of the human acid phosphatase. Amer J Med 56: 605, 1974.

12. RADIOIMMUNOASSAY FOR HUMAN PROSTATIC ACID PHOSPHATASE

B.K. CHOE, N.R. ROSE, and E.J. PONTES

I. INTRODUCTION

A. Serum acid phosphatases

Acid phosphatases (EC 3.1.3.2.) are a group of enzymes which hydrolyze various esters of ortho-phosphoric acid at pH optimum of 4.8 to 6.0. The enzyme was first identified in human erythrocytes by Martland and co-worker in 1924. However, it was the pioneering reports of Gutman and his co-workers that opened a new era of serum acid phosphatase in clinical medicine. Since the first demonstration of elevation of serum acid phosphatase in advanced prostatic cancer by Gutman and his associates, measurement of this enzyme has been employed as a biochemical aid to diagnosis of prostatic cancer. Furthermore, since Huggins and Hodges in 1941 demonstrated the effect of steroid hormones on prostatic cancer and its correlation to serum phosphatase levels, serum acid phosphatase assay has been adopted as an indicator in surgical and hormonal therapy of prostatic cancer (Batsakis et al. 1970, Bodanski 1972, Sodeman and Batsakis 1977, Townsend 1977, Yam 1974).

Serum acid phosphatase is a representation of enzymes from various tissue cells through tissue injuries and cell renewals. Therefore, the elevation of serum acid phosphatase level is not limited in prostatic disorders but also has been noted in many non-prostatic diseases. Many attempts have been made in the past to devise a specific substrate or inhibitor for the determination of acid phosphatase of prostatic origin in the hope of correlating this enzyme level with the progression of prostatic cancer, yet satisfactory specific substrates are not yet introduced (Helms et al. 1977. Townsend 1977). Numerous reports have shown an increased incidence of elevated serum acid phosphatase levels in patients with advanced prostatic cancer.

Considerable controversy exists, however, concerning the significance of spectrophotometric assay of acid phosphatase for the early stages of prostatic carcinoma (Murphy et al. 1978, Sodeman and Batsakis 1977, Townsend 1977). Therefore, a new method has been sought in recent years which is specific for the prostatic acid phosphatase in face of the bulk of other acid phosphatases in sera. Antigenic specificity of prostatic acid phosphatase has been first demonstrated by Shulman et al. (1964) and its possible clinical application was reported by Milisauskas and Rose (1972). Since then a few immunological assay methods have been proposed for prostatic acid phosphatase in recent years and commercial assay kits have become available.

The purposes of this chapter are: 1) to outline the radioimmunoassays for prostatic acid phosphatase (RIA-PAP) and 2) to evaluate the performance of RIA-PAP in given clinical situations.

B. Prostatic acid phosphatase

Recent rapid development of immunoassay methods of prostatic acid phosphatase (PAP) owes its origin not only to the antigenic study of Shulman et al. (1964), but also to the efforts of characterization of this enzyme by Ostrowski and his co-workers (Derechin et al. 1971). Earlier attemps at purification of PAP have been reviewed by Bodansky (1972) and the procedure that has been adopted by most investigators was reported by Ostrowski et al. (1970). Their method employed an initial treatment of prostatic homogenate with Tween 80 and recovery of the extracts by centrifugation. The extracts were further fractionated by $(NH_4)_2SO_4$ at pH 4.0. The enzyme fraction was subsequently chromatographed on DEAE-cellulose and filtered through Sephadex G-100 columns. The homogeneity of the purified enzyme was examined by rechromatographic procedures, polyacrylamide gel electrophoresis, and specific enzyme activity. For the development of immunological assay methods, we have modified their purification method in two aspects: the affinity chromatography step and immunochemical examination of the purified preparations. Human ejaculate was fractionated by the $(NH_4)_2SO_4$ precipitation method and the resulting enzyme fraction was chromatographed on CM-Sephadex and subsequently on concanavalin A column. The enzyme thus purified exhibited high specific activity, and homogeneity by chemical and immunological criteria (Choe et al. 1978a).

Recently, Vihko et al. (1978a) and Van Etten and Saini (1978) described a rapid and specific purification method by the use of a tartrate-affinity column. When such a specific affinity column matrix becomes available commercially, the task of PAP purification will be greatly simplified.

The PAP is a glycoprotein of molecular weight approximately 100,000 with varying amounts of carbohydrate (Derechin et al. 1971). This heterogeneity in carbohydrate content, particularly neuraminic acid residues, gives rise to several discrete electrophoretic isozymic forms in this enzyme (Ostrowski et al. 1970). The PAP exhibit a single homogenous band in SDS-polyacrylamide gel electrophoresis, or SDS-8Murea polyacrylamide gel electrophoresis which gives the estimated molecular weight of 48,000 to 50,000. Tryptic peptide mapping and other evidences suggested that the PAP consists of indistinguishable subunits of 50,000 (Luchter-Wasyl and Ostrowski 1974).

PAP does not show antigenic cross-reactivity among acid phosphatases of other tissue origins (Choe et al. 1978b, Choe et al. 1978c). The antigenic specificity of PAP seems to reside in the protein portion of the molecule rather than in the neuraminic acid residues. Therefore, electrophoretic isozymic forms of PAP are antigenically indistinguishable. To date, anti-PAP antisera prepared against prostatic acid phosphatase derived from prostatic fluid, prostatic extracts, or seminal plasma in different laboratories have been immunochemically indistinguishable. The term 'prostatic acid phosphatase' (PAP) is defined here by the antigenic specificity of this enzyme.

II. RADIOIMMUNOASSAY OF PROSTATIC ACID PHOSPHATASE

A. Immunological assay

Several immunological assays of prostatic acid phosphatase have been developed in recent years in an effort to measure a small increment of acid phosphatase of prostatic origin in sera. These methods are based either on competitive binding radioimmunoassay (RIA) or on immunologic enzyme assay (Table 1). A double antibody RIA for PAP was introduced first by Cooper and Foti (1974) as a clinically useful immunoassay. Later, they developed a solid-phase RIA for PAP (Foti et al. 1975). However, the double antibody method gained greater popularity among other investigators (Table 1). Two commercial radioimmunoassay kits (New England Nuclear, North Billerica, MA and Mallinckrodt, St. Louis, MO) for PAP are based on a double antibody method.

Another immunologic enzyme assay of PAP, counterimmunoelectrophoresis, is semi-quantitative, whereas solid-phase fluorescent immunoassay and immunoenzyme assay are quantitative methods. These immunologic enzyme assays are equally

Table 1. Clinical immunoassays for human prostatic acid phosphatase.

Method	Range of normal value mg/ml	Reference
(A) Competitive binding radioimmunoassay		
Solid-phase RIA	1-8	Foti et al. 1975
Double antibody RIA	1-8	Cooper and Foti 1974 Choe et al. 1978a Vihko et al. 1978b Belville et al. 1978 Mahn and Doctor 1979
(B) Immunologic enzyme assay		
Counterimmunoelectrophoresis	20	Chu et al. 1978 McDonald et al. 1978 Romas et al. 1978 Foti et al. 1978
Solid phase fluorescent immunoassay	0.5-8	Lee et al. 1978
Immunoenzyme assay	1-8	Choe et al. 1979

sensitive or even superior to RIA methods in their performances. However, clinical application of the RIA has been broader and it is now possible to evaluate its performance in the light of clinical context, whereas other immunoassays are still at investigative stages. Extensive reviews of theory and techniques of radioimmunoassay for diverse systems have been published (Berson and Yalow 1973, Ekins et al. 1968, Haber and Poulsen 1974, Hunter 1973, Jaffe and Behrman 1974).

B. Antigen requirements

The PAP used for immunization and as the standard should be as pure as possible. The criteria of purity are molecular weight, specific enzyme activity and the absence of degradation products or other unrelated protein contaminants. Some of the physicochemical properties of homogeneous PAP are listed in Table 2. Highly purified PAP is stable under many different storage conditions, e.g., lyophilization, freezing, and refrigeration at pH 5.0-8.0. Protein concentration of purified PAP can be determined by absorbance measurement at 280 nm, assuming $E_{1\,cm}^{1\%} = 14.4$ (Derechin et al. 1971). In RIA, antigenic identity of radioactively labeled antigen to the unlabeled standard antigen is a prerequisite. The radioactive labeling procedure should not alter the antigen to any detectable extent. Detailed discussions of labeling procedures and assessment of properties of labeled antigen is available elsewhere (Chervu and Murty 1975, Hunter 1973). For the ^{125}I-labeling of pap, both chloramine-T method (Hunter 1973) and the lactoperoxidase method (Thorell and Johnson 1971) seem equally suitable. For PAP, the cloramine-T method has been quite convenient and reliable; for oxidizing conditions and for the short incubation period, we found 4 to 5 ug chloramine-T per ug of PAP and 45 to 90 seconds of reaction period satisfactory. If we assume a modest 25 to 40% ^{125}I incorporation and Poisson statistics for the collision between ^{125}I atoms and PAP molecules, 1 mCi of ^{125}I for 5 ug PAP seems to yield 1 atom of iodine per molecule of protein. Also, a high specific activity ^{125}I-PAP preparation with good antigenicity has been obtained using 5 ug PAP and up to 4 mCi of ^{125}I. The specific radioactivities of such

Table 2. Some properties of human prostatic acid phosphatase.

Physical	
Molecular weight	102,000 at pH 7.0[a]
Sedimentation coefficient (S20,W)	5.62[a]
Isoelectric points	4.05 – 5.2[b]
Extinction coefficient, $E_{1\,cm}^{1\%}$ at 280 mm	14.4[a]
Mobility on agar electrophoresis	β mobility, pH 8.6[a]
Subunit	50,000[c]
Chemical	
Total amino acid residues	764[a]
N-Acetylneuraminic acid residues	6
Carbohydrate content	12.8%[a]
pH optimum	4.8 – 6.0[e]
Specific enzyme activity (u/mg protein)	500 – 600[e]
Immunochemical	
Antigenicity of polypeptides residues	unique, multiple determinants[d]
Antigenicity of carbohydrate residues	not demonstrated[d]
Materials cross-reacting with PAP	not clearly established yet[d]

[a] Derechin et al. (1971).
[b] Ostrowski et al. (1970).
[c] Luchter-Wasyl and Ostrowski (1974).
[d] Choe et al. (1978 a, b).
[e] Van Etten and Saini (1978).

preparations ranged between 22 uCi to 360 uCi per ug PAP. The stability of such ^{125}I-PAP preparations are approximately 2 months when stored as a solution or lyophilized. An example of typical labeling protocol is diagrammed in Figure 1.

For the activity assay of serum acid phosphatases, it has been said that the pH and temperature at storage is crucial; therefore, it has been recommended to use fresh plasma specimen buffered with citrate to a pH of 6.2 to 6.6 (Sodeman and Batsakis 1977). For the immunologic assays such as counterimmunoelectrophoresis, immunoenzyme assay, and solid phase fluorometric assay, the same recommendations may apply. However, RIA specimens are not influenced by factors such as inactivation and an unpredictable contribution of enzyme for platelets during clotting. An appropriate sample for RIA is fresh plasma or serum.

C. Antibody requirements

The techniques for immunization to obtain a high affinity for antibodies at high concentration are empirical. Generally, relatively small amounts of antigen (100 to 500 μg) with complete Freund's adjuvant have been used. Usually 40 days after the primary inoculation, animals are boosted with the same amounts of PAP with incomplete Freund's adjuvant weekly for three times. Since individual antisera vary widely in their affinity and in their heterogeneity, each batch of antisera should be investigated individually. The binding constant of the antibody is the most important factor in choosing among the different batches of antisera for RIA. One method of estimation of the average binding constant for RIA was introduced by Berson and Yalow (1973) using the Scatchard plot (1949). Aliquots of a constant antiserum dilution are saturated with increasing amounts of antigen. The bound-to-free ratio (R) is obtained and plotted against the concentrations of bound antigen. If the

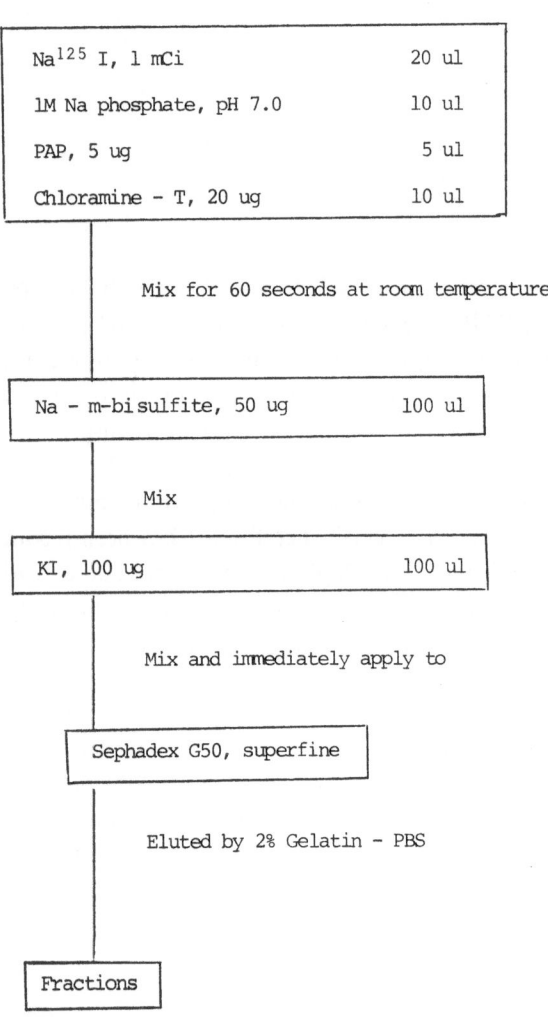

Mix for 60 seconds at room temperature

Na - m-bisulfite, 50 ug   100 ul

Mix

KI, 100 ug   100 ul

Mix and immediately apply to

Sephadex G50, superfine

Eluted by 2% Gelatin - PBS

Fractions

5 ul,   count radioactivity and assay for acid phospatase activity.

Figure 1. Radioiodination of human prostatic acid phosphatase by chloramine-T method.

antigen-combining sites of antibodies possess identical affinity to antigen, the plot is linear, and the slope equal to -K. The intercept of the graph with x-axis gives an estimation of the concentration of antigen binding sites of antibodies. An example of the estimation of average affinity constant of an anti-PAP antiserum is shown in Figure 2. The Scatchard plot of Figure 2 is not a straight line, but appears to be a graph of several components which is indicative of the inhomogeneity of antibody population.

The lowest concentration of PAP measurable by the RIA is limited by the affinity of anti-PAP antibodies. This can be seen from the basic immunochemical relationship, $\alpha = \dfrac{Kc}{Kc + 1}$, which was presented by Karush (1970), where α is the fraction of antigen reacted when c is the free equilibrium concentration of specific antibody and K is the affinity constant. For example, if anti-PAP antiserum with $K = 5 \times 10^8$ M^{-1} and the specific antibody concentration of approximately 300 $\mu g/ml$ (the IgG concentration approximately $2 \times 10^{-6}M$) is available, at 10,000-fold dilution of this antiserum a maximum of only 20% of PAP can be bound. As the basic immunochemical relationship dictates, the concentrations of free and bound PAP have to be the same order of magnitude or lower than antibody concentration. Then concentration of bound PAP will be the range of $10^{-10}M$, which is approximately 10 ng per ml or lower. Making a higher dilution of antiserum, the PAP concentrations lower than 1 ng per ml could be measured. However, the binding will become statistically very unreliable at this dilution. Through extensive mathematical analysis of the equilibrium reaction between ligand and binder, Ekins and his collaborators showed that the antibody concentration should be approximately 3/K and the concentration of the labelled antigen approximately 4/K (1968). Regardless of the value of K, with these concentrations of reactants, B/F will be 50%. These are the conditions for which Ekins has shown maximum sensitivity when the slope of the dose response curve as well as the precision of the experimental determination of B/F is taken into account for defining sensitivity. However, since the PAP is a high molecular weight protein, the use of concentration range $10^{-9}M$ (100 ng/ml) is imprac-

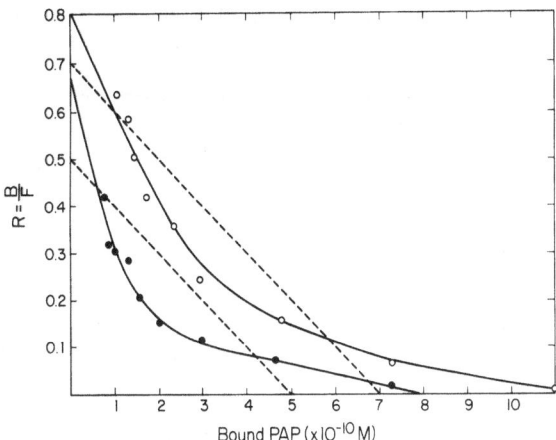

Figure 2. Scatchard plot for radioimmunoassay of human prostatic acid phosphatase. Because of the heterogeneity of antibody population the plot does not give a straight line. The calculated average slope (– – – – –), −1.0, indicate the average affinity constant K of this antiserum to be 10^9 liter/mol. Curves a) and b) represent the different antiserum dilutions used in these experiments.

tically high for RIA. As a rule of thumb, the lowest antibody concentration that will bind a measurable fraction of antigen has been used by most investigators for maximal sensitivity. The antigen concentrations measured under these conditions are 10^{-10} to 10^{-11}M (10 to 1 ng/ml). However, assays run under these conditions suffer from poor precision, a point Yalow and Berson (1973) emphasized.

D. Evaluation of the assay procedure

The rationale of RIA is to establish a stoichiometric relationship between the anti-PAP antibody and the ^{125}I-labeled PAP in the presence of various concentrations of unlabeled PAP to obtain a standard curve. The extent to which the unknown competes for anti-PAP antibody is compared with the standard curve, and the concentration of the PAP in the unknown sample is read from the curve. If the competition between labeled and unlabeled antigen is allowed to occur simultaneously until a mass equilibrium is reached between the antigen and the antibody, the technique is called as equilibrium saturation. It is possible, however, to accomplish the saturation of the antibody in two successive steps, first with the unlabeled and second with the labeled. This technique is referred to as sequential saturation or as nonequilibrium analysis. Thus far, equilibrium type RIA have been developed for PAP-RIA by many workers (Zettner 1973). Se-

quential saturation, however, can be applied where sensitivity is poor or to a system where affinities of labeled and unlabeled antigens are different (Rothenberg et al. 1972, Zettner and Duly 1974). Another crucial factor of successful radioimmunoassay is the separation of bound and free antigen. Since we are dealing with an equilibrium situation that can shift, the separation step should be as short as possible and almost identical for all samples being compared. In terms of separation of bound and free antigen, the solid-phase RIA of Foti and Cooper (1975) would be ideal. However, a double-antibody RIA is also reliable as long as the second antibody step is short and effective, and the temperature is kept low, since the equilibrium of antigen-antibody reaction is a direct function of temperature. In order to achieve effective separation of bound from free antigen in second antibody RIA, it is very important to use the proper dilutions of second antibody and carrier protein. The incubation times needed to establish equilibrium are inversely related to the concentration of reactants; the higher the concentrations, the shorther the incubation times. Therefore, to shorten the second antibody incubation stage, high concentrations of second antibody and carrier protein can be used. A double antibody RIA has, occasionally, another complex problem; i.e., an interference of human plasma in the precipitation of immune complexes during second-stage incubation. This interference particularly introduces errors in the estimation of very low concentrations of antigen. Morgan, Sorenson and Lazarow (1964) and Sheldon and Taylor (1965) have reported a variable reduction in efficiency of precipitation, possible due to the presence of complement in samples and easily prevented by the inclusion of EDTA in the diluent.

We have observed that certain plasma specimens increased the efficiency of precipitation in the immune complex separation step. This results in falsely high levels of 'antibody bound' (precipitated) radio-activity and, in extreme cases, a level of precipitated radioactivity that was higher in specimen tubes than in tubes containing the '0' standard, leading to apparently negative assay results. Buckler (1971) and Court and Hurn (1971) reported a similar type of complication of the double antibody RIA systems, and they obtained satisfactory results by the inclusion of PVP at the

136

final concentration of about 4%. However, ETDA and PVP do not seem to affect the PAP-RIA in any way. If this type of problem persists, batch of anti-PAP sera that do not cause this interference should be sought.

One of the typical double antibody RIA protocol is diagrammed in Figure 3 (also see Figure 6). Anti-PAP antibody can be diluted to cover wide concentration ranges of standard PAP (Figure 4). Since the estimation of very low concentrations (e.g., 2 to 6 ng/ml) of PAP with a high dilution of anti-PAP antiserum is statistically rather unreliable, a sequential saturation technique can be applied for this range of PAP concentrations (Figures 5 and 6).

The lowest PAP concentration detectable by the RIA method seems to be 4-5 ng/ml. This detection limit will not be lowered, unless one can produce an exceptionally high affinity antibody (e.g., 10^{10}

M^{-1}.) Clinically significant PAP concentrations are higher than 8 ng/ml (Tables 1 and 3).

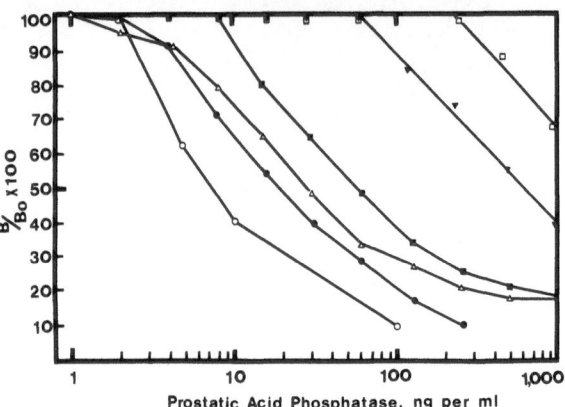

Figure 4. Antiserum delution curves using anti-PAP rabbit antiserum R22. ^{125}I-PAP, 0.2 ng/ml; unlabeled PAP, 1.0-1,000 ng/ml; dilutions of anti-PAP serum (R22), (□), 1:500; (▼), 1:1,000; (■), 1:2,500; (△), 1:5,000; (●), 1:10,000; (○), 1:20,000. Assayed by equilibrium technique as described in Figure 3.

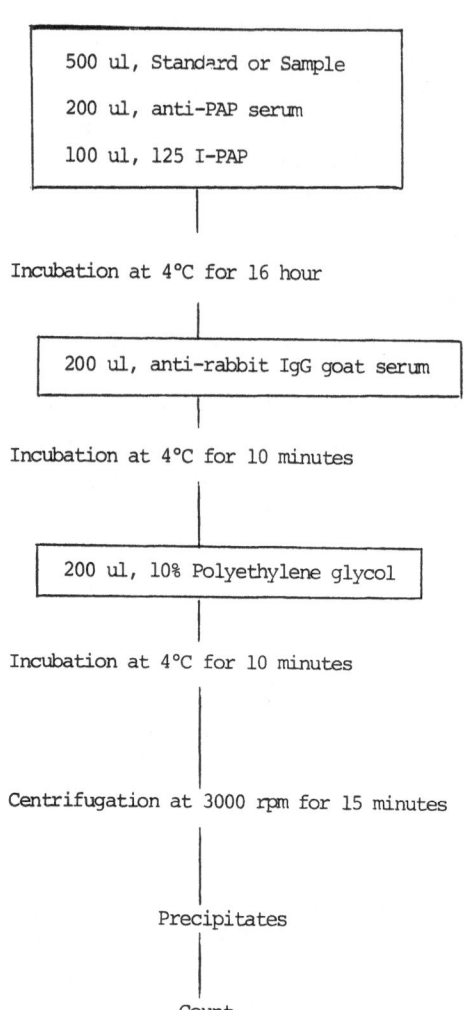

Figure 3. Protocol of equilibrium method.

III. CLINICAL SIGNIFICANCE OF IMMUNO-ASSAY VALUES OF PROSTATIC ACID PHOSPHATASE

A. Normal value

For PAP-RIA, different reference preparations are being used by different investigators and the results are expressed accordingly (Table 1). Previously reported normal values are relatively high in comparison with recent data (Choe et al. 1978b, Copper and Foti 1974, Foti et al. 1975). Because of the availability of highly purified PAP preparations, anti-PAP sensitive immunologic enzyme assay as a reference method, the normal values for serum PAP have been established (range <1 to 8 ng/ml) in our laboratory. A survey of the recent literature (Table 1), shows <1 to 10 ng/ml to be the normal range. The question of antigenic specificity of PAP is not settled; with the exception of prostatic acid phosphatase, none of the human acid phosphatases are totally purified and antigenicity has not yet been studied as a purified enzyme. However, PAP is a high moleculear weight protein with multiple antigenic determinants.

It is possible that one or two of these determinants might be crossreactive with some determinants on acid phosphatases from renal and alveolar epithelial cells. Therefore, significance of normal values of PAP in healthy females and males is not totally clear at this time.

B. Prostatic cancer

The serum acid phosphatase assay has demonstrated its usefulness over the past four decades in mostly advanced cases of carcinoma, but its usefulness seems to be limited in the early stages of carcinoma. Today, intensive efforts have been made to stage the lesion accurately in order to discover new cases at potentially curable stages and to plan the therapeutic regimens (Klein 1979). Immunological assays have been proposed in the hope of contributing to the early detection of curable lesions. To examine this wishful optimism, correlation between the acid phosphatase levels and clinical progression of the disease is summarized in Table 3. The RIA data (Foti et al. 1977) suggest that immunological assay methods have the potential to detect over half the cases of intracapsular prostatic cancer. Carroll's statistical evaluation of the data have confirmed this conclusion (1978). Other data from immunological assays such as CIEP (Chu et al. 1978, Romas et al. 1978) and IEA (Choe et al. 1979, Murphy et al. 1978) are still preliminary and could not provide comparable information at the time of this writing.

As an adjunct to pathological staging and bone surveys, immunological assays of PAP in bone marrow biopsies have been attempted (Cooper et al. 1978, Pontes et al. 1978). As discussed below, PAP levels in bone marrow and lymph node biopsies are expected to be a valuable aid for the survey of metastasis from the theoretical point of view.

However, large-scale studies showed that bone marrow acid phosphatase levels are of no added value (Boehme et al. 1978, Sadlowski 1978). Screening for asymptomatic patients with potentially curable prostatic carcinoma relies on the digital rectal

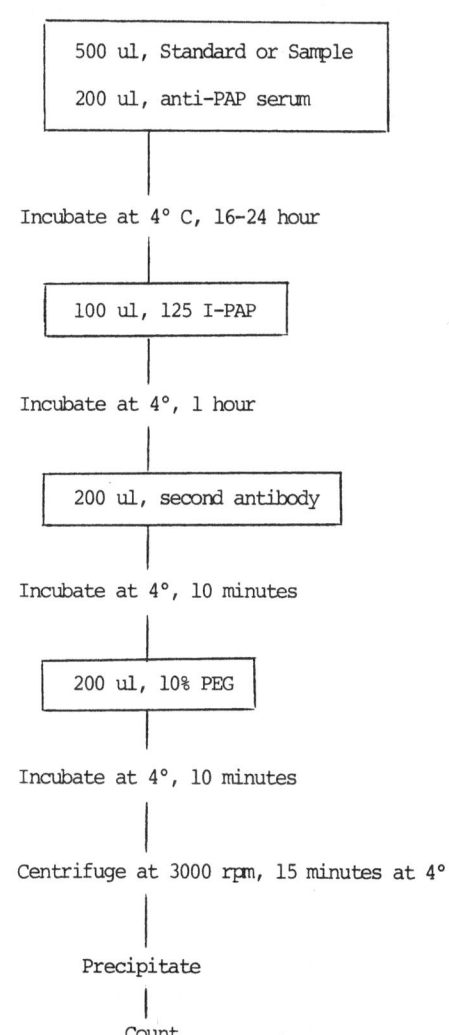

Figure 5. Protocol of modified sequential method.

Table 3. Percentage of patients with 'elevated' PAP at different clinical and surgical stages of prostatic cancer.[d]

Stage[a]	Lymph node metastasis[a] (%)	Serum acid phosphatase[b] (%)	Immunoassay for PAP[c] (%)
(A) Tumor not detected, occult	5-25	5-12	33
(B) Tumor 1.5 cm diameter, confined to 1 lobe	8.45	5-15	79 (20)
(C) Tumor locally extensive	40-80	5-15	71 (40)
(D) Any size tumor with bone metastasis	100	60-90	92 (70)

[a] Adapted from Klein (1979).
[b] Adapted from Murphy et al. (1969), Batsakis et al. (1970), Yam (1974), Foti et al (1977).
[c] Adapted from Foti et al. (1977), Chu et al. (1978); and also Choe Pontes and Rose's unpublished data are presented in parantheses.
[d] Mean (arithmetic mean of normal value + 2 SD (standard deviation) was chosen as the upper limit of normal range. Serum PAP values higher than this limit are regarded as 'elevated'.

138

examination. Then, could an immunoassay of PAP be a supplementary method for such a screening program? It seems relevant to discuss the limitations of the PAP immunoassay before answering this question.

In normal prostatic glandular epithelium, the secretory organelles are oriented toward the glandular lumen, and the leakage of prostatic acid phosphatase into the circulation is not observed. In cases of infiltrating and metastasizing prostatic cancer, tumor cells exhibit many ultrastructural anomalies which include the loss of polarity with apical distribution of secretory vacuoles and disorientation of hypertrophic Golgi apparatus, loss of basement membrane and absence of basal cells (Brandes and Kirchheim 1977). Therefore, it is believed that accumulated prostatic acid phosphatase in these cells diffuse into the interstitial space, instead of to the glandular lumen, and lead to the elevation of prostatic acid phosphatase concentration in the general circulation. As shown in Table 3, lymph node metastasis seems to occur in the early stage of carcinoma; theoretically, enzymes released from these metastatic cells are expected ultimately to appear as an elevated level of PAP. In approximately 10-20 percent of patients with prostatic carcinoma metastatic to bone, serum acid phosphatase activity remains relatively low or, more rarely, normal, despite active metastatic growth (Sodeman and Batsakis 1977, Townsend 1977). These paradoxical situations have been explained by 1) low or dedifferentiation of the neoplasm, 2) insufficient invasion of the vascular or lymphatic channels 3) some 'barrier' to egress from the metastatic loci. Therefore, the sensitivity of immunologic assay of prostatic acid phosphatase is ultimately limited by the biosynthesis, transport and leakage of this enzyme from the neoplastic cells. The basic mechanisms of biosynthesis and secretion of this enzyme are largely unknown.

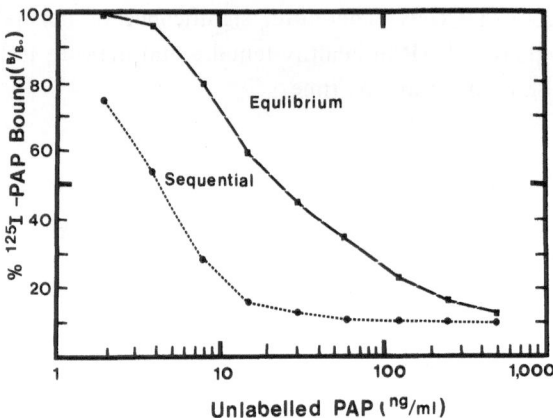

Figure 6. Comparison of PAP-RIA dose response curves by equilibrium and sequential saturation techniques.

C. Prostatic acid phosphatase in non-prostatic disorders

Moderate elevation of total serum acid phosphatases are frequently observed in a variety of non-prostatic disorders which include metabolic skeletal disease, hepatic disease, renal disease, hematologic disease, urological disease, and cancers other than prostatic carcinoma. Because of the antigenic specificity of prostatic acid phosphatase, immunoassays distinguish these acid phosphatases of non-prostatic origins from PAP. However, certain degrees of cross-reactivity have been reported. Foti et al. (1977) reported up to 11% of false positive in their solid-phase RIA, while less than 5% of false positives was experienced in our laboratory (unpublished). In a case of neoplastic acid phosphatase, we have observed true cross-reactivity with PAP (Choe et al. 1978c).

ACKNOWLEDGEMENTS

This work was supported in part by Public Health Award CA 16426 and CA 18747 from the National Cancer Institute.

REFERENCES

Batsakis JG, Briere RO, Markel SF: Diagnostic Enzymology. Chicago: American Society of Clinical Pathologists, Commission on Continuing Education, 1970, pp 1-231

Belville W, Cox HD, Mahn DE, Olmert JP, Mittemeyer BT, Bruce AW: Bone marrow acid phosphatase by radioimmunoassay. Cancer 41: 2286-2291, 1978.

Berson SA, Yalow R, eds: Methods in Investigative and Diagnostic Endocrinology. Amsterdam: North Holland Publishing Company, 1973, pp 84-135.

Bodanski O: Acid phosphatase. Adv Clin Chem 15: 43-147, 1972.

Boehme WM, Augspurger RR, Wallner SF, Danahue RE: Lack of usefulness of bone marrow enzymes and calcium in staging patients with prostatic cancer. Cancer 41: 1433-1439, 1978.

Brandes D, Kirchheim D: Histochemistry of the prostate. In: Urologic pathology: the prostate, Tannenbaum M, ed. Philadelphia: Lea and Febiger, 1977.

Buckler JMH: A comparison of the effect of human serum in two double antibody radioimmunoassay systems for the estimation of luteinizing hormone. In: Radioimmunoassay methods, Hunter WM, Kirkham KE, eds. Baltimore: Williams and Wilkins, 1971, pp 273-283.

Carrol BJ: Radioimmunoassay of prostatic acid phosphatase in carcinoma of the prostate. New England J Med 298: 912, 1978.

Chervu LR, Murty DRK: Radiolabeling of antigens: Procedures and assessment of properties. Seminars in Nucelar Medicine 5: 157-172, 1975.

Choe BK, Pontes EJ, McDonald I, Rose NR: Purification and characterization of human prostatic acid phosphatase. Prep Biochem 8: 73-89, 1978a.

Choe BK, Pontes EJ, Morrison MK, Rose NR: Human prostatic acid phosphatase II. A double antibody radioimmunoassay. Arch Andrology 1: 227-233, 1978b.

Choe BK, Pontes EJ, Rose NR, Henderson MD: Expression of human prostatic acid phosphatase in a pancreatic islet cell carcinoma. Invest Urol 15: 312-318, 1978c.

Choe BK, Rose NR, Karol M, Pontes EJ: Immunoenzyme assay for human prostatic acid phosphatase. Proc Soc Exp Biol Med, 1979.

Chu TM, Wang MC, Scott WW, Gibbons RP, Johnson DE, Schmidt JD, Leoning SA, Prout GR, Murphy GP: Immunochemical detection of serum prostatic acid phosphatase. Methodology and clinical evaluation. Invest Urol 15: 319-323, 1978.

Cooper JF, Foti A: A radioimmunoassay for prostatic acid phosphatase. I. Methodology and range of normal male serum values. Invest Urol 12: 98-102, 1974.

Cooper JF, Fot AG, Shank PW: Radioimmunochemical measurement of bone marrow prostatic acid phosphatase. J Urol 119: 392-295, 1978.

Court G, Hurn BAL: An effect of plasma and other macromolecular solutions in double antibody radioimmunoassay systems. In: Radioimmunoassay methods, Kirkham KE, Hunter WM eds. Baltimore Williams and Wilkins, 1971, pp 283-289.

Derechin M, Ostrowski W, Galka M, Barnard EA: Acid phosphomonoesterase of human prostate, molecular weight, dissociation and chemical composition. Biochim Biophys Acta 250: 143-154, 1971.

Ekins RP, Newman GB, O'Riordan JLH: Theoretical aspects of 'saturation' and radioimmunoassay. In: Radioisotopes in medicine: inv itro studies, Hayes RL, Goswitz FA, Murphy BEP, eds. Oak Ridge, Tenn: U.S. Atomic Energy Commission, 1968, p 58.

Van Etten RL, Saini MS; Selective purification of tartrate-inhibitable acid phosphatases: rapid and efficient purification (to homogeneity) of human and canine prostatic acid phosphatases. Clin Chem 24: 1525-1530, 1978.

Foti AG, Herschman H, Cooper JF: A solid-phase radioimmunoassay for human prostatic acid phosphatase. Cancer Res 35: 2446-2452, 1975.

Foti AG, Cooper JF, Herschman H, Malvaez RR: Detection of prostatic cancer by solid-phase radioimmunoassay of serum prostatic acid phosphatase. New England J Med 297: 1357-1361, 1977.

Foti AG, Cooper JF, Herschman H: Counterimmunoelectrophoresis in determination of prostatic acid phosphatase in human serum. Clin Chem 24: 140-142, 1978.

Haber E, Poulsen K: The application of antibody to the measurement of substances of physiological and pharmacological interest. In: The Antigens, II, Sela M, ed. New York: Academic Press, 1974, pp 249-275.

Helms SR, Brattain MG,Pretlow TG, Kreisberg JI: Prostatic acid phosphatase? Am J Pathol 88: 529-538, 1977.

Hunter WM: Radioimmunoassay. In: Handbook of experimental immunology, 2nd ed, Weir DM, ed. Philadelphia: F.A. Davis Co., 1973, pp 17.1-17.36.

Jaffe BM, Behrman HR, eds: Methods of hormone radioimmunoassay. New York: Academic Press, 1974.

Karush F: Affinity and the immune process. Ann N Y Acad Sci 169: 56-71, 1970.

Klein LA: Prostatic carcinoma, New England J Med 300: 824-833, 1979.

Lee C, Wang MC, Murphy GP, Chu TM: Solid-phase fluorescent immunoassay for human prostatic acid phosphatase. Cancer Res 38: 2871-2878, 1978.

Luchter-Wasyl E, Ostrowski W: Subunit structure of human prostatic acid phosphatase. Biochim Biophys Acta 365: 349-359, 1974.

Mahan DE, Doctor PP: A radioimmunoassay for human prostatic acid phosphatase. Clin Biochem, 1979.

McDonald I, Rose NR, Pontes EJ, Choe BK: Human prostatic acid phosphatase III. Counterimmunoelectrophoresis for rapid identification. Arch Androl 1: 234-239, 1978.

Milisauskas V, Rose NR: Immunochemical quantitation of prostatic acid phosphatase. Clin Chem 18: 1529-1931, 1972.

Morgan CR, Sorenson RL, Lazarow A: Studies of an inhibitor of the two antibody immunoassay system. Diabetes 13: 1-5, 1964.

Murphy GP, Reynoso G, Kenny GM, Gaeta JF: Comparison of total and prostatic fraction serum acid phosphatase levels in patients with differentiated and undifferentiated prostatic carcinoma. Cancer 23: 1309-1314, 1969.

Murphy GP, Karr J, Chu TN: Prostatic acid phosphatase: where are we? Ca–A Cancer Journal for Clinicians 28: 258-264, 1978.

Ostrowski W, Wasyl Z, Weber M, Guminska M, Luchter E: The role of neuraminic acid in the heterogeneity of acid phosphomonoesterase from the human prostate gland. Biochim Biophys Acta 221: 397-406, 1970.

Pontes EJ, Choe BK, Rose NR, Pierce JM Jr: Bone marrow acid phosphatase in staging of prostatic cancer: How reliable is it? J Urol 119: 772-776, 1978.

Romas NA, Hsu KC, Tomashefsky P, Tannenbaum M: Counterimmunoelectrophoresis for detection of human prostatic acid phosphatase. Urology 12: 79-83, 1978.

Rothenberg SP, Dacosta M, Rosenberg Z: A radioimmunoassay for serum folate: use of a two-phase sequential incubation, ligand-binding system. New England J Med 286: 1335, 1972.

Sadlowski RW: Early stage prostatic cancer investigated by pelvic lymph node biopsy and bone marrow acid phosphatase. J Urol 119: 89-93, 1978.

Scatchard G: The attractions of proteins for small molecules and ions. Ann N Y Acad Sci 51: 660-672, 1949.

Sheldon J, Taylor KW: The immunoassay of insulin in human serum treated with sodium ethylene diamine tetra-acetate. J Endocrinol 33: 157-158, 1965.

Shulman S, Mamrod L, Gonder M, Soanes WA: The detection of prostatic acid phosphatase by antibody reactions in gel diffusion. J Immunol 93: 474-480, 1964.

Sodeman TM, Batsakis JG: Acid phosphatase. In: Urologic pathology – the prostate, Tannenbaum M, ed. Lea and Philadelphia: Lea and Febiger, 1977, pp 129-139.

Thorell JI and Johansson BG: Enzymatic iodination of polypeptides with ^{125}I to high specific activity. Biochim Biophys Acta 251: 363-369, 1971.

Townsend RM: Enzyme tests in diseases of the prostate. Annals Clin Lab Sci 7: 254-261, 1977.

Vihko P, Kontturi M, Korhonen LK: Purification of human prostatic acid phosphatase by affinity chromatography and isoelectric focusing. Part I. Clin Chem 24: 466-470, 1978a.

Vihko P, Sajanti E, Janne O, Peltonen L, Vihko R: Serum prostate-specific acid phosphatase: development and validation of a specific radioimmunoassay. Clin Chem 24: 1915-1919, 1978b.

Yam YT: Clinical significance of the human acid phosphatases: a review. Amer J Med 56: 604-616, 1974.

Zettner A: Principles of competitive binding assays (saturation analyses). I. Equilibrium techniques. Clin Chem 19: 699-705, 1973.

Zettner A, Duly PE: Principles of competitive binding assays (saturation analyses). II. Sequential saturation. Clin Chem 20: 5-14, 1974.

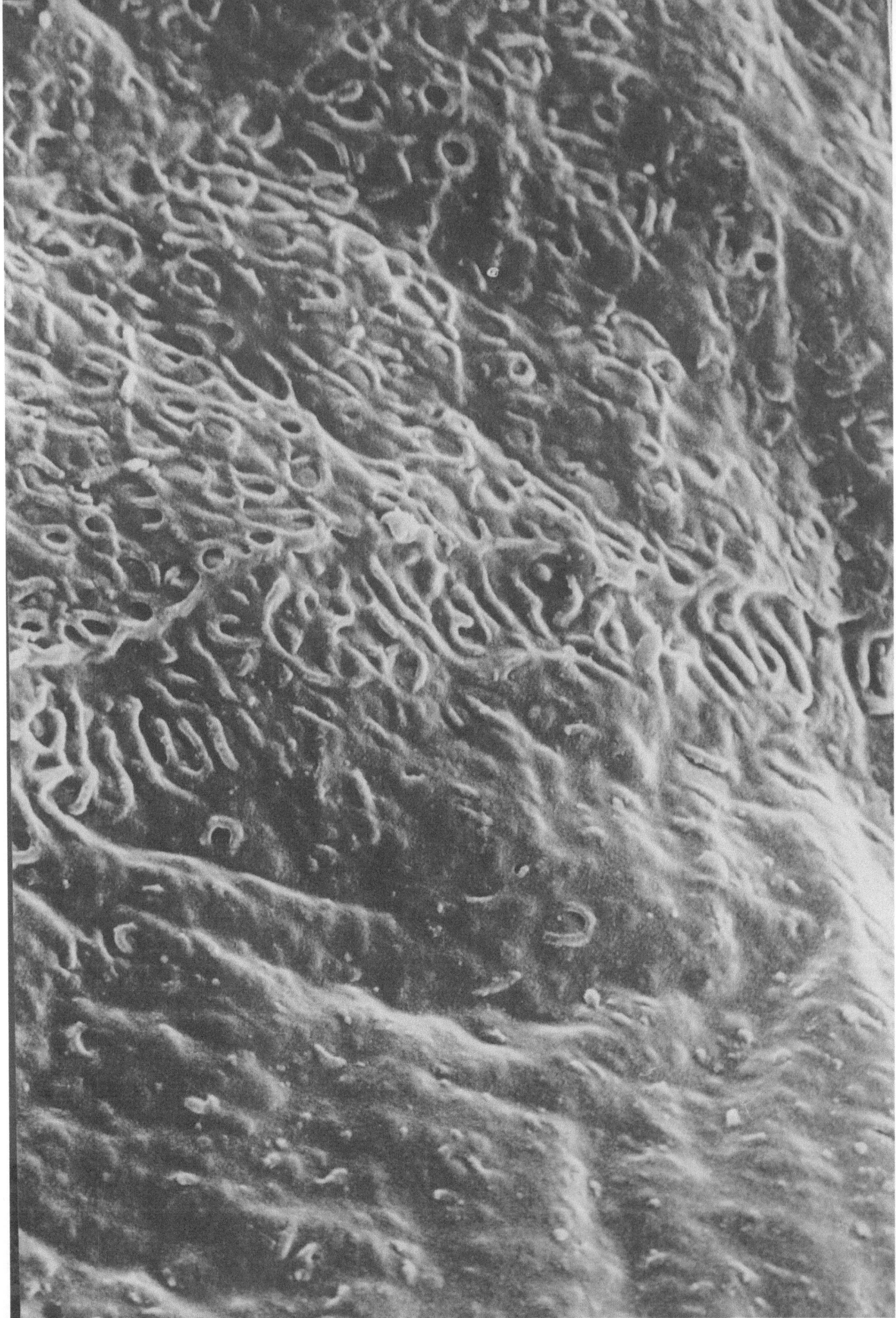

III. IN VITRO STUDIES AND ANIMAL MODELS

13. IN VITRO MODELS

M. M. WEBBER

I. INTRODUCTION

Adenocarcinoma of the prostate is the third leading cause of death in the adult human male cancer patient, after cancers of the lung and colon/rectum. The incidence of prostatic cancer has increased by more than 25% in the last 25 years. The number of deaths from prostatic carcinoma in the U.S.A. in 1979 is estimated to be 21,000 and 64,000 new cases are estimated during the same period (American Cancer Society, Facts and Figures 1979). Yet, we know very little about the etiology of prostatic cancer. Investigations on the etiology, mechanism of carcinogenesis and on the modes of treatment for prostatic cancer can be made using in vitro and in vivo model systems. Considerable progress has been made in the last five years in developing such models. In this chapter I will discuss in vitro models for prostatic cancer.

The in vivo animal models are useful for studies on tumor progression, metastasis and modes of treatment. However, there may be important differences between the prostate of man and other animals. The in vitro cell models derived from normal human cells are particularly well suited for studies on the etiology and on the mechanism of carcinogenesis. Normal cell models further provide a basic understanding of the physiology of normal cells and of the various growth regulating mechanisms. Models using malignant human cells are useful for testing different modes of treatment.

Studies on the etiology of prostatic cancer and on the mechanism of carcinogenesis have been hampered primarily by the rarity of spontaneous prostatic cancer in common laboratory animals and by difficulties in inducing the same. In view of this, the importance of in vitro cell models for the prostate has been recognized and great emphasis is being placed on the development of in vitro systems using normal prostatic epithelial cells. In order to understand the malignant prostatic epithelial cell, it is important first to have a thorough understanding of the physiology, i.e., of growth controls, cell interactions and hormone responses of the normal prostatic epithelial cell.

II. NORMAL CELL MODELS

The major objective of my studies is to develop an in vitro cell model using post-pubertal, normal human prostatic epithelium, which could be used 1) to study early steps in prostatic carcinogenesis; 2) to identify specific carcinogens for these target cells; 3) to elucidate the metabolic activation of carcinogens and their organ specificity; and 4) to examine the mechanism of transformation.

The value of establishing an in vitro model using normal human cells is based on the following facts: 1) In an isolated cell system, one is more likely to be able to pinpoint the specific changes involved in carcinogenesis. 2) Until recently, long-term experiments with animals provided the only means for detecting the potential of various agents as carcinogens. The bio-assay of compounds by in vivo testing seems to be an insurmountable task. Therefore, in vitro models have proved to be very useful for screening potential carcinogens for man. Also, such in vitro procedures can provide results in a shorter period of time, are less costly, and are reliable, sensitive and practical. 3) Concern and doubts have been expressed on the usefulness and applicability of animal model systems for studying problems of human disease. Although it is difficult to obtain and culture normal human epithelial cells, it is believed that the ultimate answer to the question of cancer etiology can only be provided by testing various agents on human cells. Therefore the use of cells derived from man is naturally appropriate for studies on human cancer.

Current information suggests that 80% of all human cancers may be caused by environmental carcinogens. Hence, considerable emphasis is being placed on the identification of these carcinogens and on the methods of interfering with the process of malignant transformation. Nearly 85% of all human tumors arise from epithelial cells. It is therefore important to identify and determine the mechanism of carcinogen-target cell interaction in organs which show a high incidence of cancer. The incidence of benign tumors of the prostate may be as high as 80% in men over the age of 40 (Walsh 1976). Also, at least 30% of all men over 50 years may have histological carcinoma and this figure increases to 50% after the age of 70 (Franks 1976). In view of this, it is important to understand the mechanism of carcinogenesis in the prostate. Because of these reasons, it is necessary to develop an in vitro model using human prostatic epithelium. In order to develop such a model, it is necessary to meet certain basic requirements, which are: to isolate normal epithelium, to establish its growth and maintenance requirements in vitro and to characterize it to establish its prostatic epithelial origin (Figure 1).

Very few studies have been made on the isolation and growth and maintenance of normal human prostatic epithelium in vitro. One of the major problems has been the acquisition of normal viable tissue. Our major source of normal tissue has been cadaver organ transplant donors and autopsies. Neonatal, human prostatic epithelium has been sucessfully grown in culture (Lechner et al. 1978). The use of explant cultures of normal human prostate for carcinogenesis studies has been explored (Sanefuji et al. 1978, Webber et al. 1974). No other work than that done in my laboratory and which is the subject of this and other forthcoming papers (Webber 1979a, 1980a, b, Webber and Chaproniere-Rickenberg 1980, Webber a, Webber and Bouldin b, Webber et al. c, Webber and Jankowsky, Webber and Prasad), has been reported on the successful isolation, cultivation and maintenance of normal, post-pubertal, human prostatic epithelium. The significance of using post-pubertal prostate

must be emphasized. Since prostatic carcinomas arise from adult, androgen responsive epithelium, it is important to use such epithelium for developing an in vitro model. All other studies on in vitro cultivation of human prostatic epithelium have used benign or malignant prostate.

It has generally been difficult to grow and maintain normal, human epithelial cells in vitro. This is paradoxical when one realizes that the majority of human cancer are of epithelial origin. One of the reasons for this failure has been the general dependence on standard commercially available media and the failure to recognize that prostatic epithelial cells are specialized secretory cells whose growth, maintenance and differentiation in vivo are controlled by several hormones, vitamins and other growth controlling factors. It is, therefore, logical to assume that these cells would have certain specific requirements of the above substances for their growth and maintenance in vitro. My investigations were therefore based on the premise that since prostatic cells did not grow well under the environmental tissue culture conditions provided so far, the first logical step would be to suitably modify the environment for their optimum growth and survival, i.e., to design a special medium to satisfy growth requirements of normal prostatic epithelium in vitro.

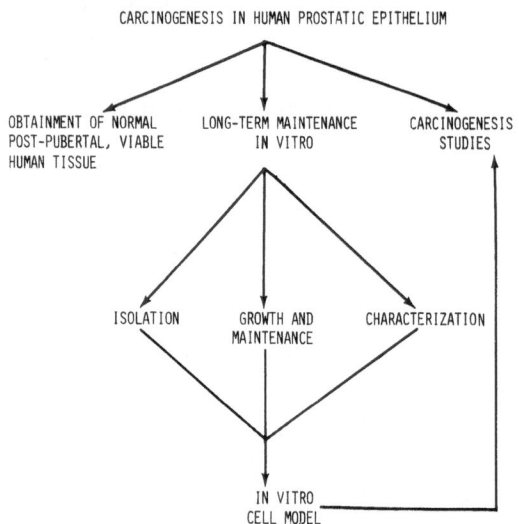

Figure 1. A diagram showing the basic requirements for developing an in vitro cell model using normal, human prostatic epithelium for studies on prostatic carcinogenesis (Webber 1980a).

One of the basic requirements for establishing this in vitro model is to establish pure cultures of prostatic epithelium and for this, one must first isolate the cells.

A. Isolation of normal prostatic epithelium for in vitro cultivation

1. Introduction   Cultures of animal prostatic epithelium to date have primarily been established from explant cultures (see Webber 1979a). Human prostatic epithelium has also primarily been grown in vitro using explant cultures (Webber 1974, Webber and Stonington 1975, Webber et al. 1974, for other references see Webber 1979a). Enzymatic digestion of prostatic tissue has also been tried (see Webber 1979a). One of the major problems in culturing human epithelial cells has been the contamination with fibroblasts. When ordinary tissue culture methods are used, prostatic epithelial cultures are generally contaminated with stromal fibroblasts. My investigations on the usefulness of collagenase in establishing pure monolayer cultures of prostatic epithelium began in 1974 on both normal and benign human prostatic tissue (Webber and Batts 1977). Physiological breakdown of collagen in many mammals and amphibians is accomplished by the action of specific collagenases, produced in very small amounts as needed. The same enzyme might also be used for isolation of cells from tissues after digestion with collagenase. Collagenases are enzymes capable of dissolving fibrous collagen by peptide bond cleavage under physiological conditions of pH and temperature. The specific substrate, collagen, comprises 33% of the total protein in mammalian organisms (Mandl 1972). Lasfargues (1957) pioneered the use of collagenase for digestion of tissue for cell dispersal in the preparation of primary cultures of mouse mammary epithelium. Since prostate has a histological composition similar to that of the mammary glands, I have used collagenase for the isolation of prostatic epithelium. Stromal elements form a major part prostatic tissue. Separation of epithelial cells from the stroma, using collagenase, is an interesting phenomenon. Electron microscopy was used to pinpoint the site of action of collagenase which facilitates isolation of acini (Webber 1979a).

2. Methods   Specimens of normal prostatic tissue were collected from cadaver organ transplant donors and autopsies. In earlier experiments explant cultures were used (Webber et al. 1974). Later experiments employed collagenase digestion of tissue. Viable acini can be isolated from digested tissue and primary cultures of prostatic epithelium initiated from these acini (Webber 1979a). In earlier experiments $CMRL_{1066}$ medium containing 10% fetal bovine serum (FBS), 10% horse serum (HS), 100 U/ml penicillin, 100 μg/ml streptomycin, 10 μg/ml gentamicin and 2mM L-glutamine was used. Recent experiments were conducted using $RPMI_{1640}$ plus the supplements listed above (Webber and Jankowsky).

For transmission electron microscopy, cells were prepared according to the method described earlier (Webber and Bouldin 1977). Sections were examined with a Philips EM-300 transmission electron microscope. For scanning electron microscopy cells were prepared according to the method described by Porter et al. (1973). The cells were examined with a Cambridge S-4 stereoscan electron microscope operated at 20 kV. For light microscopy, cells were fixed and stained by a Giemsa method (Poché et al. 1974).

3. Results   Collagenase, when incorporated into culture medium does have cytotoxic and growth inhibitory effects on fibroblasts. Cultures containing 50 U/ml collagenase show vigorously growing epithelium with no fibroblasts or only minute colonies of fibroblasts. Fibroblasts can thus be eliminated to some extent from mixed cultures by the use of collagenase as a component of the tissue culture medium (Webber 1979a).

Prostatic acini were isolated according to the method described earlier (Webber 1979a). Using this procedure, intact acini can be isolated. Plating of these acini results in pure cultures of vigorously growing epithelium. Occasional colonies of fibroblasts do appear in some cultures. Cells isolated from the supernate and washings are predominantly fibroblasts.

Normal prostatic epithelium rests on a basal lamina which separates it from the underlying stromal elements. When prostatic tissue is exposed to collagenase, the basal lamina is one of the sites of its action, in addition to the collagen in the stroma.

148

As a result, the epithelial cells separate from the underlying stromal elements. Collagenase is toxic to fibroblasts but the epithelial cells remain viable and have a clean outer epithelial surface (Figure 2).

It has generally been difficult to initiate cultures from explants prepared from autopsy tissue specimens or samples obtained from transurethral resection of the prostate (TURP). However, good epithelial cell growth has been initiated from acini isolated from these tissues after collagenase digested (Webber 1979a). TURP is fast replacing open prostatectomies as the mode of surgery. Using this method, epithelial cultures can be initiated from TURP specimens. Cultures from TURP specimens may contain some fibroblast colonies due to incomplete separation of acini from the stroma. This results from incomplete digestion by collagenase of denatured tissue caused by electro-cauterization during surgery.

4. Discussion   Growth of epithelial cells is en-

hanced when 50 U/ml collagenase is incorporated into the culture medium, while growth of fibroblasts is inhibited. For isolation of acini, crude collagenase is most effective in prostatic tissue digestion. It is a mixture of hydrolytic enzymes containing some peptidase and trypsin-like proteinase in addition to collagenase. Pure collagenase is not as effective. The effectiveness of digestion of tissue with collagenase partly depends upon the age of the donor, which may be related to the amount of collagen present. Since collagenase is not toxic to epithelial cells, organs with heavy collagen matrices like the prostate, can therefore be incubated for several hours without loss of cell viability.

Post-pubertal prostatic epithelium of normal human origin has been successfully isolated for in vitro cultivation, using the collagenase dispersal technique (Webber 1979a). Isolated acini give rise to vigorously growing epithelial cultures. A certain number of acini is required per culture in order to obtain a vigorously growing culture and increase

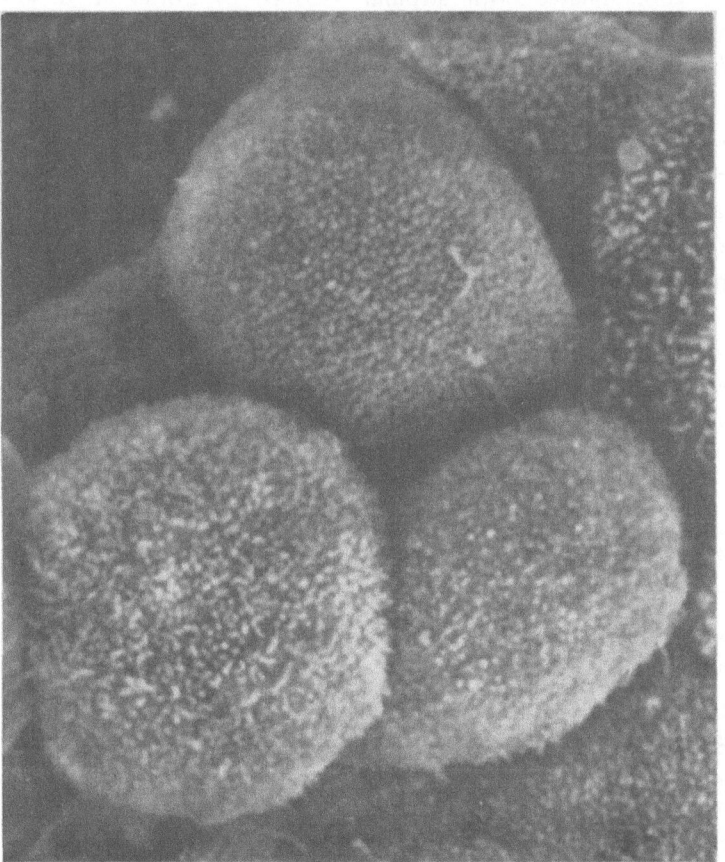

Figure 2. Scanning electron micrograph of the surface of a prostatic acinus isolated from tissue dispersed with collagenase. The surface is free of stromal elements and has numerous microvilli. ×6,720.

their lifespan (Webber 1979a). This behavior may be related to the ability of cells to condition media. Also, cells in primary cultures tend to grow better when plated in large number.

B. Growth and maintenance of normal prostatic epithelium in vitro

1. Introduction   After isolation, the next objective is to grow and maintain prostatic epithelial cells in culture for long periods of time. Limited studies have been made on the maintenance of human prostatic organ cultures, derived from benign and malignant prostate. However, no concerted effort had been made to define nutrient and growth requirements of normal prostatic cells in vitro.

Lasnitzki (1963) has been a pioneer in the studies on the maintenance of mouse prostatic tissue organ cultures. However, when the present studies began, successful cultivation and maintenance of normal prostatic epithelium had never been accomplished.

Criteria for adequacy of growth and nutrition for prostatic cells in vitro are only now being established. Culture media commonly used for established cell lines have been used in the past for prostatic cell cultures with disappointing results. Since prostatic epithelial cells are specialized secretory cells and since their growth is affected directly by certain hormones and vitamins in vivo, a tissue culture medium must be designed to satisfy their specific growth requirements. In order to achieve this, a number of different serum types and media were first tested for their growth supporting properties for these cells. In vivo, testosterone, insulin and vitamin A control growth, secretory activity, differentiation and cell morphology of prostatic epithelium. On this basis, these three agents were selected for an extensive study of their effects on the growth and maintenance of prostatic epithelium in monolayer cultures.

2. Methods   Primary cultures derived from explants or from collagenase-isolated acini were used for testing the effects of serum, media, insulin, vitamin A and 5α-dihydrotestosterone (5α-DHT), on the growth and maintenance of prostatic epithelium (Webber 1980a). A wide range of insulin levels (0.01 IU/ml-100 IU/ml), of vitamin A (0.01-200 U/ml) and DHT (0.01 μg-100 μg/ml) were tested. At the end of the experimental period, cells were fixed and stained by a Giemsa method (Poché et al. 1974).

Quantitation of cell growth in vitro is necessary in order to establish the growth enhancing effects or toxicity of the test substances. When using fibroblasts or other cells which can be easily dissociated and dispersed into single cell suspensions, it is easy to determine the extent of growth on the basis of cell number. However, many epithelial cells in primary culture, e.g. prostatic epithelium, do not dissociate easily into single cells but remain as sheets or clumps after enzymatic treatment. Assessment of growth on the basis of cell counts is, therefore, not reliable. A Datacolor Scanning Densitometer (Webber and Webber 1979) was used for quantitation of growth in cell cultures. Growth measurements are based on the measurement of the dish area covered with cells.

3. Selection of serum and medium   Serum in the culture medium may act as a selection factor and favor the multiplication of one cell type over another (Webber 1974). Horse serum favors the growth of prostatic epithelial cells in culture (Webber 1974). We have examined the effects of horse serum (HS), fetal bovine serum (FBS) and calf serum. (CS) on the growth of prostatic epithelium. The best and purest growth of prostatic epithelium occurred in cultures maintained on medium containing 10% FBS + 10% HS (Figure 3), while cultures maintained on fetal bovine serum contain many fibroblast colonies (see Webber 1980a, Webber et al. c).

Effects of $CMRL_{1066}$, $RPMI_{1640}$, medium 199, Eagle's minimum essential medium, (EMEM), Medium F-12 and Eagle's basal medium (BME), containing 10% FBS and 10% HS, were examined on the growth and maintenance of prostatic epithelium (Webber and Jankowsky). Both $CMRL_{1066}$ and $RPMI_{1640}$ stimulate good growth of epithelial cells while F-12 gives the poorest growth (Figure 4). Cell growth in RPMI was however the best and cells could also be maintained in this medium longer than in CMRL. Hence $RPMI_{1640}$ has been selected for growing normal and benign prostatic epithelium in vitro.

150

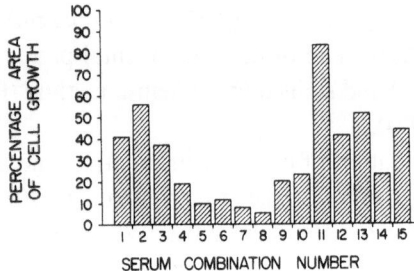

Figure 3. Effects of different serum types individually and in combination, on the growth of normal human prostatic epithelium in vitro. The following serum combinations and concentrations were tested. Numbers refer to those shown on the histogram. CS, calf serum; FBS, fetal bovine serum; HS, horse serum.

1. 5% FBS	9. 20% CS
2. 10% FBS	10. 5% FBS + 5% HS
3. 20% FBS	11. 10% FBS + 10% HS
4. 5% HS	12. 5% FBS + 5% CS
5. 10% HS	13. 10% FBS + 10% CS
6. 20% HS	14. 5% HS + 5% CS
7. 5% CS	15. 10% HS + 10% CS
8. 10% CS	

It is clear that serum combination No. 11 (10% FBS + 10% HS) supports the best growth of prostatic epithelial cells. Fetal bovine serum stimulates better growth than horse or calf sera on their own. Low levels (5%) of serum are not sufficient for good growth in the medium used, however, horse and calf serum can be toxic at high levels. Age of donor - 21 years. (From Webber, Donohue and Jankowsky).

4. *Effects of insulin*

Introduction: Insulin occasionally has been added to tissue culture media because it was thought to stimulate the uptake of glucose and increase cell growth (see Webber and Prasad). There are however very few commercially available media, e.g., Trowell's T-8 and Waymouth's MAB 87/3, which contain insulin.

Very few studies on the in vitro cultivation of prostatic epithelium have used insulin in the culture medium (Ichihara 1977, Johansson 1975). No detailed work, except for the present study, has been done on its effects on normal human prostate. Insulin stimulates carbohydrate metabolism, protein, RNA and DNA synthesis and cell multiplication (Rillema and Linebaugh 1977); potentiates the effect of fibroblast growth factor (Gospodarowicz and Moran 1974) and increases pinocytosis and uptake of glucose by increasing the cell membrane permeability (see Webber and Prasad). Insulin is particularly important because of its specific effects on prostatic epithelium and on the accessory sex organs. Severe diabetes in rats results in a failure of descent of testes, a failure in the development of germinal epithelium and in castrate type accessory glands (Hunt and Bailey 1961). Treatment with insulin corrects all the deleterious effects of diabetes on the reproductive system. Insulin therefore must be considered a hormone which seems to modify the action of testosterone on the accessory sex organs. The importance of insulin in growth regulation of prostatic epithelium has been discussed elsewhere (Webber and Prasad).

Results: The increased pinocytotic activity induced in cells exposed to insulin in vitro is well demonstrated in Figure 5. The number of pinocytotic vesicles and microvilli increases dramatically in exposed cell. Formation of these vesicles and their movement to the interior of the cell can be demonstrated by the addition of a ferritin tracer to the culture medium. Ferritin is picked up during pinocytosis and the movement of vesicles can be followed through the cell (Webber an Prasad).

Studies on the effects of insulin on the growth of normal human epithelium grown in vitro show that insulin has a distinct and pronounced stimulatory effect on the growth and lifespan of prostatic epithelium in vitro (Figure 6). At a level as low as 0.01 IU/ml, insulin slightly increases the growth of prostatic epithelium in vitro. Growth increases steadily with increase in the level of insulin, reaching a peak at 1.0 IU/ml. Beyond this concentration, growth declines and toxicity is evident at a level of 5.0 IU/ml. Insulin also increases the lifespan of human prostatic epithelium in vitro (Webber and Prasad). Cultures maintained on insulin not only show better growth but they can also be maintained in a healthy state for a longer period of time than cultures without insulin.

Another interesting and significant observation made in the course of these investigations was that explant cultures maintained on media containing insulin were devoid of fibroblasts while the control cultures has some fibroblast colonies. This observation suggests that insulin may have specific, selective growth enhancing effects on prostatic epithelium and inhibitory effect on fibroblasts. These observation were confirmed by repeated experiments on several tissue specimens. These results are of particular importance in light of the idea that insulin may have specific effects on growth and differentiation of prostatic epithelium. This

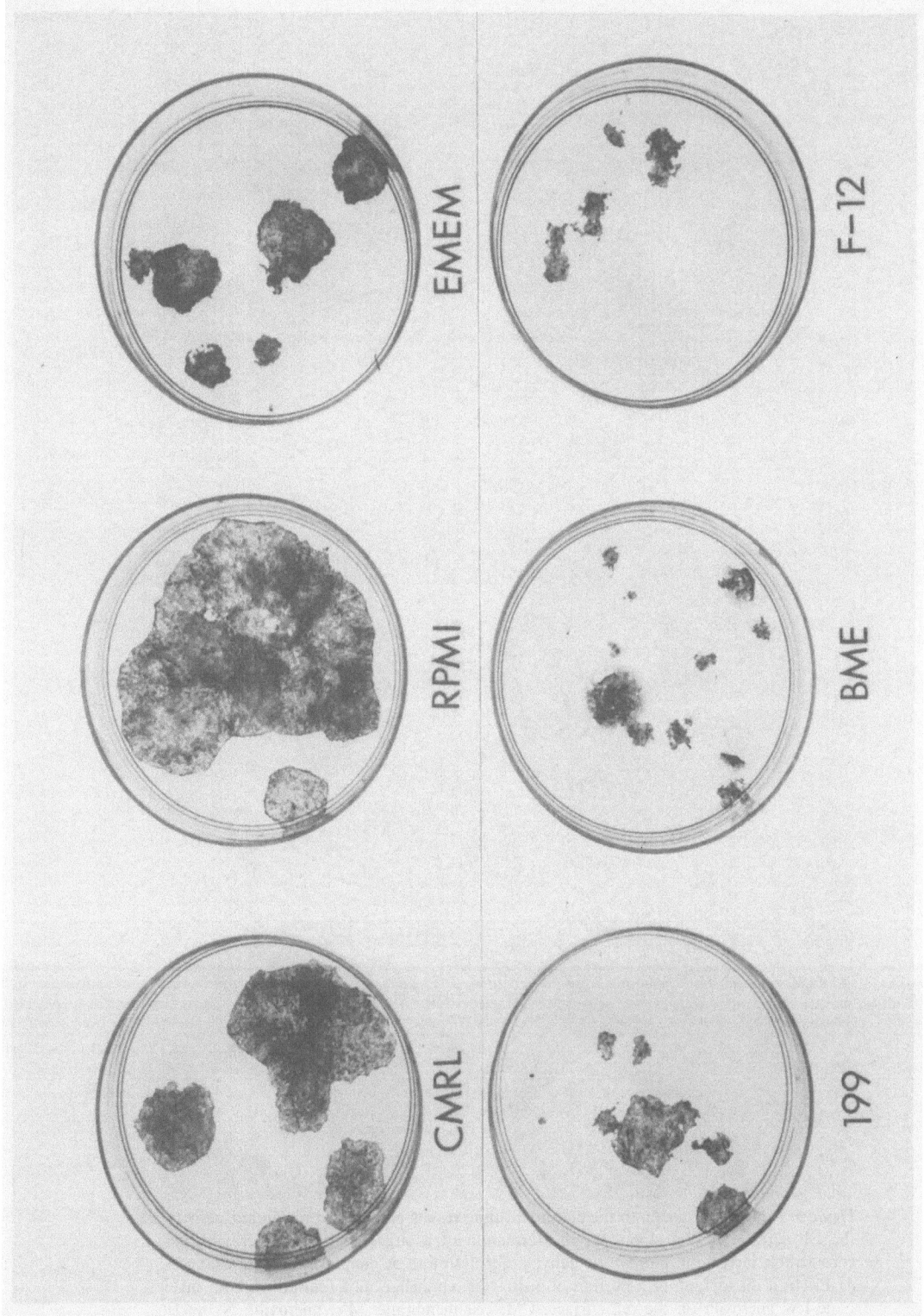

Figure 4. Effects of six different media on the growth of human prostatic epithelium in vitro. All media contain 10% FBS+10% HS. Results show that RPMI supports the best growth. Media used were CMRL$_{1066}$ RPMI$_{1640}$, EMEM (Eagle's minimum essential medium), medium 199, Basal medium (Eagle's) and Ham's F-12, Giemsa stain. (From Webber and Jankowsky.)

152

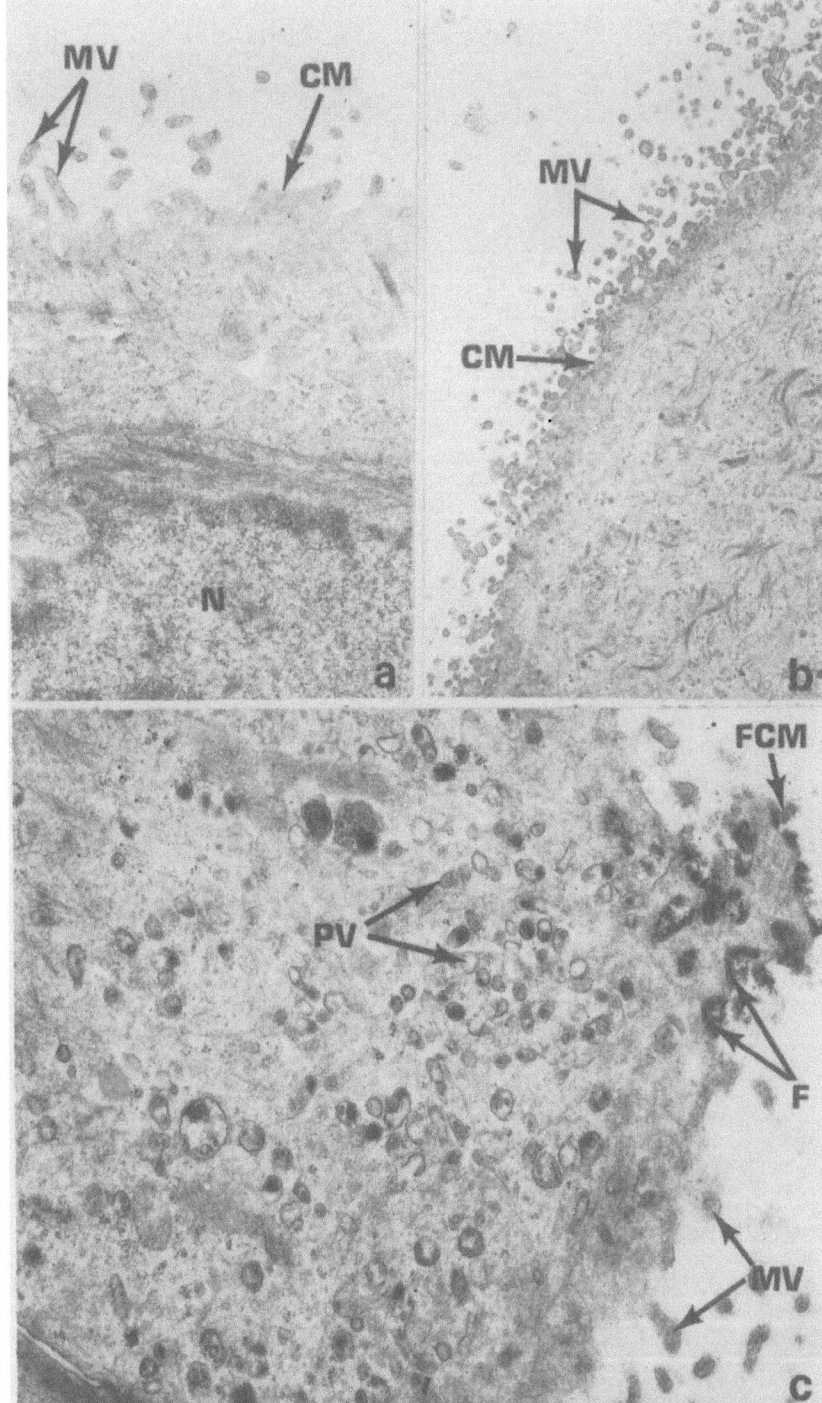

Figure 5. Addition of insulin to the culture medium results in increased membrane activity at the cell surface. Insulin stimulates the formation of a large number of microvilli and a considerable increase in pinocytotic activity. Figures 5a to 5c demonstrate these changes.

a) Electron micrograph of a portion of a prostatic epithelial cell in culture without insulin. Note few microvilli on the cell surface. CM, cell membrane; MV, microvilli; N, nucleus. ×12,755 (From Webber and Prasad).

b) Electron micrograph of a prostatic epithelial cell from a culture exposed to insulin, showing a marked increase in cell membrane activity. Note the large number of microvilli (MV) on the cell surface. CM, cell membrane. ×7,250 (From Webber and Prasad.)

c) Portion of a cell exposed to insulin and ferritin in the culture medium. Ferritin is picked up during pinocytosis and is enclosed in the vesicles. Note a very large number of pinocytotic vesicles (PV) in the area underlying the cell membrane. F, ferritin enclosed in a forming vesicle; MV, microvilli. ×15,750 (From Webber and Prasad.)

matter is worth further consideration (Webber and Prasad).

Discussion: Griffith (1970) studied the effects of insulin on confluent cultures of Wl-38 human embryonic lung fibroblasts. His observations suggest that these cells are unresponsive to growth stimulating effects of insulin. This is interesting in view of the fact that human fibroblasts have been shown to possess specific binding sites for insulin on their cell surface (Hollenberger and Fryklund 1977). It is believed that although fibroblasts have binding sites that interact with insulin, it is possible that these receptor sites are intended really for another chemically related peptide. Further, very high concentrations of insulin are required to elicit a response in fibroblasts, indicating the relatively low affinity of the receptors for insulin, hence these cells are not considered to be primary target cells for insulin.

In conclusion, it can be stated that cultured human fibroblasts, arising from lung, skin and the prostate are relatively insensitive to insulin (Webber and Prasad). Thus, either in vivo or while in vitro, they lose their ability to respond to insulin in terms of cyclic AMP metabolism, glucose oxidation and promotion of growth. This phenomenon is particularly useful in selectively stimulating growth of prostatic epithelium while inhibiting fibroblasts in mixed cultures. This helps in achieving pure cultures of prostatic epithelium.

The growth promoting effects of insulin on epithelial cells and its growth inhibiting effects on fibroblasts can be summarized as follows: insulin alters the cell membrane permeability and increases glucose and amino acid uptake. It also decreases intracellular levels of cyclic AMP and stimulates protein, RNA and DNA synthesis and cell division in target cells (Cuatrecasas 1974, Johansson 1975). Many cell types have receptor sites on their surface for insulin and its effects are thus mediated through the cell membrane (Cuatrecasas 1974). It is however interesting to note that although human fibroblasts possess receptor sites where insulin may bind, they are unresponsive to its growth stimulating effects. Because of this unresponsiveness, our cultures when exposed to insulin, did not show any fibroblastic growth.

5. Effects of vitamin A

Introduction: Vitamin A plays an important role in the maintenance of secretory epithelial cells (Lasnitzki 1963). Vitamin A deficiency causes loss of secretory activity, squamous metaplasia and keratinization while hypervitaminosis results in mucous transformation of epithelial cells. This is also true for prostatic epithelium (see Webber a). Apart from the present studies, no other work appears to have been reported on the effects of vitamin A on growth and maintenance of normal human prostatic epithelium in vitro.

Results; Effects of vitamin A on growth of normal prostatic epithelium in vitro show that vitamin A at low levels stimulates growth (Figure 7). The best growth is observed in cultures containing 0.1 U/ml vitamin A in culture medium, while levels above 5.0 U/ml are clearly toxic (Figure 7).

Ultrastructural changes observed in vitamin A exposed and control cultures are interesting. Prostatic epithelium when grown in commercial media lacking vitamin A, undergoes squamous metaplasia. At the ultrastructural level, these changes manifest themselves in the form of increased number of filaments and filament bundles. However, when vitamin A is added to the culture medium, the cells revert to a more glandular type of ultrastructure with abundant Golgi complex and fewer filaments (Webber a). This configuration is similar to the ultrastructure of normal epithelium in vivo. A study of the ultrastructure has been a very useful tool for assessing the physiological well-being of the cell and changes induced in the ultrastructure can be correlated with the treatment to which the cells are exposed (Webber 1975). Effects of vitamin A at

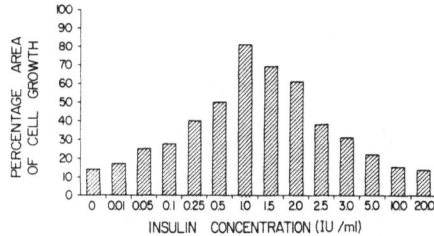

Figure 6. Histogram showing the effects of insulin on the growth of normal human prostatic epithelium in vitro. Thirteen different concentrations of insulin were tested. Results show a classic dose response. Growth of cells increases with the increase in the amount of insulin and reaches a peak at 1.0 IU/ml. Levels greater than 5.0 IU/ml insulin are toxic. Age of cell donor - 21 years. (From Webber and Prasad.)

154

the ultrastructural level have been described in detail elsewhere (Webber a).

Discussion: Results show that vitamin A clearly stimulates growth of normal human prostatic epithelium at low doses, prevents metaplasia and regulates the normal course of differentiation. Vitamin A possibly controls the rate of cell multiplication and differentiation in secretory epithelium and restores the normal balance of the two processes (Lasnitzki 1963).

There is considerable interest currently in the possible therapeutic use of retinoids (vitamin A and its synthetic analogs) against tumors of epithelial origin. Certain retinoids have the ability to inhibit carcinogenesis, to reverse preneoplastic hyperplasia induced by carcinogens and to inhibit growth of tumor cells. However, it is important to remember that the effects of vitamin A on mitotic activity and DNA synthesis vary and depend on the dose level. Generally lower doses stimulate and higher doses inhibit mitosis. Growth stimulation in prostatic epithelium at very low doses has been observed and optimum stimulation occurred at 0.1 U/ml level (1.0 U = 0.3 μg retinyl acetate) (Webber a). However. inhibition of DNA synthesis occurred in mouse epidermal cells at 12.5 μg/ml (Yuspa and Harris 1974), which is 416 times greater than the level where stimulation is observed. Consideration should be given to differences between species and cell types. It should also be kept in mind that the increased growth may be the result of a combination of increased mitotic activity and reduced rate of cell death. Further work must be done to establish the effects of vitamin A, using a wide range of dose levels, on DNA, RNA and protein synthesis in normal human prostatic epithelium and

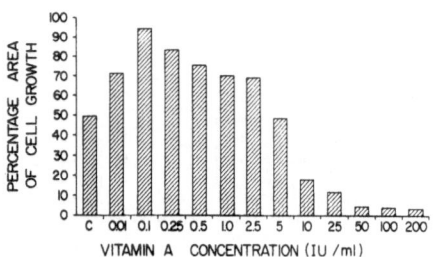

Figure 7. Histogram showing the effects of vitamin A (retinol acetate) on the growth of normal, human prostatic epithelium in vitro. C refers to control cultures. Results show that vitamin A at a level of 0.1 U/ml stimulates good growth of these cell in vitro. 5.0 U/ml and higher levels of vitamin A are toxic. Age of cell donor - 21 years. (From Webber a.)

the complex interactions of vitamin A with other growth factors.

6. Effects of 5α-dihydrotestosterone (5α-DHT).

Introduction: Prostatic epithelium in vivo, is under the growth control exerted by testosterone. Testosterone is required for its growth, renewal, maintenance and secretory activity. Certain testosterone metabolites, particularly 5α-DHT, actively affect these target cells and control their cell division.

Almost all of the experimental work in vivo and in vitro, on the effects of testosterone on the prostate, has been done on mice and rats (Edwards et al. 1976, Webber 1980a). Lasnitzki (1963) was one of the earliest investigators who made detailed studies on the effects of testosterone in organ cultures of mouse prostate. In the absence of testosterone, the cultures showed regressive changes in alveolar epithelium which were prevented if the medium was supplemented with testosterone propionate. It restored the secretory activity and the morphology to normal and also induced a mild epithelial hyperplasia.

In vitro studies on the effects of testosterone on the human prostate are recent and few (see Webber 1980a), Webber and Bouldin b). All of these studies were made on benign or malignant epithelium, primarily, to determine tumor sensitivity for therapeutic purposes. Studies on the use of testosterone or its metabolites for growth and maintenance of normal prostatic epithelial cells were not made. Hence, the present observations on normal human prostatic epithelium may be considered pioneer studies.

Results: 5α-DHT has a distinct and well marked stimulatory effect on prostatic epithelium (Figure 8). Results consistently show that 0.1 μg/ml 5α-DHT in culture medium induces growth of prostatic epithelial cells. Concentrations above 10 μg/ml are toxic. This toxicity is indicated at the ultrastructural level by a large number of autophagosomes (Webber and Bouldin b).

Discussion: When 5α-DHT is added to the culture medium, increase in cell growth occurs. Many animal studies support the present observations made on the effects of 5α-DHT in prostatic epithelial cells. It is the active metabolite of testosterone, and is a potent androgen and mitogen for target cells. It induces cell proliferation in animal and human prostatic epithelium.

7. Effects of other growth factors Effects of epidermal growth factor (EGF) and polyamines have also been investigated. Due to limited space these will not be discussed in detail here. It would suffice to say that EGF enhances the growth of prostatic epithelium at levels of 10 to 30 ng/ml. Beyond this level, there was no further enhancement. EGF also increases the lifespan of prostatic epithelial cultures.

Another area of major interest to us at the present time is growth regulation of prostatic epithelium by polyamines and their possible role in the etiology of benign and malignant disease of the prostate. It should be noted that prostate produces large amounts of two polyamines, spermine and spermidine. Effects of putrescine and spermine on the growth of prostatic epithelium in vitro are currently being investigated (Webber and Chaproniere-Rickenberg 1980).

C. Characterization

Once the cells have been isolated and established in vitro, it is necessary to prove that these cells indeed are of prostatic epithelial origin. Efforts have been made to characterize prostatic epithelial cells on the basis of a variety of their unique physiological, secretory and morphological characteristics. Our methods for characterization of prostatic epithelium by cytochemical localization of prostatic acid phosphatase were described earlier (Stonington et al. 1975, 1978, Webber 1979a). One of these methods is based on the greater resistance to inhibition of prostatic acid phosphatase by 10% neutral buffered formaldehyde, than other acid phosphatases. Results show (Webber 1979a) that even after 24 hour immersion in cold 10% formalin, the acid phosphatase activity in prostatic epithelium is still present.

III. MALIGNANT CELL MODELS

It was mentioned earlier that in vitro models using malignant cells are useful for testing the effectiveness of different modes of treatment: for developing

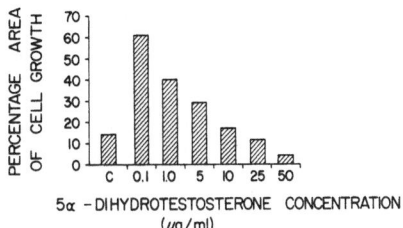

Figure 8. Histogram showing the effects of 5α-dihydrotestosteron (5α-DHT) on the growth of normal, human prostatic epithelium in vitro. 0.1 μg/ml DHT stimulated good growth of these cells in vitro. With increasing levels, growth declines and levels above 25 μg/ml DHT in culture medium are toxic. (From Webber and Bouldin b.)

more effective drugs for chemotherapy of prostatic cancer; for predicting the response of a given tumor to treatment, and for studying the biology of cancer cells.

Treatment of prostatic cancer, until recently, has primarily been based on surgical removal of the prostate when the tumor is localized within the prostate and anti-androgen therapy, when the tumor has spread beyond the capsule. The discovery of anti-androgen therapy was a major milestone in the treatment of prostatic cancer. However, we now know that although hormone therapy has great palliative value for the patient, it is not effective in all forms of prostatic cancer and it does not cure the disease. In fact, almost all patients on hormone therapy eventually become resistant to this mode of treatment, due to progression of the disease. Twenty percent of prostatic cancer cases do not respond to hormone therapy at all and the remaining 80% eventually become hormone resistant and the tumor continues to grow inspite of the anti-androgen therapy including orchiectomy, adrenalectomy and hypophysectomy (Franks 1976). We do not have adequate systems as yet to assess the response of the tumor to a certain treatment and thus establish the appropriate course of therapy. In vitro cell models can be of great use in this area.

The significance of developing in vitro human cell models is obvious since this is the closest we can get to the in vivo situation in man (see Webber 1980b). In vitro models, using human prostatic cancer cells, have not been available until very recently. Three human cell lines (Lubaroff 1977, Kaighn et al. 1979, Stone et al. 1978) are now available but their usefulness as a test system still must be established. A brief discussion of these and earlier cell lines is appropriate here.

The MA-160 cell line first became available for investigations in 1970. This cell line was reported to have arisen from tissue cultures of a human benign prostatic adenoma. The cells were thought to have undergone transformation in vitro. This cell line is, however, suspected to have been contaminated with HeLa cells (Nelson-Rees and Flandermeyer 1976, Webber et al. 1977). Then in 1974, EB33 cell line, derived from a human prostatic carcinoma came into existence (Okada et al. 1974). However, doubts still exist as to the fidelity of this cell line and its true origin. It has been suggested that EB33 may also have been contaminated with HeLa cells.

HPC-36 cell line was derived from a tissue specimen removed from a patient at the time of cryosurgical treatment. The isolated cells showed acid. phosphatase activity. Although these cells in culture showed loss of contact inhibition, considerable work still needs to be done to establish their human, prostatic, malignant epithelial origin. Cells derived from primary site of the tumor, i.e., the prostate, are not the most reliable, since one is likely to obtain a mixture of normal, benign and malignant cells from the prostate. Cell line PC-3 (Kaighn et al. 1979) was derived from a poorly differentiated adenocarcinoma of the prostate from a 62 year old Caucasian man, at the time of autopsy. The cells form colonies in soft agar, indicating their transformed nature. Karyotypic analysis shows that the cells are aneuploid with a modal number of 58 chromosomes at passage 30. The karotype and quinacrine banding patterns are different from those of HeLa cells although the Y chromosome is absent (Nelson-Rees personal communication). Cells produce subcutaneous tumors in nude mice. In culture, these cells have reduced serum requirement and do not respond to androgens. With further characterization, if fidelity of this cell line can be established, then it can be used for the evaluation of various modes of therapy for prostatic cancer. The cell line DU-145 (Stone et al. 1978) was derived from a metastatic lesion in the brain, from a 69 year old patient with widespread metastatic carcinoma of the prostate. The pathological diagnosis of the removed brain lesion was prostatic adenocarcinoma. These cells have been kept in culture for over two years. Cells grow in soft agar and form colonies. This cell line is not hormone sensitive and shows a weakly positive staining reaction for acid phosphatase. In passage 57, the modal chromosome number was 64, and Y chromosome was present with a translocated fragment from another chromosome.

The metastatic origin of DU-145 and PC-3 cell lines removes any doubt about the malignant origin of these cells. Both DU-145 (Mickey et al. 1977) and PC-3 (Kaighn et al. 1979) have been transplanted into nude mice. The resulting tumors show the same cell morphology as the tumor of origin. This provides another model system for studying therapy and tumor progression.

IV. COMMENTS, CONCLUSIONS AND FUTURE RESEARCH

1. Normal cell models The findings presented here, on a human cell model using normal prostatic epithelium, may be summarized as follows:

i. Isolation of normal, viable, post-pubertal, human prostatic epithelium has been accomplished. Vigorously growing cultures can be obtained from isolated acini.

ii. Medium $RPMI_{1640}$ containing a combination of horse and fetal bovine serum supports good growth and maintenance of these cells in vitro.

iii. Insulin selectively enhances growth of prostatic epithelium but inhibits growth of fibroblasts. This effect is useful for selection of epithelial cells. Insulin is an important growth regulator for prostatic epithelium and it potentiates the effects of testosterone.

iv. Vitamin A is necessary for growth and maintenance of normal ultrastructural morphology of prostatic epithelium and it selectively enhances growth of these cells at low dose levels.

v. 5α-dihydrotestosterone induces cell division in prostatic epithelium in culture. Its role in cell differentiation is being investigated.

vi. Epidermal growth factor increases growth and lifespan of prostatic epithelium in culture. Spermine also selectively enhances growth and lifespan of prostatic epithelium but indirectly inhibits growth of fibroblasts.

vii. Cells grown from explants and isolated acini have been characterized by cytochemical localization of prostatic acid phosphatase. The test is based on the greater stability of prostatic acid phosphatase in neutral buffered formalin than other acid phosphatases.

Studies described in this paper were all made on primary cultures. Efforts are now being made to subculture these cells. Subcultivation will be greatly facilitated by what we now know about the growth requirements of these cells in vitro. Studies on the importance of stromal-epithelial interaction are in progress. Considerable effort is also needed in finding additional specific markers for characterization of prostatic epithelium.

The next goal in the development of this model system is to develop a totally defined medium. It must be kept in mind that we are dealing with post-pubertal, hormone responsive cells. Thus, media which may support growth of fetal or neo-natal prostatic epithelium will not necessarily be adequate for the adult epithelium. Considerable amount of work still needs to be done in order to develop a completely chemically defined medium. However, such defined media should be designed not just for rapid growth but also for maintenance.

It is hoped that studies using the described in vitro cell model will make it possible to examine the early steps in human prostatic carcinogenesis; the carcinogen-target cell interaction; metabolic activation of specific carcinogens and the role of multiple agents and co-carcinogens in transformation. Such human cell models can also be used for screening suspected carcinogenic and toxic environmental agents. The use of these cells for studies on cell nutrition, metabolism, growth and aging in hormone dependent cells is promising.

2. Malignant cell models The usefulness of in vitro cell models for testing modes of treatment, for predicting response to therapy and for screening drugs for their effectiveness against prostatic cancer has already been emphasized. When developing a malignant cell system, be it an in vivo or in vitro system, it is important to bear in mind that the maintenance of biological and physiological characteristics of the tumor is important. Otherwise, investigations may lead to misleading conclusions. The in vitro human cell systems do have several advantages over the in vivo systems because they are more practical, economical and reliable and their use is preferred and is logical since they are of human origin. Thus one does not have the problem of species differences.

Most therapeutic agents like hormones, drugs and x-rays do not destroy all tumor cells. This results in a population of cells which is insensitive to the treatment and is responsible for the growth of the tumor and recurrences, which are resistant to that treatment. This population could be killed by increasing the dose of the drug or x-rays. However, higher doses are also lethal to normal cells. In vitro models can be used to determine and select the mode of treatment to which the tumor is most sensitive. Studies that seem promising at the present time include the effectiveness of the synergism between drugs. Even more promising and worthwhile are investigations on the use of non-toxic substances which may potentiate the effect of drugs or x-rays even when they are used at low dose levels. This would eliminate the need for using large doses of toxic chemotherapeutic agents while still achieving greater toxicity for tumor cells and lower toxicity for the patient as a whole.

An important observation on DU-145 and PC-3 cell lines is that they were both shown to be unresponsive to hormones. This feature is significant because although a majority of prostatic carcinomas are initially responsive to hormone therapy, they eventually become unresponsive. It is these unresponsive cells that are responsible for recurrence of the disease, for widespread metastases and for death of the cancer patient. Therefore, a study of these cells is of utmost importance. In order to bring about an effective control of these cells, it is particularly important to find the drugs to which these cells are sensitive. Therefore, the fact that these cells are unresponsive to hormones, should not in anyway distract from the usefulness of these cell models.

Another point worth noting is that cell lines PC-3 and DU-145 have been derived from metastatic tumors from sites other than the prostate. This essentially makes them pure cultures of malignant prostatic epithelial cells since there is no possibility of contaminating them with normal or benign cells, which can occur, if the tissue specimen for culture was taken from the primary site.

Cell lines described above (DU-145, PC-3, HPC-36) have not so far been used for evaluating the effectiveness of different modes of treatment; for testing synergism between drugs or for testing new drugs. This work remains to be done in the future and it is hoped that these model systems will make significant contributions in the area of treatment for prostatic cancer.

Interest in chemotherapy of prostatic cancer is a recent development and only 10% of the currently available drugs have been tested against prostatic cancer (Murphy and Merrin 1976). Considerable amount of work, therefore, needs to be done in this area. Also, continued major effort is needed in the development of several in vitro and in vivo models because no single model will be adequate for all the answers we need on the etiology, carcinogenesis, progression and treatment of prostatic cancer in man.

ACKNOWLEDGEMENTS

The author wishes to thank Thomas Bouldin, Lucy Jankowsky and Robert McGrew for their assistance in completing this work; Dr. Robert Donohue for supplying normal tissue; the Veterans' Administration Hospital for the use of their electron microscopy facility; the Department of Molecular Cellular and Developmental Biology for the use of their Scanning electron microscope; Richard Carter for his help in the preparation of photographs and Fidelia Maez and Carol Williams for their help in the preparation of this manuscript.

This work was supported by the Division of Cancer Cause and Prevention, National Cancer Institute, DHEW Contract No. NO 1-CP-65849.

REFERENCES

Cuatrecasas P: Insulin receptors, cell membranes and hormone action. Biochem Pharmacol 23: 2353, 1974.

Edwards WD, Bates RR, Yuspa SH: Organ cultures of rodent prostate: Effects of polyamines and testosterone. Invest Urol 14: 1, 1976.

Franks LM: The natural history of prostatic cancer. In: Marberger H, Haschek H, Schirmer HKA, Colston JAC, Witkin E, eds. New York: In: Prostatic disease, progress in clinical and biological research. Alan R Liss 6: 103, 1976.

Gospodarowicz D, Moran JS: Stimulation of division of sparse and confluent 3T3 cell populations by a fibroblast growth factor, dexamethasone and insulin. Proc Nat Acad Sci 71: 4584, 1974.

Griffith JB: The effect of insulin on the growth and metabolism of the human diploid cell, WI-38. J Cell Sci 7: 575, 1970.

Hollenberg MD, Fryklund L: Insulin and somatomedins A and B: comparison of biological activities in cultured human skin-derived fibroblasts. Life Sciences 21: 943, 1977.

Hunt EL, Bailey DW: The effects of alloxan diabetes on the reproductive system of young male rats. Acta Endocrinol 38: 432, 1961.

Ichihara I: Some ultrastructural effects of testosterone and insulin on the ventral prostate of rats in organ culture. Cell Tiss Res 181: 327, 1977.

Johansson R: RNA, protein and DNA synthesis stimulated by testosterone, insulin and prolactin in the rat ventral prostate cultured in chemically defined medium. Acta Endocrinol 80: 761, 1975.

Kaighn ME, Narayan S, Ohnuki Y, Lechner JF: Establishment and characterization of a huma prostatic carcinoma cell line (PC-3). Invest Urol 17: 16, 1979.

Lasfargues EY: Cultivation and behavior in vitro of the normal mammary epithelium of the adult mouse. Anat Rec 127: 117, 1957.

Lasnitzki I: Growth patterns of the mouse prostate glands in organ cultures and its response to sex hormones, vitamin A and 3-methylcholanthrene. In: Biology of the prostate and related tissues, Vollmer EP, ed. Nat Cancer Inst Monogr 12: 381, 1963.

Lechner JF, Narayan KS, Ohnuki Y, Babcock MS, Jones LW, Kaighn ME: Replicative epithelial cell cultures from normal human prostate gland: brief communication. J Nat Cancer Inst 60: 797, 1978.

Lubaroff DM: Development of an epithelial tissue culture line form human prostatic adenocarcinoma. J Urol 118: 612, 1977.

Mandl I: Collagenase comes of age. In: Collagenase, 1st Interdiscip. Symp. on Collagenase. Mandl I, ed. New York: Gordon and Breech Science 1972, pp 1-15.

Mickey DD, Stone KR, Wunderli H, Mickey GH, Vollmer RT, Paulson DF: Heterotransplantation of a human prostatic adenocarcinoma cell line in nude mice. Cancer Res 37: 4049, 1977.

Murphy GP, Merrin CE: Chemotherapy of advanced prostatic cancer today. In: Prostatic Disease, Progress in Clinical and Biological Research. Marberger H, Haschek H, Schirmer HKA, Colston JAC, Witkin E, eds. New York: Alan R Liss. 6: 285, 1976.

Nelson-Rees WA, Flandermeyer RR: HeLa cultures defined. Science 191: 96, 1976.

Okada K. Schröder FH: Human prostatic carcinoma in cell culture: preliminary reports on the development and characterization of an epithelial cell line (EB33). Urol Res 2: 111, 1974.

Porter KR, Todaro GJ, Fonte V: A scanning electron microscope study of surface features of viral and spontaneous transformants of mouse BALB/3T3 cells. J Cell Biol 59: 633, 1973.

Poché PA, Webber MM, Jankowsky L: A rapid method for in situ staining of prostatic and other tissue culture cells. Stain Technol 49: 229, 1974.

Rillema JA, Linebaugh BE: Characteristics of the insulin stimulation of DNA, RNA and protein metabolism in cultured human mammary carcinoma cells. Biochim Biophys Acta 475: 74, 1977.

Sanefuji H, Heatfield BM, Trump BF: Studies on carcinogenesis of human prostate. I. Technique for long-term explant cultures. TCA Manual 4: 855, 1978.

Stone KR, Mickey DD, Wunderli H, Mickey GH, Paulson DF: Isolation of a human prostate carcinoma cell line. Int J Cancer 21: 274, 1978.

Stonington OG, Szwec N, Webber M: Isolation and identification of the human malignant prostatic epithelial cell in pure monolayer culture. J Urol 114: 903, 1975.

Stonington OG, Szwec N, Webber M: Identification of cultured, human malignant prostatic epithelial cells. Nat Cancer Inst Monogr 49: 31, 1978.

Walsh PC: Benign prostatic hyperplasia: etiological considerations. In: Prostatic disease, progress in clinical and biological research. Marberger H, Haschek H, Schirmer HKA, Colston JAC, Witkin E, eds. New York: Alan R Liss. 6: 1, 1976.

Webber MM: Effects of serum on the growth of prostatic cells in vitro. J Urol 112: 798, 1974.

Webber MM: Ultrastructural changes in human prostatic epithelium grown in vitro. J Ultrastruct Res 50: 89, 1975.

Webber MM: Normal and benign human prostatic epithelium in culture. I. Isolation. In Vitro 15: 967, 1979a.

Webber MM: Growth and maintenance of normal prostatic epithelium in vitro – a human cell model. In: Models for Prostate Cancer. Murphy GP, ed. New York: Alan R Liss. 1980a, pp 181-216.

Webber MM: In vitro models for prostate cancer. In: Models for Prostate Cancer. Murphy GP, ed. New York: Alan R. Liss. 1980b, pp 133-147.

Webber MM: Growth and maintenance of normal human prostatic epithelium in vitro. IV. Effects of vitamin A. In preparation, a

Webber MM, Batts AF: Cultivation of human prostatic epithelium – present status. In Vitro 13: 143, 1977.

Webber MM, Bouldin TR: Ultrastructure of human prostatic epithelium – secretion granules or virus particles? Invest Urol 14: 482, 1977.

Webber MM, Bouldin TR: Growth and maintenance of normal human prostatic epithelium in vitro. V. Effects of testosterone and 5α-dihydrotestosterone, In preparation, b.

Webber MM, Chaproniere-Rickenberg, D: Spermine oxidation products are selectively toxic to fibroblasts in cultures of normal human prostatic epithelium. Cell Biol Internat Rep 4: 185, 1980.

Webber MM, Donohue RE, Jankowsky L: Growth and maintenance of normal human prostatic epithelium in vitro. I. Effects of serum In preparation, c.

Webber MM, Horan PK, Bouldin TR: Present status on MA-160 cell line - prostatic epithelium or HeLa cells? Invest Urol 14: 335, 1977.

Webber MM, Jankowsky L: Growth and maintenance of normal human prostatic epithelium in vitro. II. Effects of different media and glutamine. In preparation.

Webber MM, Prasad KN: Growth and maintenance of normal human prostatic epithelium in vitro. III. Effects of insulin. In preparation.

Webber MM, Stonington OG: Hypocellularity in organ cultures of human prostate - application in epithelial cell isolation. J Urol 114: 246, 1975.

Webber MM, Stonington OG, Poché PA: Epithelial outgrowth from syspension cultures of human prostatic tissue. In Vitro 10: 196, 1974.

Webber MM, Webber PJ: The use of a television scanning densitometer for measuring growth in stained cell cultures, in preparation.

Yuspa SH, Harris CC: Altered differentiation of mouse epidermal cells treated with retinyl acetate in vitro. Exp Cell Res 86: 95, 1974.

14. ANDROGEN REGULATION IN THE PROSTATE OF RHESUS MONKEY (MACACA MULATTA)

R. GHANADIAN

I. INTRODUCTION

The search for a suitable animal prostate similar to that of the human to be employed as an experimental model for prostatic research has been most desirable. The lack of an appropriate animal model to produce results relevant to the human prostate has seriously hampered the progress towards the elucidation of many aspects of hormonal manipulation and drug treatment. Much attention has recently been given to the prostate of the rhesus monkey and its potential in prostatic research. This is mainly due to the significant resemblance between the prostate in this primate and that of the human. The prostate gland of the rhesus monkey lies on the dorsal aspect of the urethra and the neck of the bladder. It consists of two discrete lobes; a cranial and a caudal (Figure 1) (Price 1963, Blacklock and Bouskill 1977). The surface of the cranial entity is deeply furrowed, which closely resembles the seminal vesicles of the monkey in external appearance. The caudal lobe is more closely associated with the urethra and has a smooth surface. The cranial and caudal lobes are separated peripherally, but anteromedially the two lobes merge where the duct from the caudal lobe in company with the common ejaculatory ducts penetrates the flat surface of the caudal lobe before passing through the wall of the urethra at the level of the verumontanum. The cranial lobe is easily separable from the seminal vesicles above and surrounds the terminal vas deferens and the duct of the seminal vesicles on each side, as these pass downwards and forwards to the urethra (Blacklock and Bouskill 1977). Price (1963) has reported significant differences in the histological appearance of the cranial and caudal lobes. These differences have been studied in more detail by Blacklock and

Bouskill (1977) and Battersby et al. (1977).

A comparative study of the prostates in both monkey and man has revealed remarkable similarities between the prostates of these two species. Blacklock (1977) compared the cranial and caudal lobes of the monkey prostate with that of central and peripheral zones of the human prostate. The latter regional subdivision of the human prostate was originally suggested by McNeal (1968). Based on anatomical and histological observations, Blacklock and Bouskill (1977) suggested that the cranial lobe in the monkey prostate could be equated to the human peripheral zone. This anatomical and histological resemblance of the human to the monkey tissues provides a reasonable basis for using the monkey prostate in prostatic research. However, many of the hormonal aspects of the monkey prostate have not yet been fully investigated, and information regarding the mechanism of action of steroid hormones in this prostate is limited.

In this chapter an attempt has been made to review the available data on the regulation of androgens in the prostate of the rhesus monkey (macaca mulatta).

II. ANDROGENS IN CIRCULATING BLOOD AND PROSTATIC TISSUES

In the studies of production and secretion of androgens in the male rhesus monkey, primary consideration must be given to the seasonal rhythm of the hormone levels. There is now good evidence to suggest that both the production rate (Wickings and Nieschlag 1977) and plasma level (Gordon et al. 1976) of testosterone reach a peak during October, this being the breeding season. Wickings and Nieschlag (1977) reported the production rate to be 3.1 mg/day during October whilst in April and August it was constant at 1.2 mg/day. These values would appear to be lower than those observed in adult men, which range from 5-7 mg/day. When differences in weight between the monkey and man are taken into consideration the apparent production rate in monkey becomes 0.5 mg testosterone/kg/day, whilst that in man is 0.1 mg/kg/day. In the same group of monkeys the plasma testosterone

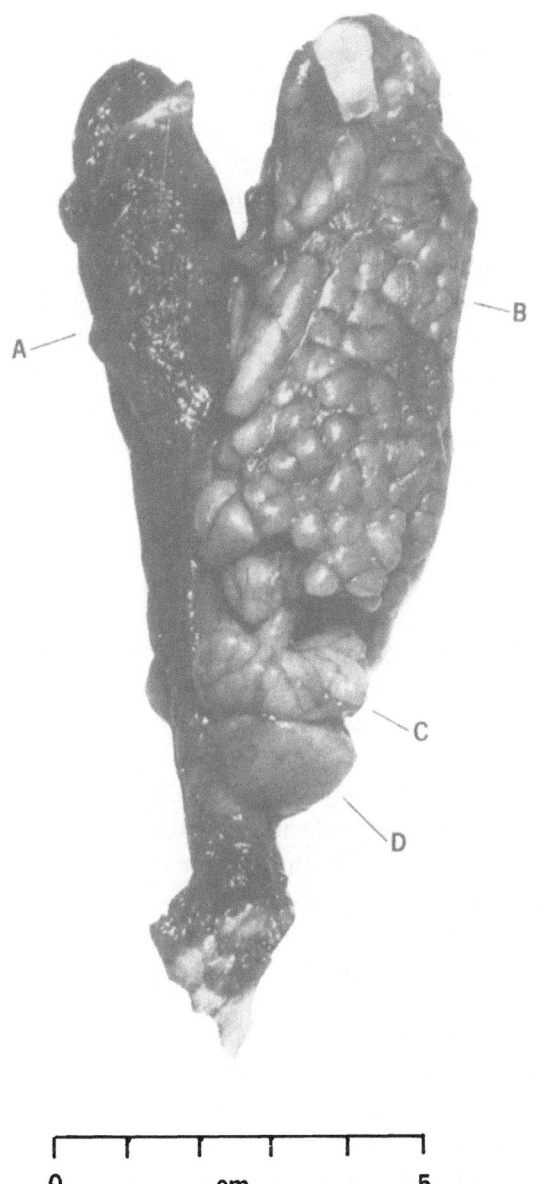

Figure 1. Lateral view of the lobes of the rhesus monkey prostate which lies on the posterior aspect of the urethra. A) bladder B) seminal vesicles C) cranial lobe of the prostate D) caudal lobe of the prostate. The two lobes are easily separable peripherally and the duct of the seminal vesicle with the vas deferens can be seen to pass into the upper aspect of the cranial lobe.

levels increased from 162 ng/100 ml in April to 253 ng/100 ml in August and finally reached its peak of 371 ng/100 ml in October (Wickings and Nieschlag 1977). Other reports have indicated the lowest levels during April (Gordon et al. 1976, Plant et al. 1974, Michael and Bonsall 1977). Apart from the seasonal factor, environmental as well as social consideration should be taken into account. Notable amongst the latter is the presence or absence of a female partner (Rose et al. 1972, Bernstein et al. 1977, Phoenix et al. 1977).

In a three year study of the seasonal rhythm in plasma level on a breeding group of rhesus monkeys, the level of plasma testosterone in the male animals showed considerable variation (Gordon et al. 1976). The mean testosterone values for seven monkeys peaked in October or November of each year at 1200 ng/100 ml whereas in the spring and summer months the mean testosterone value dropped to 200 ng/100 ml. Furthermore, there is a distinctive diurnal variation in serum testosterone level in monkeys characterised by a lower value during the day and a marked increase in the early evening with the maximum level in the early hours of the morning (Michael et al. 1974, Perachio et al. 1977, Rose et al. 1978). Apart from the aforementioned changes, account must be taken of the variation between the individual animals. Aso et al. (1976) reported a range of 317-1030 ng/100 ml in ten monkeys age range 7-22 years. Other serum androgens reported by this group included dihydrotestosterone (132-227 ng/100 ml), androstenedione (76.5-121 ng/100 ml) and dehydroepiandrosterone (746-1790 ng/100 ml).

A trend towards seasonal variation which is similar to that of testosterone has been reported for plasma dihydrotestosterone levels by Robinson et al. (1975). They found plasma dihydrotestosterone levels to be between 20-30 per cent of the plasma testosterone. However, these investigators did not determine whether or not the dihydrotestosterone concentration was a result of direct testicular secretion, target tissue metabolism or the combined effects of these two. The level of dihydrotestosterone reported for monkey appears to be considerably higher than human (Lewis et al. 1976, Vermeulen 1976).

There is a paucity of information with regard to the androgen levels within the monkey prostate.

However, preliminary studies on a series of eight monkeys in the author's laboratory have indicated the level of dihydrotestosterone to be between 7-15 ng/g tissue in caudal lobe and 6.9-13.0 ng/g tissue in the cranial (Ghanadian and Papadopoulos 1980).

III. METABOLISM OF ANDROGENS IN THE PROSTATE

The available data on the metabolism of androgens in the monkey prostate is limited. Arora-Dinakar et al. (1977) studied the in vitro metabolism of ^{3}H-testosterone in the prostate and other sex accessory organs. They found 5α-dihydrotestosterone to be the main radiometabolite in the prostate, seminal vesicles, epididymis, bulbo-urethral gland and ductus deferens. In this study no reference was made to the lobal differences of the prostate gland in this primate.

In our studies, when caudal and cranial lobes of the prostate were incubated with ^{3}H testosterone at 37°C for 90 mins without added cofactors, the major radiometabolite in both lobes of the gland was 5α-dihydrotestosterone. This is shown in Table 1. Initial separation of radiometabolites were obtained by thin layer chromatography, which was subsequently confirmed by gas liquid chromatography (Smith and Ghanadian 1979). It appears from this data that there is remarkable similarity in the ability of the caudal and cranial lobes of the gland to metabolise testosterone to its major 5α-reduced metabolite.

In this study a comparison was made between the metabolism of ^{3}H testosterone in the caudal and cranial lobes of the prostate with that in the liver as control tissue. However, no attempt was made to determine the actual concentration of the enzyme, nor their localisation with the lobes of the prostate or liver. The finding that both lobes of the monkey prostate have an active 5α-reductase system for the conversion of testosterone to 5α-dihydrotestosterone appears to suggest that the metabolism of testosterone within these tissues could be an essential pre-requisite to the binding of androgens and the subsequent action of androgens in this target organ. It was interesting to note that in the monkey liver the main radiometabolite was androstenedione (56.7%) whilst approximately 25% of the ^{3}H testosterone remained unmetabolised. The conversion of testosterone to 5α-dihydrotestosterone and further to androstanediols was only 5-6% of the total radiometabolites in the liver. This result would suggest negligible 5α-reductase activity in the monkey liver. Data on the activity of this enzyme in the liver of other species is very limited although the presence of this enzyme in rat liver has been reported (Tomkins 1957).

IV. UPTAKE OF ANDROGENS BY THE PROSTATE

An in vitro uptake study has been performed on the caudal and cranial lobes of the prostate which has indicated a differential ability for these tissues to take up and retain androgens (Ghanadian et al. 1977a). In this study slices of prostate and other tissues were incubated with ^{3}H testosterone at 37°C for one hour, and subsequently for a further hour in hormone free media. The uptake of radioactivity by the two lobes of the prostate was measured, and the results were compared with those of seminal vesicle, urethra and liver (Figure 2). These results showed a significantly higher ($p < 0.001$) uptake of radioactivity by the caudal lobe when compared with the cranial lobe. The cranial lobe appeared to take up radioactivity in the same order of magnitude as the seminal vesicles. It is interesting to note that the seminal vesicle resembles the cranial lobe in its appearance. The uptake of the tritiated androgen by the liver was also high. However, we have shown in metabolic studies that the radioactivity retained in this tissue is almost exclusively confined to

Table 1. Metabolites of ^{3}H testosterone recovered from rhesus monkey tissues, following in vitro incubation of tissues (250 mg) with 100 nM ^{3}H testosterone for 90 min at 37°C and subsequent extraction and analysis by G.L.C. (Smith and Ghanadian 1979).

Steroid recovered	% steroid recovered (mean $\pm$ SEM)		
	Caudal prostate	Cranial prostate	Liver
Dihydrotestosterone	46.2$\pm$6.2	48.6$\pm$4.7	3.9$\pm$1.0
Androstanediols	30.0$\pm$5.1	27.1$\pm$4.2	2.3$\pm$0.5
Testosterone	8.8$\pm$5.1	8.6$\pm$6.5	25.1$\pm$3.6
Androsterone	5.8$\pm$0.1	6.4$\pm$0.4	2.2$\pm$1.1
Androstanedione	3.7$\pm$0.4	4.9$\pm$0.5	5.3$\pm$1.7
Androstenedione	1.2$\pm$0.4	1.3$\pm$0.6	56.7$\pm$3.8
Unidentified	4.2$\pm$0.6	3.1$\pm$0.2	4.5$\pm$1.1

androstenedione and testosterone, but not dihydro-testosterone as is the case for caudal and cranial tissues. Previous studies using liver from other species as a control tissue have shown that prolonged washing of the liver tissue tends to remove the radioactivity far more effectively than in androgen target tissues (Ghanadian et al. 1976). Furthermore, in this study, when excess unlabelled testosterone (100 fold) was introduced in the incubation media, the uptake of radioactive hormone by caudal and cranial lobes of the prostate was significantly reduced, whereas the uptake of radioactivity by the liver or muscle was unaffected. This could be considered as an indication for the presence of specific binding sites within both lobes of the prostate and its absence in the liver. When 1000-fold excess of unlabelled testosterone was included in the incubation media, the uptake of radioactivity by the caudal lobe of the gland was further suppressed, whereas no increased suppression was observed with the cranial lobe, suggesting a greater responsiveness of the caudal lobe to androgenic stimulation.

Karr et al. (1978) has reported the uptake of ³H oestradiol-17β by the cranial lobe of the baboon prostate to be 2-3 times higher than by caudal lobe. Although this study was carried out in baboons, it

is interesting to note that the response to oestradiol-17β in the caudal and cranial lobes is converse to that of testosterone in the rhesus monkey. However, further studies with other steroids are required to substantiate this pattern within the rhesus monkey prostate.

V. ANDROGEN RECEPTORS IN THE PROSTATE

Attempts have been made to investigate whether or not the mechanism of action of androgens in the monkey prostate was comparable to that reported for prostatic tissues in other species. The available data is restricted to the presence of a cytoplasmic androgen binding component. Ghanadian et al. (1977b) reported on the presence of an androgen binding protein in the cytosol fraction of both caudal and cranial lobes of the monkey prostate. In this study androgen receptors have been measured using synthetic androgen, Methyltrienolone (R 1881) which has been shown to be specific for androgen receptors in both human and rat prostates (Ghanadian et al. 1978, Bonne and Raynaud 1976). This study has shown that there is a marked difference between the receptor levels of the two lobes. They measured bound and free receptors and found the receptor content of the caudal lobe to be higher than that in the cranial lobe. This study was performed on a limited series of monkeys. The first two mature animals showed a significantly higher receptor population in the caudal lobe than that of the cranial lobe, whereas much smaller differences were observed between the two lobes of the third and fourth monkeys. The total receptor population in the third monkey was low but the free receptor was comparatively high. Although this monkey was a mature animal they noted that the testes were small. Finally the fourth monkey was an immature animal and demonstrated low receptor content in both lobes (Table 2).

It was interesting that there was a remarkable similarity between this study and the ³H testosterone uptake study, in that the results obtained for the caudal lobe were consistently higher than those in the cranial lobe.

Characterisation of the androgen receptor component has only been performed in the caudal lobe of the gland. The molecular weight of this

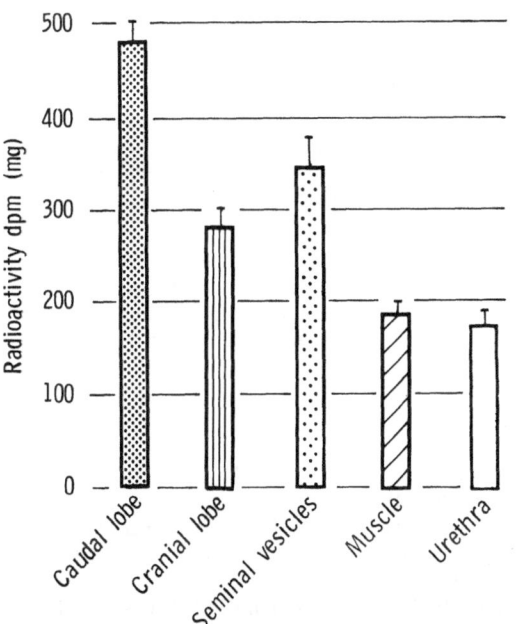

Figure 2. In vitro uptake of ³H testosterone (2.5 nM) by caudal and cranial lobes of the prostate and other tissues obtained from ten adult rhesus monkeys (Ghanadian et al. 1977a).

Table 2. Concentration of free and bound androgen receptors in the cytoplasmic fraction of the caudal and cranial lobes of the prostate from four rhesus monkeys. (Ghanadian et al. 1977b)

Monkey		Cranial lobe fmol/mg protein			Caudal lobe fmol/mg protein		
No	Age (year)	total	free	bound	total	free	bound
1	9	39.7	2.0	37.9	112.7	3.7	109.0
2	9	41.5	2.6	38.9	101.3	6.6	94.7
3	6	55.0	7.7	47.3	67.0	23.7	43.3
4	2	21.2	2.1	19.1	36.0	6.3	29.7

androgen binding protein has been reported to be $2.8\text{-}2.9 \times 10^5$ daltons which is of the same order of magnitude as that of the rat (Mainwaring 1969) and human prostate (Ghanadian et al. 1978). At the present time it appears that data on androgen receptors within the lobes of the rhesus monkey prostate is limited to the reference discussed above. However, Karr et al. (1978) have reported the presence of an oestrogen binding component having the characteristic features of a receptor within both lobes of the baboon prostate. These workers have not yet quantified the level of this oestrogen receptor in the individual lobes. Hence, at this stage, it is not possible to see whether the oestrogen receptor pattern in the two lobes of the baboon prostate will follow their reported uptake of oestradiol by these tissues. Based on the data reported for the uptake and binding of androgens in the rhesus monkey (Ghanadian et al. 1977a, Ghanadian et al. 1977b) it might be speculated that a similar situation might exist in the baboon, which would lead to the assumption that there is a higher level of oestrogen receptor in the cranial lobe of the gland. This being converse to the situation observed for the androgens in the rhesus monkey. However, more studies must be carried out to establish the relationship of the different classes of steroid hormones within these two lobes.

VI. CONCLUDING REMARKS

The present available data on the mechanism by which steroid hormones interact with prostatic tissue and thereby exert their biological action in the monkey prostate is limited. The primary information on the metabolism of testosterone in the prostatic tissue and the binding of androgens to cytoplasmic components suggest some similarities between the prostate of rhesus monkey and that reported for the human. This information is by no means sufficient to provide a basis for considering these tissues to be homologous in this respect. However, more comprehensive data on the anatomical and histological characters of the gland would indicate that there are major similarities between the caudal and cranial lobes of the rhesus monkey prostate when compared to the peripheral and central zones of the human prostate. Biochemical information regarding the zonal differences within the human prostate is an essential requirement if an homology with the lobes of the monkey prostate is to be further established. This information as yet has not been forthcoming. Despite the present paucity of information, the monkey prostate appears to present us with an appropriate model for prostatic research. However, the compound rhythmic variation of plasma androgen levels in this primate would indicate that some degree of caution must be taken for studies which involve androgens.

ACKNOWLEDGEMENT

I wish to express my appreciation to the members of the Prostate Research Laboratory and in particular to Mr. C.B. Smith for discussion and time spent in the preparation of this review. Thanks are also due to Mrs. Lynette Sofra for her secretarial assistance.

REFERENCES

Arora-Dinakar R, Dinakar N, Prasad MRN: Metabolism in vitro of ^{3}H testosterone in testis, epididymis and sex accessories of the rhesus monkey Macaca Mulatta: effects of cyproterone acetate on androgen metabolism. Indian J Exp Biol 15: 953-958, 1977.

Aso T, Concharov N, Cekan Z, Diczfalusy E: Plasma levels of unconjugated steroids in male baboons (Papio Hamadryas) and rhesus monkeys (Macaca Mulatta). Acta endocr (Kbh) 82: 644-651, 1976.

Battersby S, Chandler JA, Harper ME, Blacklock NJ: The ultrastructure of rhesus monkey prostate. Urol Res 5: 175-183, 1977.

Bernstein IS, Rose RM, Gordon RP: Behaviour and hormonal responses of male rhesus monkeys introduced to females in the breeding and non-breeding seasons. Anim Behav 25: 609-614, 1977.

Blacklock NJ: The morphology of the parenchyma of the prostate. Urol Res 5: 155-158, 1977.

Blacklock NJ, Bouskill K: The zonal anatomy of the prostate in man and in the rhesus monkey (Macaca Mulatta). Urol Res 5: 163-167, 1977.

Bonne C, Raynaud JP: Assay of androgen binding sites by exchange with methyltrienolone (R 1881). Steroids 27: 497-507, 1976.

Ghanadian R, Holland JM, Chisholm GD: Uptake and distribution of ^{3}H testosterone in tissues of male Praomys (mastomys) Natalensis: An in vivo and in vitro study on the prostate. Urol Res 4: 77-81, 1976.

Ghanadian R, Smith CB, Chisholm GD, Blacklock NJ: Differential androgen uptake by the lobes of the rhesus monkey prostate. Brit J Urol 49: 701-704, 1977a.

Ghanadian R, Auf G, Smith CB, Chisholm GD, Blacklock NJ: Androgen receptors in the prostate of rhesus monkey. Urol Res 5: 169-173, 1977b.

Ghanadian R, Auf G, Chaloner PJ, Chisholm GD: The use of methyltrienolone in the measurement of the free and bound cytoplasmic receptors for dihydrotestosterone in benign hypertrophied human prostate. J Steroid Biochem 9: 325-330, 1978.

Ghanadian R, Papadopoulos A: Testosterone and dihydrotestosterone levels in caudal and cranial lobes of the rhesus monkey prostate. 1980 (in preparation).

Gordon TP, Rose RM, Bernstein IS: Seasonal rhythm in plasma testosterone level in the rhesus monkey (Mucaca Mulatta): a three year study. Horm Behv 7: 229-243; 1976.

Karr JP, Sufrin G, Kirdani RY, Murphy GP, Sandberg AA: Prostatic binding of oestradiol-17β in the baboon. J Steroid Biochem 9: 87-94, 1978.

Lewis JG, Ghanadian R, Chisholm GD: Serum 5α-dihydrotestosterone and testosterone changes with age in man. Acta endocr (Kbh) 82: 444-448, 1976.

Mainwaring WIP: A soluble androgen receptor in the cytoplasm of rat ventral prostate. J Endocr 45: 531-541, 1969.

McNeal JE: Regional morphology and pathology of the prostate. Amer J clin Path 49: 347, 1968.

Michael RP, Setchell KDR, Plant TM: Diurnal changes in plasma testosterone and studies on plasma corticosteroids in non-anaesthetised male rhesus monkey (Macaca Mulatta). J Endocr 63: 325-335, 1974.

Michael RP, Bonsall RW: A 3 year study of an annual rhythm in plasma androgen levels in male rhesus monkey (Macaca Mulatta) in a constant laboratory environment. J Reprod Fertil 49: 129-131, 1977.

Perachio AA, Alexander M, Marr LD, Collins DC: Diurnal variation of serum testosterone level in intact and gonadectomised male and female rhesus monkey. Steroids 29: 21-33, 1977.

Poenix CH, Dixson AF, Resko JA: Effects of ejaculation on levels of testosterone, cortisol and luteinizing hormone in peripheral plasma of rhesus monkeys. J Comp Physiol Psychol 91: 120-127, 1977.

Plant TM, Zumpe D, Sauls M, Michael RP: An annual rhythm in the plasma testosterone of adult male rhesus monkeys maintained in the laboratory. J Endocr 62: 403-404, 1974.

Price D: Comparative aspects of development and structure in the prostate. Monogr nat Cancer Inst 12: 1, 1963.

Robinson JA, Scheffler G, Eisele SG, Goy RW: Effects of age and season on sexual behaviour and plasma testosterone and dihydrotestosterone concentrations of laboratory housed male rhesus monkeys (Macaca Mulatta). Biol Reprod 13: 203-210, 1975.

Rose RM, Gordon TP, Bernstein IS: Plasma testosterone levels in the male rhesus monkey: influences of sexual and social influence. Science 178: 643, 1972.

Rose RM, Gordon TP, Dernstein IS: Diurnal variation in plasma testosterone and cortisone in rhesus monkey living in social groups. J Endocr 76: 67-74, 1978.

Smith CB, Ghanadian R: Androgen metabolism within the lobes of rhesus monkey prostate. Europ Urol. (In press.)

Tomkins GM: The enzymatic reduction of Δ^4-3-Ketosteroid. J biol Chem 225: 13, 1957.

Vermeulen A: Testosterone and 5α-androstan-17β-ol-3-one (DHT) levels in man. Acta endocr (Kbh) 83: 651-644, 1976.

Wickings EJ, Nieschlag E: Testosterone production and metabolism in laboratory maintained rhesus monkey. Int J Fertil 22: 56-59, 1977.

15. EFFECTS OF CARCINOGENS AND RETINOIDS ON PROSTATIC EXPLANTS

D.P. CHOPRA and L.J. WILKOFF

I. INTRODUCTION

Prostate cancer is one of the leading causes of cancer related deaths in men over 50 years of age (Jackson et al. 1975). It is apparent that with an increasing number of older men in this country, more prostatic cancer patients will be seen and carcinima of the prostate will become the leading cause of death in men over 75 years of age. This prediction is further supported by the fact that an increasing number of chemicals, the long-term effects of which are not known, are being introduced into our already less-than-desirable environment. Inspite of its seriousness, the etiology of the carcinoma of the prostate remains unknown and treatment and prevention are inadequate.

Current evidence indicates that chemical agents are responsible for a majority of human cancers (Higginson and Muir 1973, Higginson 1977). Therapy of prostatic cancer has been limited to conventional treatments that include radiation therapy, orchiectomy, and estrogen therapy (Scott and Schirmer 1966). But the persistence of the lesions and the limited survival times of patients receiving these types of therapy indicate that these modalities may be primarily palliative. More recently, studies with antiandrogen and chemotherapeutic agents have been initiated (Scott and Wade 1969, Flocks and Cheng 1968, Eagan and Utz 1975), but evaluation of many pertinent drugs has been hampered by the reluctance of investigators to initiate clinical trials. Further, there is no adequate animal model either to test putative carcinogens for causing prostate cancer or to select drugs which may be effective against prostate lesions.

Cell and organ culture models have been extensively used in studying a variety of biological problems. Cell culture systems consisting primarily of fibroblasts have been employed for testing the carcinogenic potential of chemicals (Berwald and Sachs 1965, Dipaolo et al. 1965, Chen and Heidelberger 1969). However, studies using fibroblasts in vitro may have some inherent limitations since most chemicals are metabolized to a greater extent by epithelial cells than by stromal fibroblasts (Williams et al. 1973). This is consistent with the observations that approximately 80% of cancers are epithelial in origin. The organ culture methods overcome the limitations of the cell culture models, since in explant culture tissue organization and specific cellular susceptibilities are retained. Further in contrast to the expensive and time consuming animal models in which the response of a test agent may be modified by the hosts' biochemical and immunological factors, in organ culture the effects of an agent can be studied in an organized tissue under controlled and reproducible conditions. Prostate gland from several animal species can be maintained as organ culture for a prolonged period without significant alteration in its morphology (Lasnitzki 1974). Treatment of prostate explants with certain carcinogens leads to hyperplastic and anaplastic alterations similar to those of preneoplasia (Roller and Heidelberger 1967, Lasnitzki 1954, 1974, Chopra and Wilkoff 1977b).

Vitamin A and certain synthetic analogs (retinoids) have prophylactic and therapeutic effects on various premalignant and malignant epithelial lesions (Sporn et al. 1976). Retinoids also inhibit and reverse carcinogen-induced hyperplastic and anaplastic lesions in mouse prostate organ cultures (Chopra and Wilkoff 1976, 1977a, Lasnitzki 1976). However, the utility of retinoids in the prevention of carcinogenic lesions is limited because of toxic side effects when administered in effective doses (Sporn et al. 1976). Currently attempts are being made to synthesize new retinoids which may be effective against carcinogenic alterations without appreciable toxicity (Sporn et al. 1976).

In this chapter, I will describe the use of the mouse prostate organ culture model for studying the abilities of chemicals to induce hyperplastic and anaplastic changes and for evaluating the anti-carcinogenic effects of synthetic retinoids.

II. PROSTATE ORGAN CULTURE: AN EXPERIMENTAL MODEL

The procedure for culturing prostate explants has been described (Lasnitzki 1954, Franks 1959, Chopra and Wilkoff 1977a, b). In earlier studies, mouse and rat prostate explants were cultured in a complex medium of clotted plasma and chick embryo extract (Lasnitzki 1954). Later the explants were grown on strips of lens paper supported by stainless steel grids placed in Petri dishes containing tissue culture medium supplemented with serum and/or chick embryo extract (Roller and Heidelberger 1967, Lasnizki 1976, Chopra and Wilkoff 1978). The level of the medium in the dish was such that it touched the explants. The gas phase varied from 95% O_2 + 5% CO_2 to air + 5% CO_2. The viabilities of the explants were usually determined by histological examination of the tissues. More recently prostate explants were cultured on the bottoms of scratched 35 mm Petri dishes containing 2 ml medium (Chopra and Wilkoff 1977a). The Petri dishes containing explants were perfused with 95% O_2 + 5% CO_2, in a rocker chamber that was rocked 8-10 times per minute to expose the explants alternatively to gas and culture medium. The scratched dish technique allowed excellent maintenance of the morphology of prostate explants for prolonged periods, although some explants became loose by the rocking action and were lost. Nevertheless the results obtained by culturing prostate explants in scratched dishes or on grids were comparable.

Several different culture media supplemented with different animal sera have been used for long-term survival of prostate explants (Roller and Heidelberger 1967, Chopra and Wilkoff 1977a, b, Lasnitzki 1976, Bal and DeLustig 1976). It is important to point out that inclusion of sera in the culture medium, although beneficial for long-term

explant survival has certain disadvantages. For instance, the concentration of various enzymes and hormones vary significantly in different batches of sera (Hon et al. 1975). Further carcinogenic and hyperplastic effects of test chemicals on cultured tissue may be influenced by serum in the medium (Bertram 1977, Lane and Miller 1976).

The method used in our laboratory for culturing mouse prostate has been described (Chopra and Wilkoff 1977a, b, 1978). Prostate gland was obtained from 8- to 12-week-old BDF1 or C3H mice. The gland was freed of fatty tissue and teased into explants of approximately 1.5 × 1.5 mm. Special precautions were taken to avoid excessive damage to the tissue which could cause a regenerative response. Explants were cultured on lens paper supported by stainless grids and also on scratched Petri dishes. Each dish contained 6-8 explants in CMRL 1066 medium supplemented with 10% fetal bovine serum or horse serum, penicillin (100 U/ml), streptomycin (100 μg/ml) and amphotericin B (2.5 μg/ml). The cultures were incubated at 37°C on a rocker platform in an atmosphere of 95% O_2 + 5% CO_2 or on grids in an atmosphere of 50% O_2 + 45% N_2 + 5% CO_2. Culture medium was changed every 48 hours.

The morphology of the prostate explants cultivated for up to 12 days in the control medium remained essentially similar to that seen in vivo. The explants consist of a number of finger shaped alveolar glands. At eight days after incubation the alveoli were lined by a single layer of epithelial cells that showed a low degree of proliferative activity (Figure 1). Prolonged cultivation resulted in the loss of glandular appearance and the epithelial folds characteristic of the gland in vivo became less evident. Some newly formed alveoli were seen, although the secretory activity appeared negligible in these alveoli. There was no significant change in the stromal elements of the explants and the morphology was similar for explants maintained for twelve days in the control medium.

At the ultrastructural level, the nuclei of secretory cells often occupied basal position and contained large nucleoli (Figure 2). The mitochondria that were distributed throughout the cytoplasm were usually oval to elongated in shape with moderately developed cristae. The cytoplasm contained moderate amounts of free ribosomes although the rough endoplasmic reticulum was poorly developed. The supranuclear cytoplasm usually contained well developed golgi complexes associated with secretory vacuoles that occupied large parts of the cytoplasm Lipid droplets, lysosomal elements, and dense bodies were frequently seen in the epithelial cells.

This method of explant culture has been applied to the maintenance of the tissues from trachea (Harris et al. 1978), lung (Stoner et al. 1978), colon (Autrup et al. 1978), and pancreatic duct (Jones et al. 1977). These explant culture systems are being utilized in many diverse studies in the fields of carcinogenesis and anticarcinogenesis.

III. EFFECTS OF CARCINOGENS AND NON-CARCINOGENS

The advantages of explant cultures for the studies of in vitro carcinogenesis have been mentioned above. Treatment of prostate explants with 3-methylcholanthrene caused hyperplastic and anaplastic changes similar to those of preneoplasia in the prostatic epithelium (Lasnitzki 1974). Similarly, other investigators have also reported the indiction

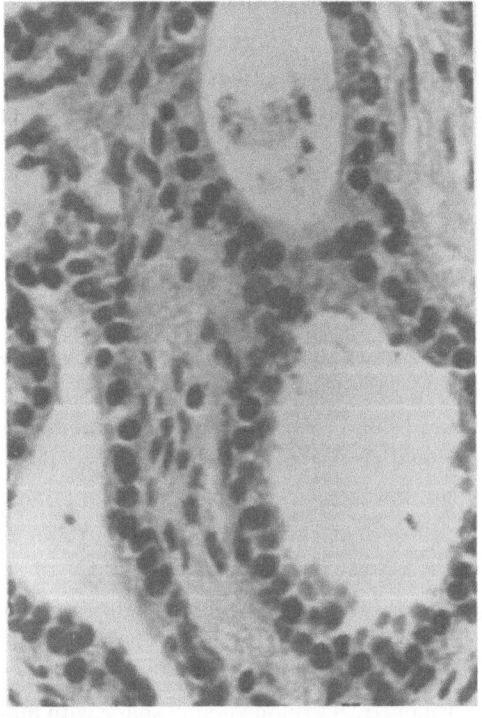

Figure 1. Light micrograph of a prostate explant cultivated for 8 days × 200.

of hyperplasia and anaplasia in the prostate explants treated with carcinogens (Roller and Heidelberger 1967, Chopra and Wilkoff 1977b, Bal and DeLustig 1976). The hyperplastic changes were accompanied by a loss of normal differentiation and the appearance of numerous mitotic cells in the epithelium of explants treated with carcinogens. In some alveoli the rapid cellular proliferation resulted in the development of squamous metaplasia (Lasnitzki 1974). Similar preneoplastic changes in explants of human prostate treated with 3-methylcholanthrene have been reported (Noyes 1975).

The prostate explant system was employed to test the carcinogenic potential of selected chemicals. (carcinogens and noncarcinogens) to induce hyperplastic and anaplastic changes. These chemicals included 3-methylcholanthrene (MCA), benzo (*a*) pyrene (BP), 11-12-epoxide of methylcholanthrene (Ep.MCA, an activated metabolite of MCA), pyrene (Py), phenanthrene (Phe), and N-methyl-N-nitro-N-nitrosoguanidine (MNNG) (Chopra and Wilkoff 1977b).

Explant cultures of the mouse prostate gland were treated with test chemicals at different concentrations. The degree of hyperproliferation produced by suspected chemicals at different intervals after treatment was determined by estimating mitotic indices using the colcemid metaphase arrest technique (Chopra and Flaxman 1973). It was found that all known carcinogens examined in these studies (MCA, BP, Ep.MCA, and MNNG) stimulated proliferation while noncarcinogens (Py and Phe) had no effect (Chopra and Wilkoff 1977b). The mitotic stimulatory effect of the carcinogens was concentration-dependent, the maximum stimulation being produced at 1, 2, 4 and 8 μg/ml of MNNG, Ep.MCA, MCA, and BP respectively. When added at optimum concentrations, the carcinogens initiated hyperproliferation by 4 days and extensive hyperplasia was present at 8 days after treatment (Chopra and Wilkoff 1977b).

The stimulation of cell proliferation by carcinogens produced concomitant alterations in the epithelial morphology of the carcinogen-treated explants. The epithelium of the carcinogen-treated explants became five to six cell layers thick and exhibited high degrees of proliferative activity (Figure 3). In contrast to the untreated explants where mitotic cells were localized in the basal

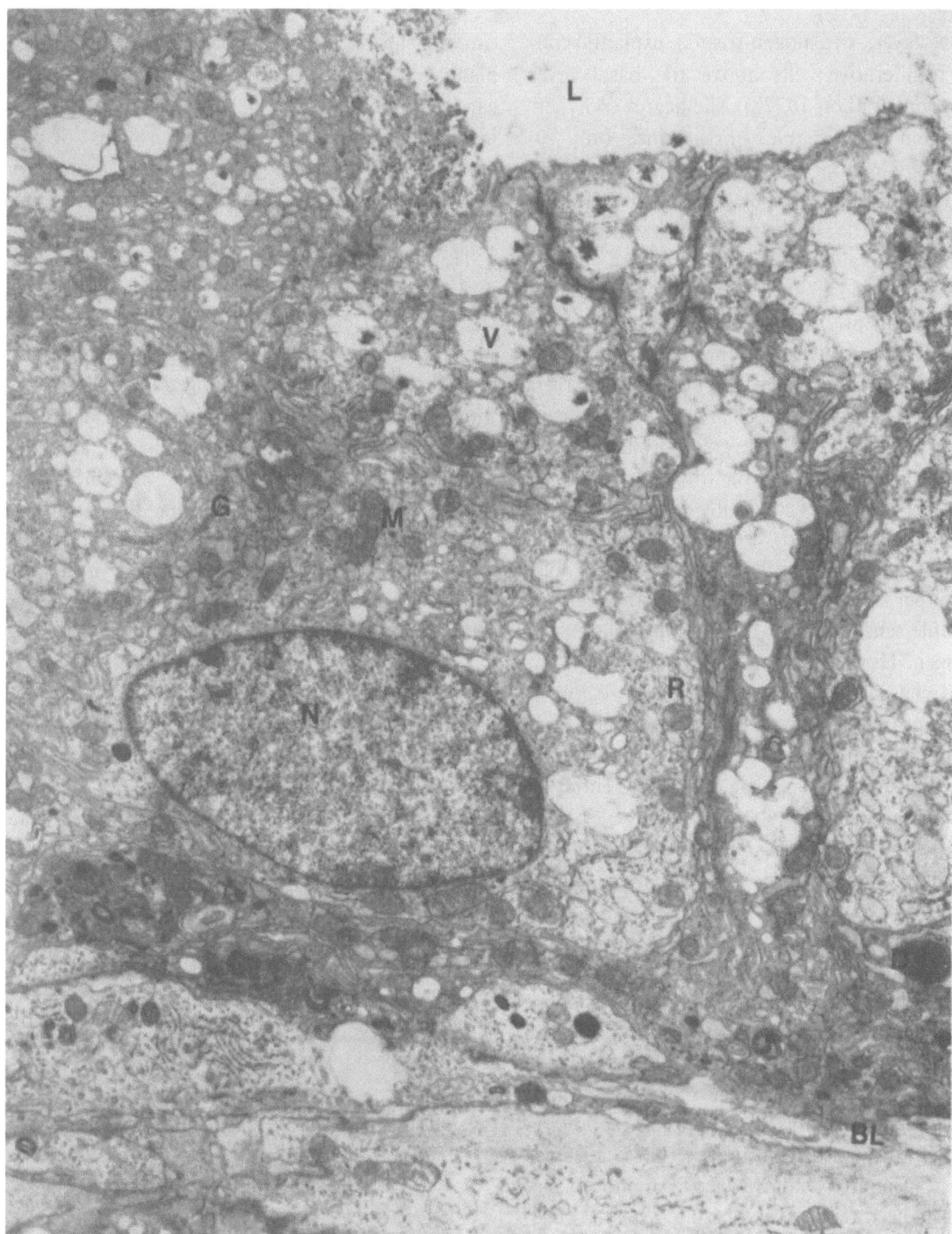

Figure 2. Electron micrograph of prostate explant × 7200 basal lamina (BL) dense body (D), Golgi (G), lumen (L). mitochondria (M), nucleus (N), ribosomes (R), vacuole (V).

170

epithelial layer, carcinogen-treated explants contained proliferative cells above the basal layer (Chopra and Wilkoff 1977b). The degree of hyperproliferation was variable. For instance, only 70-75% of the carcinogen-treated explants responded to the carcinogen treatment. Among the affected explants 50 to 60% showed hyperplastic alterations in 80-95% of the alveoli; in the remaining 40-50% of the explants approximately 30% of the alveoli were affected. Frequently, only a part of the alveolar wall was involved in contrast to the remainder of the epithelium which still consisted of one to two layers of cells. By 12 days after the carcinogen treatment, the hyperplastic alveoli were pleomorphic and the cells were polygonal with large irregular basophilic nuclei. At this time foci consisting of anaplastic cells of irregular shape and size were present. This diversity of response within the same explant may be due either to the availability of the carcinogen or to variable sensitivities of the prostate cells to the carcinogen. However, since the affected and non-affected cells were present in the same region, it would appear that some cells remained refractory to the carcinogen action. The refractory cells may have been at a particular stage of the differentiation pathway from which thay could not be reverted to the growth phase. The reason for the failure of 25-30% of the explants to respond to carcinogens is not clear.

Withdrawal of certain carcinogens from the medium after 8 days of treatment of the explants, and reincubation of the treated explants in carcinogen-free medium produced no reduction of hyperplastic lesions (Chopra and Wilkoff 1977b). In fact, hyperplasia in these explants became more pronounced and some alveoli showed squamous metaplasia after withdrawal of the carcinogen. The persistence of hyperplasia after withdrawal of carcinogen had previously been reported in prostate explants (Lasnitzki 1974) and in tracheal organ cultures (Croker and Sanders 1970). The persistence of hyperplasia after withdrawal of the carcinogen is probably not due to the accumulation of carcinogen or its metabolite in the tissue. For instance. MNNG has a half-life of approximately 30 minutes at pH 7.4 (Lawley and Thatcher 1970) and 80% of the carcinogen was reported lost from the tissue within 48 hours after its withdrawal (Lasnitzki and Goodman 1974). Further the metabolites derived from the activated

carcinogen are vary unstable. The most likely explanation for the persistent hyperplasia is that the carcinogen induces relatively permanent alterations in the target molecule (DNA or proteins) of cells and that the synthesis of enzymes required for hyperplasia continues until it is inhibited by some antagonizing factors.

Tranplantation of carcinogen-treated explants into isologous hosts failed to produce any tumors (Roller and Heidelberger 1967, Heidelberger and Iype 1967). However, the inoculation of cell suspensions prepared from carcinogen treated explants, into isogeneic mice resulted in the formation of sarcomas and carcinomas (Heidelberger and Iype 1967). Treatment of aneuploid cell lines from mouse prostate with carcinogenic hydrocarbons produced transformed colonies (Mondel 1970) which on inoculation into isogeneic mice also produced fibrosarcomas (Chen and Heidelberger 1969).

IV. REVERSAL OF CARCINOGEN INDUCED LESIONS BY RETINOIDS

Retinoids have been shown to produce prophylactic and therapeutic effects against several epithelial

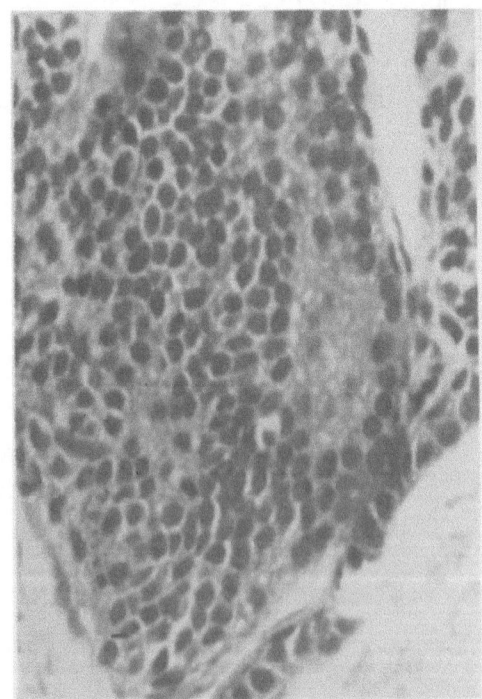

Figure 3. Light micrograph of a prostate explant treated with benzo (*a*) pyrene for 8 days × 200. Note hyperplasia.

lesions. Deficiency of vitamin A in experimental animals leads to metaplastic changes similar to those of preneoplasia in the bronchus, trachea, intestine, stomach, uterus, pancreatic duct and skin (Sporn et al. 1976). Development of these preneoplastic changes can be prevented and reversed by the administration of high doses of vitamin A (Sporn et al. 1976). Clinical studies have shown that patients with established skin keratosis or basal cell carcinomas can be successfully treated with topical application of retinoic acid (Bollag and Ott 1971, Bollag and 1973). Oral treatment with retinoic acid caused regression of leukoplakias of the mouth, tongue and larynx as well as papillomas of the urinay bladder (Bollag 1973, Ryssell et al. 1971). However, the utility of retinoids as prophylactic and therapeutic agents is limited because of their undesirable side effects that include headaches, desquamation of the skin and alopecia when applied in high doses (Spron et al. 1976, Bollag 1975). Currently new retinoids are being synthesized in an effort to find highly active and less toxic analogs. Since carcinogens produce hyperplastic and anaplastic changes in prostate explants and these preneoplastic alteration are reversed by β-retinoic acid (Chopra and Wilkoff 1976), this system has been extensively used to compare the antihyperplastic activity of new retinoids relative to their ability to reverse carcinogen-induced hyperproliferation (Chopra and Wilkoff 1977a).

For evaluating the effects of retinoids (Figure 4)

prostate explants were treated with BP for 8 days. After this time when most carcinogen-treated explants had developed lesions, they were divided into different groups. One group of explants continued to receive BP. Three more groups were simultaneously treated with BP and different concentrations of a retinoid for an additional 4 days. Explants were processed for histology and mitotic indices and standard deviations determined for each group of explants. The activity of the retinoids was compared with β-retinoic acid.

Table 1 shows that several retinoids were significantly more active than β-retinoic acid. It is not essential that retinoids contain a six-carbon ring to retain important biological activity. The two cyclopentenyl retinoids, in which the six-carbon ring is substituted by a five-carbon ring were significantly more active than β-retinoic acid in reversing carcinogen-induced lesions. Of the three trimethylmethoxyphenyl (TMMP) analogs tested, the TMMP analog of β-retinoic acid appeared to be less active whereas the TMMP analogs with side chain modification and estrified terminal carboxyl group were either as active or more active than β-retinoic acid. If, however, the double bond of the ring is shifted from the 5-6 to the 4-5 position, so that it is not in conjugation with the double bond system in the side chain of the molecule, the resulting retinoid (α-retinyl acetate) was devoid of any of the antihyperplastic activity in the carcinogen-treated explants (Chopra and Wilkoff

Table 1. Comparative activities of retinoids against benzo (a) pyrene (BP) induced hyperplasia in the mouse prostate explants. Explants treated with BP for 8 days followed by simultaneous treatment with BP and a retinoid for an additional four days.

Retinoids more active than β-retinoic acid	Retinoids as active as β-retinoic acid	Retinoids less active than β-retinoic acid
13-cis-retinoic acid	lactone of 13-cis-retinoic acid	12-(Z)-fluororetinoic acid ethyl ester
methylketo cyclopentenyl analog of retinoic acid	retinyl methyl ether	
1-methoxyethyl cyclopentenyl analog of retinoic acid	N-retinoylglycine ethyl ester	TMMP analog of retinoic acid
N-retinoylglycine	10-fluoro derivative of TMMP analog of all-trans-retinoic acid methyl ester	β-retinyl sulfone
14-fluoro derivative of TMMP analog of retinoic acid ethyl ester	10-fluoro derivative of TMMP analog of 13-cis-retinoic acid methyl ester	
	12-(E)-fluororetinoic acid ethyl ester	
	trimethylthiophene analog of retinoic acid ethyl ester	

172

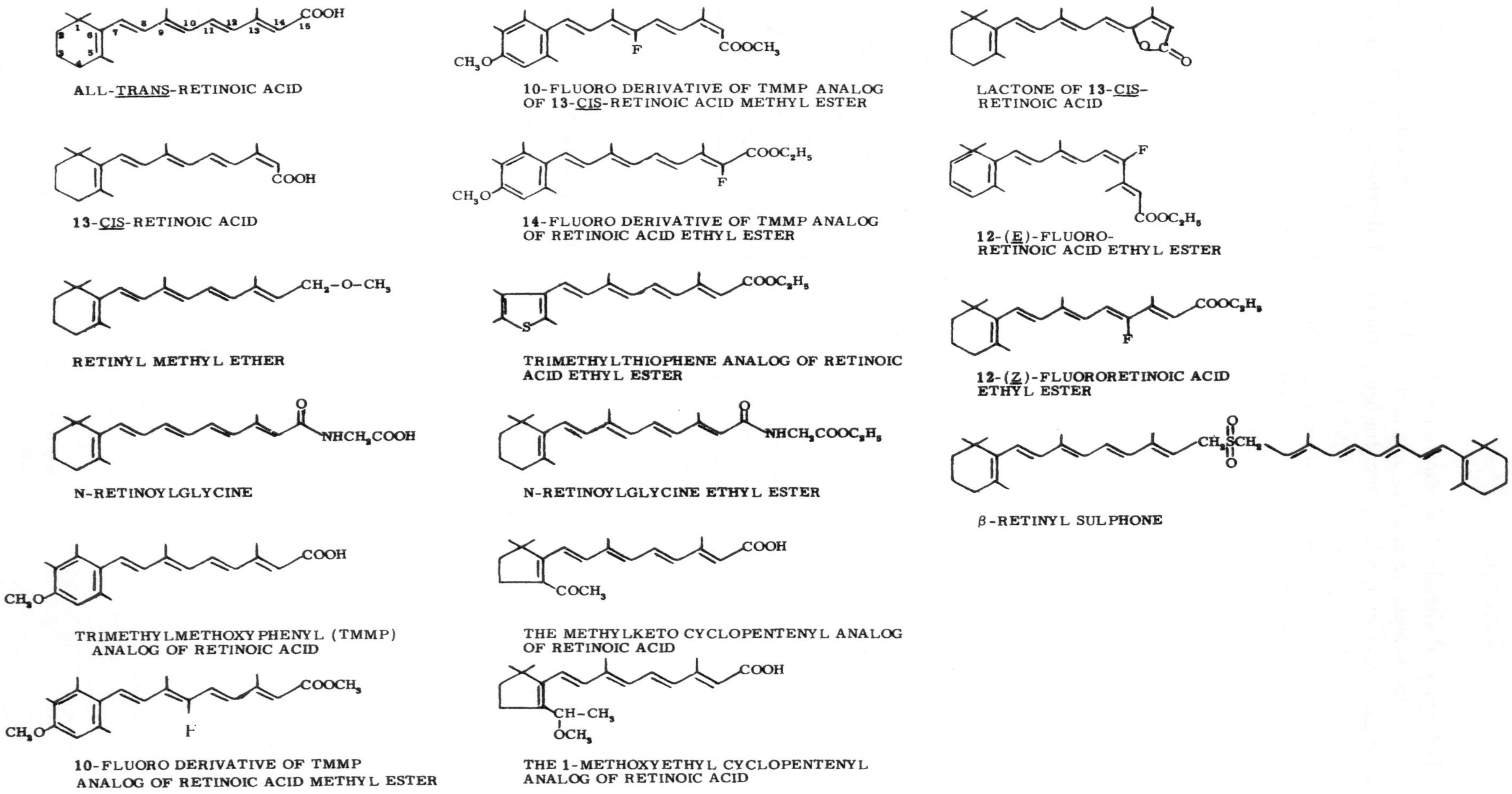

Figure 4. Structure of retinoids.

1977a).

Among the retinoids with side chain modifications only 13-cis-retinoic acid was more active than β-retinoic acid. This analog reportedly was very active in preventing hydroxybutyl-butyl-nitrosamine induced lesions in the rat bladder (Sporn et al 1977) and was significantly less toxic than β-retinoic acids in the mouse (Hixson and Denine 1978).

Toxic effects of retinoids are associated with the terminal carboxyl group (Goodman et al. 1974. Bard and Lasnitzki 1977). Therefore, retinoids with a less polar terminal group were synthesized. Retinyl methyl ether and N-retinoylglycine ethyl ester were as active as β-retinoic acid while N-retinylglycine was substantially more active than β-retinoic acid in reversing BP-induced hyperplastic changes. In other studies retinyl methyl ether. that was significantly less toxic than retinol or retinyl acetate, was also active in preventing the induction of mammary tumors in 7-12-dimethylbenz (a) anthracene treated rats (Grubbs et al. 1977).

In conclusion, the prostate explant model is an excellent system to prescreen carcinogens and anticarcinogens and compounds that are found to be positive may then be further evaluated in an in vivo system. The important advantage of the organ culture system is that it could markedly accelerate the testing of suspected carcinogens and potential anticarcinogens for their activity. Several retinoids that were found more active than β-retinoic acid in reversing carcinogen-induced lesions of prostate explants, are already being tested for toxicity and anticarcinogenecity in animal models.

ACKNOWLEDGEMENT

Supported by Public Health Service Contract No 1-CP-22064 from the Lung Cancer Segment, Division of Cancer Cause and Prevention. National Cancer Institute.

REFERENCES

Autrup H, Stoner GD, Jackson F, Harris F, et al.: Explant culture of rat colon in vitro: A model system for studying metabolism of chemical carcinogens. In Vitro 14: 868, 1978.

Bal E, DeLustig ES: Prostate carcinogenesis in vitro, unresponsiveness to ascorbic acid. Medicina (Buenos Aires 36: 23, 1976.

Bard DR, Lasnitzki I: Toxicity of anticarcinogenic retinoids in organ culture. Brit J Cancer 35: 115, 1977.

Bertram JS: Effects of serum concentration on the expression of carcinogen induced transformation in the C3H/10T 1/2 CL8 cell line. Cancer Res 37: 514, 1977.

Berwald Y, Sachs L: In vitro transformation of normal cells to tumor cells by carcinogenic hydrocarbons. J Natl Cancer Inst 35: 641, 1965.

Bollag W: Prophylaxis of chemically induced benign and malignant epithelial tumors by vitamin A acid (retinoic acid). Europ J Cancer 8: 689, 1972.

Bollag W: Therapy of epithelial tumors with an aromatic retinoic acid analog. Chemotherapy 21: 236, 1975.

Bollag W, Ott F: Therapy of active keratoses and basal cell carcinoma with local application of vitamin A acid. Cancer Chemother Rep 55: 59, 1971.

Chen TT, Heidelberger C: Quantitative studies on the malignant transformation of mouse prostate cells by carcinogenic hydrocarbons in vitro. Int J Cancer 4: 166, 1969.

Chopra DP, Flaxman BA: Mitotic inhibition of epidermal cells from psoriasis lesions in vitro by extracts from normal human skin. J Natl Cancer Inst 50: 281, 1973.

Chopra DP, Wilkoff LJ: Inhibition and reversal by β-retinoic acid of hyperplasia induced in cultured mouse prostate tissue by 3-methylcholanthrene or N-methyl-N'-nitro-N-nitroso-guanidine. J Natl Cancer Inst 56: 583, 1976.

Chopra DP, Wilkoff LJ: Reversal by vitamin A analogues (retinoids) of hyperplasia induced by N-methyl-N'-nitro-N-nitrosoguanidine in mouse prostate organ cultures. J Natl Cancer Inst 58: 923, 1977a.

Chopra DP, Wilkoff LJ: Induction of hyperplasia and anaplasia by carcinogens in organ cultures of mouse prostate. In vitro 13: 260. 1977b.

Chopra DP, Wilkoff LJ: Organ culture of mouse prostate for evaluating the antihyperplastic activity of retinoids. Tissue Culture Association Manual 4: 893, 1978.

Chopra DP, Wilkoff LJ: Activity of retinoids against benzo (a) pyrene induced hyperplasia in the mouse prostate organ cultures. Europ J Cancer 15: 1417. 1979.

Crocker TT, Sanders LL: Influence of vitamin A and 3,7, dimethyl 2,6-octadienal (citral) on the effect of benzo (a)-pyrene on hamster trachea in organ culture. Cancer Res 30: 1312, 1970.

DiPaolo JA, Donovan PJ, Nelson R: Quantitative studies of in vitro transformation by chemical carcinogens. J Natl Cancer Inst 42: 867, 1969.

Eagan RT, Utz DC, Myers RP, Furlow WL: Comparison of adriamycin (NSC 123127) and combination of 5-fluorouracil (NSC 19893) and cyclophosphamide (NSC 26271) in advanced prostatic cancer: a preliminary report. Cancer Chemother Rep 59: 203, 1975.

Flocks RH, Cheng SF: Combination therapy for prostatic carcinoma with special emphasis on the role of chemotherapy. J Iowa Med Soc 58: 125, 1968.

Franks LM: The effects of age on the structure and response to oestrogens and testosterone of the mouse prostate in organ culture. Brit J Cancer 13: 59, 1959.

Goodman DS, Smith JE, Hembry RM, Dingle JT: Comparison of the effects of vitamin A and its analogs upon rabbit ear cartilage in organ culture and upon growth of the vitamin A deficient rats. J Lipid Res 15: 406, 1974.

Grubbs CJ, Moon RC, Sporn MB, Newton DL: Inhibition of

174

mammary cancer by retinyl methyl ether. Cancer Res 37: 599, 1977.

Harris CC, Autrup M, Stoner GD, Trump BF: Carcinogenesis studies in human respiratory epithelium: an experimental model system. In: Pathogenesis and Therapy of Lung Cancer, Harris CC, ed. New York and Basal: Marcel Dekker 1978, pp 559.

Heidelberger C, Iype PT: Malignant transformation in vitro by carcinogenic hydrocarbons. Science 155: 214, 1967.

Higginson J: The role of the pathologist in environmental medicine and public health. J Am J Pathol 86: 459, 1977.

Higginson J, Muir CS: Epidemiology. In: Cancer Medicine, Holland JF, Frei E. eds. Philadelphia: Lea and Febiger 1973, pp 241-307.

Hixson EJ, Denine EP: Comparative subacute toxicity of all-trans and 13-cis-retinoic acid in Swiss mice. Toxicol and Pharmacol 44: 29, 1978.

Hon KV, Singley JA, Chavin W: Fetal bovine serum: a multivariate standard. Proc Soc Exp Bio Med 149: 344, 1975.

Jackson MA, Ahluwalia BS, Attah EB, et al: Characterization of prostatic carcinoma among blacks: a preliminary report. Cancer Chemother Rep 59: 3, 1975.

Jones RT, Barrett LA, vanHaaften C, Harris CC, Trump BF: Carcinogenesis in the pancreas. I. Long term explant cultures of human and bovine pancreatic ducts. J Natl Cancer Inst 58: 557, 1977.

Lane BP, Miller SL: Carcinogen induced changes in tracheal epithelium cultured in serum free, chemically defined medium. J Natl Cancer Inst 56: 991, 1976.

Lasnitzki I: The effect of estrone alone and combined with 20-methylcholanthrene on mouse prostate gland grown in vitro. Cancer Res 14: 632, 1954.

Lasnitzki I: Prostate gland in organ culture. In: Male Accessory Sex Organs, Brardes D. ed. New York: Academic Press 1974, pp 34-282.

Lasnitzki I: Reversal of methylcholanthrene induced changes in mouse prostates in vitro by retinoic acid and its analogues. Brit J Cancer 34: 239, 1976.

Lasnitzki I, Goodman DS: Inhibition of the effects of methylcholanthrene on mouse prostate in organ culture by vitamin A and its analogs. Cancer Res 34: 1564, 1974.

Lawley PD, Thatcher CJ: Methylation of deoxyribonucleic acid in cultured mammalian cells by N-methyl-N-nitro-N-nitroso-guanidine. Biochem J 116: 693, 1970.

Mondel S: Hydrocarbon carcinogenesis in vitro. Proc Int Cancer Congress, 10th 1970, Clark RL, Ed. Yearbook of Medicine, Chicago.

Noyes WF: Effect of 3-methylcholanthrene on human prostate in organ cultures. Cancer Chemother Rep 59: 67, 1975.

Roller MR, Heidelberger C: Attempts to produce carcinogenesis in organ culture of mouse prostate with polycyclic hydrocarbons. Int J Cancer 2: 509, 1967.

Ryssel HJ, Brunner KW, Bollag W: Die perorale Anwendung von Vitamin A. Säure bei Leukeplakien, Hyperkeratosen und platten Epithelkarzinomen: Ergebnisse und Verträglichkeit. Schweiz Med Wochenschr 101: 1027, 1971.

Scott WW, Schirmer HKA: A new oral progestational steroid effective in treating prostatic cancer. Trans Am Assoc Genitourin Surg 58: 54, 1966.

Scott WW, Wade JC: Medical treatment of benign modular prostatic hyperplasia with cyproterone acetate. J Urol 101: 81, 1969.

Sporn MB, Dunlop NM, Newton DL, Smith JM: Prevention of chemical carcinogenesis by vitamin A and its synthetic analogs (retinoids). Fed Proc 35: 1332, 1976.

Sporn MB, Squire RA, Brown CC, Smith JM, Wenk ML, Springer S: 13-cis Retinoic acid: inhibition of bladder carcinogenesis in the rat. Science 195: 487, 1977.

Stoner GD, Harris CC, Autrup H, Trump BF, Kingsbury EW, Myers GA, Newkirk R: Explant culture of human peripheral lung tissue. I. Metabolism of benzo (a) pyrene. Lab Invest 38: 685, 1978.

Williams GM, Elliott JM, Weisburger JH: Carcinoma after malignant conversion in vitro of epithelial like cells from rat livers following exposure to chemical carcinogens. Cancer Res 33: 606, 1973.

16. EPILOGUE

E.S.E. HAFEZ

Prostatic carcinoma has familial incidence. It has a relatively high frequency in the black population in U.S.A. and a relatively low frequency amongst Jews and Japanese. Mortality from prostatic carcinoma constitutes the second most frequent cause of deaths from cancer in the male population in the U.S.A. Extensive investigations are being conducted by the National Prostatic Cancer Project in the U.S.A. to determine if a high-risk group can be further identified.

Prostatic carcinoma is not associated with characteristic distinct symptoms which are often indistinguishable from those of benign hyperplasia of the prostate. Advanced stages of prostatic carcinoma are associated with back pain and anemia, which indicates bone metastasis. Rectal examination for the detection of prostatic carcinoma of the prostate is indicated in patients over 50 years of age. A hard nodule or an area of induration in the prostate gland is cancer unless proved otherwise. Several cytological, biochemical, radiological and pathological techniques have been employed for the diagnosis of prostatic carcinoma.

Prostatic carcinoma is detected unexpectedly and incidentally in some 30-50% of autopsy examinations of patients who have died from some other cause. The pathological diagnosis of prostatic carcinoma falls into two categories: a) incidental detection either in tissue removed for a clinically benign enlargement of the prostate or at autopsy of a patient who has died of other causes and b) clinically symptomatic cancer of the prostate. Recent improvements in the diagnostic techniques may increase this percentage.

Since the discovery in 1933 by Gutmann and Gutman where the presence of acid phosphatase was found in the serum of patients with metastasizing cancer of the prostate, numerous studies of rather conflicting results have been reported. Further research is needed to correlate serum acid phosphatase levels to the histologic-cytologic differentiation of prostatic carcinoma. Prostatic carcinoma is usually a slow-growing tumor and with proper treatment and sometimes even without treatment patients may live for many years. Despite numerous clinical advances and innovations with hormonal therapy, age-adjusted death rates for prostatic cancer have not significantly changed in the past 40 years.

Prostatic carcinoma in man remains an enigma. The results of primary treatment, such as surgery or irradiation from an interstitial or external source, are at a clinical plateau. Further investigations through cooperative, randomized clinical trials are needed for the development of additional chemotherapeutic agents. Extensive fundamental research is needed on the biochemistry and physiology of the prostate to correct historically-conditioned errors of concept and terminology.

Extensive investigations have been conducted on the occurrence, etiology, mortality (Table 1); structure, ultrastructure, endocrinology, metabolism, enzymology, immunology, microbiology (Table 2); classification, grading, diagnosis (Table 3); pathology, physiopathology, complications (Table 4); chemotherapy, radiotherapy, surgical therapy (Table 5); and animal models (Table 6) for human prostatic carcinoma.

Table 1. Summary of some recent research on occurrence, etiology and mortality from human prostatic carcinoma (1976-78).

Parameter	Studies, concepts and techniques	Author
Occurrence	incidence rates by race and social class	Ernster et al. 1978
	misleading reports: Japanese incidence of prostatic cancer	Ravich 1978
	prostatic obstruction	Kambal 1977
	epidemiology	Rotkin 1977, Tulinius 1977
	pattern of tumors	Naik 1977
	recurrent benign prostatic hypertrophy	Steg et al. 1976
	latent carcinoma	Breslow et al. 1977
Etiology	role of hormonal factors	Baranowska et al. 1977
	primary transitional cell carcinoma	Green et al. 1976
	malacoplakia following urinary tract infection	Rhodes et al. 1977
	granulomatous prostatitis with Mycobacterium kansasii and Mycobacterium fortuitum	Lee et al. 1977
	congestion, T-mycoplasma infection	Frick et al. 1976
	prostatic mycosis: nonsurgical diagnosis	Bissada et al. 1977
	sexuality & prostatitis	Drach 1976
Survival mortality	biologic and pathophysiologic prognosticating indices	Madduri et al. 1978
	cohort mortality: U.S. nonwhites	Ernster et al. 1978
	survival after open prostatectomy	Dias et al. 1978
	prognosis judged on clinical classification into stages and histological grading	Nissen et al. 1977
	long-term survival from Müllerian duct carcinoma	Hodgson 1975
	survival of child with rhabdomyosarcoma	Burke et al. 1976
	evolution of treatment at a comprehensive center	Murphy et al. 1976

Table 2. Summary of some recent research on the structure, ultrastructure, endocrinology, metabolism, enzymology, immunology and microbiology of human prostatic carcinoma (1976-78).

Parameter	Studies, concepts and techniques	Author
Structure and ultra-structure	scanning electron microscopy	Gaeta et al. 1977
	transmission electron microscopy	Stone et al. 1977
	morphology and immunology	Mickey et al. 1977
	adenoma and carcinoma in cell culture & heterotransplantation	Schroder et al. 1976
	exfoliative cytology	Ramzy et al. 1977
	histochemistry and electromicroscopy	Kirchheim 1976
	tumor morphology and hormone treatments in untreated and estrogen-treated	Sinha et al. 1977
	freeze-fracture membranes and junctions	Sinha et al. 1977
	antiandrogenic effects of spironolactone	Baba et al. 1978
Secretion	placental proteins and their subunits as tumor markers	Broder et al. 1977
Endocrinology	sex hormone binding, globulin binding testosterone, estradiol and prolactin	Bartsch et al. 1977, Dennis et al. 1977
	hormone levels and type of carcinoma growth differentiation	Bartsch et al. 1977, Frick et al. 1976
	castration and adrenal testosterone	Sanford et al. 1977
Metabolism	steroid receptors	Gustafsson et al. 1978, Bashirelahi et al. 1976, Ghanadian et al. 1978, Hawkins et al. 1977
	androgen binding, androgen tissue and sex hormone-binding globulin	Shain et al. 1978, Krieg et al. 1977, 1978, Snochowski et al. 1977, Sirett et al. 1977, 1978
	androgen receptor cytosol using protamine sulphate precipitation	Mobbs et al. 1978
	androgen and estrogens	Mawhinney et al. 1976, Habib et al. 1976, Ishimaru et al. 1977

Table 2. (continued)

Parameter	Studies, concepts and techniques	Author
	androgen glucuronide	Chung et al. 1978
	steroid levels from birth to old age	Hammond 1978
	C19-steroid	Morfin et al. 1977
	testosterone, 5 alpha-dihydrotestosterone & 5 alpha-adrostane-3beta, 17beta-diol diethylstilbestrol and medroxyprogesterone acetate on kinetics and production of testosterone and dihydrotestosterone	Morfin et al. 1978 Nolten et al. 1976
	estradiol on metabolism of androgens	Bard et al. 1977
	crystalloids: relationship to Bence-Jones crystals	Holmes 1977
	monodispersal and deoxyribonucleic acid of cell nuclei	Goerttler et al. 1977
	serum levels and urine excretion of corticoids	Migdalska et al.1977
	bromocriptine; plasma kinetics; production and tissue uptake of 3H-testosterone in vivo	Jacobi et al. 1978
	estramustine phosphate	Kadohama et al. 1978
	in vitro uptake of 3H testosterone and conversion to dihydrotestosterone	Prout et al. 1976
	3H-thymidine incorporation in tissue culture	Boileau et al. 1978
	6β-and 7α-hydroxylations of 5α-androstane-3β, 17β-diol	Morfin et al. 1977
	polyamine profiles	Dunzendorfer et al. 1978
	androphilic proteins in cytosols	Kodama et al. 1977
	cysteinesulfinic acid and 2-aminoethanesulfinic acid	van Sande et al. 1978
	prostatic secretion in benign hyperplasia, prostatitis and adenocarcinoma	Anderson et al. 1976
	prostatic antibacterial factor	Fair et al. 1976
	physical and chemical determinations of prostatic secretion	Anderson et al. 1976
	absorption metabolism and excretion of Estracyt	Forshell et al. 1976
	bone marrow enzymes and calcium	Boehme et al. 1978
	castration; catecholamine and 5-hydroxytrayptamine	Agarwal et al. 1977
	acute phase reactant proteins	Ward et al. 1977
	minocycline diffusion	Hensle et al. 1977
Enzymology	bone marrow acid phosphatase	Little et al. 1978
	bone marrow acid phosphatase by RIA	Belville et al. 1978
	immunohistochemistry for formalin-fixed embedded tissue	Jobsis et al. 1978
	immunochemistry of acid phosphatase	Chu et al. 1978
	isozymes of acid phosphatase	Foti et al. 1977
	DNA polymerase activity (2-o-methylcytidylate) oligodeoxyguanylate	Gerard et al. 1978
	acid phosphatase	Dounis 1977
	solid-phase fluorescent immunoassay for acid phosphatase	Lee et al. 1978
	acid phosphatase by N,N-p-di-2-chloroethyl-aminophenol, N,N-p-di-2-chloro-ethylaminophenyl phosphate and other dysfunctional nitrogen mustards	Workman 1978
	serum alkaline phosphatase isoenzyme	Wajsman et al. 1978
	histochemistry of glycosidases	Sinowatz et al. 1978
	creatine kinase isozyme	Hoag et al. 1978, Feld et al. 1977
Immunology	serum antibody	Ablin 1976
	experimental cellular allergic reaction	Robinson et al. 1976
	tumor specificity	Brannen et al. 1977
	immunostaging and immunocompetence	Ablin et al. 1976, Adolphs et al. 1977
	reductions of responder and stimulator capacities of peripheral lymphoid cells in mixed lymphocyte culture following external radiotherapy	Blomgren et al. 1977
	carcinoembryonic antigen in vitro	Williams et al. 1977
	immunosuppression and rejection of methylcholanthrene tumor isografts	Jacobs et al. 1977
	immunological tests	Evans et al. 1977
	immunological responsiveness in clinical management: inhibition of leukocyte migration and leukocyte adherence inhibition	Ablin et al. 1976
	monocytes in patients with malignant solid tumors	Kjeldsberg et al. 1978
	immunologic reactivity of lymph nodes regional to prostatic cancer	Herr 1977
	leukocyte adherence inhibition and immunoreactivity	Ablin et al. 1977
	antigens on fetal cells and viral transformed adult prostatic tissue	Javadpour et al. 1978
	hormonal and cellular immune response to cytomegalovirus-related antigens	Sanford et al. 1978
	effect of transurethral resection on lymphocyte response	Alsheik et al. 1977

Table 2. (continued)

Parameter	Studies, concepts and techniques	Author
	leukocyte migration by extracts of malignant prostatic tissue, in vitro sensitization	Ablin et al. 1978
	isotope release cytotoxicity	Frost et al. 1977
	thymic-dependent lymphocytic blastogenesis	Ablin et al. 1976
	serum proteins: alterations in immunoglobulins and clinical responsiveness following cryoprostatectomy; reduction of suppressive (blocking) properties	Ablin et al. 1977
	responsiveness of lymphocytes to soluble extracts of prostatic tumors	Bhatti et al. 1977
	serial carcinoembryonic antigen essays after chemotherapy	Kane et al. 1976
	immunoglobulin A in split ejaculates	Nishimura et al. 1977
Microbiology	RNA tumor virus-like activities	Arya et al. 1977
	oncogenic viruses	Dmochowski et al. 1977, McCombs 1977
	cytomegalovirus: in vitro transformation of human cells	Geder et al. 1977, Sanford et al. 1977
	virus-like particles	Ohtsuki et al. 1976
	herpes simplex virus type 2	Herbert et al. 1976
Blood	disseminated intravascular coagulation	Deutsch 1976
	blood group	Wajsman et al. 1977
	gland arteriography, vascular supply	Goerttler 1977
	blood vascular invasion	Kwart et al. 1978
Urine	testosterone excretion in prostatis	Yunda et al. 1977

Table 3. Summary of some recent reports on classification, grading and diagnosis of human prostatic carcinoma (1976-78).

Parameter	Studies, concepts and techniques	Author
Classification	TNM system in region of urogenital tract	Hufstetter 1978
	classification and grading	Dhom 1977
	histological prognosis	Harada et al. 1977
Radiography	retrograde urethrography with double contrast medium	Cauda et al. 1977
	lymphangiography: are nodes surrounding obturator nerve visualized?	Merrin et al. 1977
	objective interpretation of pneumocystograms	Scerbakov 1978
Radionuclide imaging	osseous scintigraphy	Louis et al. 1976
Diagnosis	natural history and adenocarcinoma	Franks 1976, Boxer 1977
	ultrasonography of the bladder and prostate	Resnick et al. 1976, 1977
	transrectal ultrasono-tomography	Hallemans et al. 1977
	transurethral resection, transrectal needle biopsy	Bissada et al. 1977, Bissada 1977, Kline et al. 1977, O'Donoghue et al. 1977, Moller 1977, Ventura et al. 1977
	supravital staining of the epithelial cells of urine	Pytel et al. 1978
	pelvic lymph node, serum and bone marrow acid phosphatase (RIA and counterimmunoelectrophoresis)	Kahn et al. 1977, Sadlowski 1978, Foti et al. 1977, 1978, Veenema et al. 1977
	serum acid phosphohydrolase (phosphatase) and ribonuclease	Chu 1978
	sex hormone binding globulin	Houghton et al. 1977
	androgen receptor assay using protamine sulphate precipitation	Mobbs et al. 1978
	serum lactic dehydrogenase and its isoenzyme V fraction levels following hyperglycemia	Ishibe 1977

Table 3. (continued)

Parameter	Studies, concepts and techniques	Author
	lactate dehydrogenase isoenzymes	Ishibe 1976, Grayhack et al. 1977
	DNA flow-through fluorescence cytophotometry	Springer et al. 1976
	urine hydroxyproline excretion, a marker of bone metastases	Bishop et al. 1977
	serial bone scanning using cyclotron-produced 18-fluorine	Buck et al. 1977
	indium chloride bone-marrow scanning	Catane et al. 1977
	therapeutic and prognostic aspects detected incidentally in adenoma enucleation	Leisering 1978
	primary lymphosarcoma	Hampel et al. 1977
	extraosseous multiple myeloma stimulating primary prostatic neoplasm	Hollenberg 1978
	embryonal rhabdomyosarcoma	King et al. 1977
	diagnosed initially as carcinoma of the rectum	Sweitzer et al. 1977
	cancer data service	Holmes et al. 1977
Prostatitis diagnosis	prostatitis: confusion clinically with carcinoma of the prostate	Taylor et al. 1977, Lapides 1976, Schwarz 1976

Table 4. Summary of some recent studies on the pathology, prostatic neoplasm, physiopathology and complications of human prostatic carcinoma (1976-78).

Parameter	Studies, concepts and techniques	Author
Pathology	needle, transrectal and perineal punch biopsies	Epstein 1976, Ackerman et al. 1977, Sonnenschein 1975, McMillen et al. 1976, Bishop et al. 1977, Nienhaus 1977, Bartsch et al. 1977
	perineal seeding after needle biopsy	Addonizio et al. 1976
	weight, stroma to gland ratio, and mitotic activity	Pietila et al. 1977
	organ, tissue and cell culture	Dilley et al. 1977, Schroder et al. 1976, Sanford et al. 1977.
	staging and grading	Barzell et al. 1977, Bruce et al. 1977
	mucinous adenocarcinoma	Chica et al. 1977
	basal cell proliferation and adenoma	Dermer 1978, Lin et al. 1978
	freeze-fracture on the membranes and junctions	Sinha et al. 1977
	origin and evolution	McNeal 1978
	particle - lamella complexes	Ohtsuki et al. 1978
	lymphocele: complication of surgical staging	Morin et al. 1977
	lymphography, pelvic lymphadenectomy and lymphangiography	Loening et al. 1977, O'Donoghue et al. 1976, Wilson et al. 1977, Nicholson et al. 1977
Pathology	testicular metastasis	Silverton 1976
	leukemic infiltration	Dajani et al. 1976
	separation and cytomorphology of epithelial cells	Epstein 1976, Pretlow et al. 1977, Brandhauer et al. 1976
	papillary carcinoma	Scott et al. 1976, Epstein 1977, Hara et al. 1977
	primary yolk-sac (endodermal sinus)	Benson et al. 1978
	urodynamic evaluation of prostatic obstructions	Elhilali et al. 1977
	indirect immunofluorescence	Pontes et al. 1977

Table 4. (continued)

Parameter	Studies, concepts and techniques	Author
	irradiation therapy of stage B and C	Schirmer et al. 1976
	enzyme, clinical, radiographic, and radionuclide for detecting bone metastases	Crisp et al. 1976, Kane et al. 1977, Schafferet et al. 1976
	relationship between primary tumor, histologic grade, and response to chemotherapy	Gibbons et al. 1976
	phosphorus-32 for intractable pain: androgen priming, parathormone rebound and combination therapy	Johnson et al. 1977
	atypical stromal hyperplasia	Attah et al. 1977
	stereology	Bartsch 1977
Physiopathology	detrusor and urethral dysfunction	Anderson et al. 1976
	urodynamics	Anikwe 1976, 1977, 1978
	combined cystomeric, sphincter electromyographic and uroflowmetric studies before and after transurethral resection	Andersen et al. 1976
	blood testosterone	Szymanoski et al. 1976
	liver function	Ishibe 1976
Prostatic neoplasm	isolation of carcinoma cell line	Stone et al. 1978
	carcinoma and leiomyoma of prostate	Catalona et al. 1978, McRoberts et al. 1978, Vassilakis 1978
	(32P) diphosphonate dose determination with bone metastases	Potsaid et al. 1978
	sarcoma of the bladder and prostate	Narayana et al. 1978
	metastatic prostatic adenocarcinoma of male breast	Lo et al. 1978
		Pervaiz et al. 1978 cutaneous metastases
Complications	intermittent cholestatic jaundice	Reddy et al. 1977
	pericardial tamponade	Quinnan et al. 1977
	hypercalcemia, corrected by orchiectomy	Olsson et al. 1977, Landgarten et al. 1978
	penile Paget's disease	Merino et al. 1978
	ureteral obstruction: response to endocrine and radiation therapy	Michigan et al. 1977
	urinary obstruction	Rao et al. 1977, Peison et al. 1977
	ectopic bone formation	Perlstein 1978
	rectal invasion and leiomyosarcoma of rectum	Herr et al. 1977, Stallwood et al. 1977
	ectopic ACTH and marked hypernatremia	Wenk et al. 1977
	hematomas	Morganstern et al. 1977
	adenocarcinoma in paraplegics	Ito et al. 1976

Table 5. Summary of some recent research on therapy, chemotherapy and radiotherapy of human prostatic carcinoma (1976-78)

Parameter	Studies, concepts and techniques	Author
Therapy (general)	standardized, controlled, prospective trials	Ray 1977
	health services delivery	Owen et al. 1977
	therapeutic concepts	Nagel 1978, Hohenfellner 1978
	subcapsular orchidectomy for carcinoma	Clark et al. 1977
	adjuvant immunotherapy	Robinson et al. 1977
	endocrine ablation for carcinoma of breast and prostate	Robin
	radiotherapy, hormone therapy and palliative therapy	Kongtawng et al. 1978, Oka et al. 1977, Frick 1977, Altwein 1978
	orchiectomy and related responses	Houghton et al. 1978, Jordan et al. 1977

Table 5. (continued)

Parameter	Studies, concepts and techniques	Author
	hypophyseal neuroadenolysis and hypophysectomy	Pasqualucci et al. 1978, Levin et al. 1978
	pelvic rhabdomyosarcoma	Brecher et al. 1977
	limitations of model systems	Handelsman 1977
Surgery	radical surgery	Pond et al. 1978 Burkman et al. 1977 Denis et al. 1978, Mathes et al. 1978, McDuffie et al. 1978
	extended total excision of prostatic adenocarcinoma	Spaulding et al. 1978
	prostatic and transurethral adenomectomy	Gregoir 1978, Donohue et al. 1977, Leisering 1978, Witherington 1977
	prostatectomy and prostatic dissection	Christoffersen et al. 1976, Abrams 1977, Rummelhardt 1976, Nicolescu et al. 1978
	selection of patients for transurethral prostatic resection	Greene 1978
	transurethral resection with a dysfibrinogen	Forman et al. 1977
	freezing index: clinical course	Haschek 1976, Petersen et al. 1978, Shiraiwa et al. 1977
	hematologic screening tests	Rader 1978
	septicemic states and infections after transurethral resection and adenomectomy	Dunzendorfer et al. 1976
Drug therapy	randomized clinical trials	Staquet 1976
	national randomized trial for chemotherapy	Johnson et al. 1977
	potential test systems	Sandberg et al. 1977
	evaluation of chemotherapy	Scott et al. 1976
	chemotherapy	Murphy et al. 1976, Murphy 1977
	estramustin phosphate (Estracyt), prednimustine	Benson 1976, Catane et al. 1976, 1977, Andersson et al. 1977, Chisholm et al. 1977, Murphy et al. 1977, Gustafson et al. 1977, von Hoff et al. 1977, Johnson et al. 1977, Fossa et al. 1977, Nagel et al. 1976, 1977
	flutamide (SCH-13521) and diethylstilbestrol	Airhart et al. 1978, Jacobo et al. 1976, Hellman et al. 1977, Lerner et al. 1977
	89 strontium	Firusian et al. 1976
	candicidin: double-blind trial	Abrams 1977
	2,6-cis-diphenylhexamethylcyclotetrasiloxane (Cisobitan)	Krarup et al. 1978, Blomback et al. 1978, Merrin 1978
	melphalan (ICRF-159) and Hydroxyurea	Houghton et al. 1977, Kvols et al. 1977
	agents activated specifically by prostatic acid phosphatase	Paul et al. 1977
	cyclophosphamide (NSC-26271)	Pollard et al. 1976
	bone marrow metastases with diethylstilbestrol	Bioorneklett et al. 1976
	doxorubicin hydrochloride, cyclophosphamide, and 5-fluorouracil combination	Collier et al. 1976
	comp-F regimen	Buell et al. 1978
	balsam pear	Clafin et al. 1978
	5α-reductase as target enzyme for antiprostatic drugs in organ culture	Kadohama et al. 1977

Table 5. (continued)

Parameter	Studies, concepts and techniques	Author
	adriamycin (NSC-123127); 5-fluorouracil (NSV-19893) and cyclo phosphamide (NSC-26271)	DeWys et al. 1977, Bonard et al. 1976, Caine et al. 1975, Eagan et al. 1976, Toljada et al. 1977
	endocrine therapy	Heaney et al. 1977
	alpha adrenergic blockers	Caine et al. 1976
	prolactin	Farnsworth
	stilboesterol and thyrotrophin-releasing hormone (TRH)	Smyth et al. 1977
	androgen	Mainwaring 1976
	antiandrogens	Neumann et al. 1976, Geller et al. 1977
	cyproterone acetate	Jameson 1976
	scanning with Stilbostate-1311	Zimel et al. 1977
	estrogen	Anikwe 1977, Schnorr et al. 1976, Beck et al. 1978
	progestogen	Denis et al. 1978
	steroidal alkylating agents	Mittelman et al. 1977
	chemotherapy of skeletal metastases	Cadman et al. 1976
	multiple chemotherapy for hormonally unresponsive carcinoma	Kane et al. 1977
	conservative treatment	Palanca et al. 1977
	rosamicin for bacterial prostatitis	Baumueller et al. 1977
	bacterial prostatitis	Pfau et al. 1976
	symphatectomy with phenol for prostatic pain	Johansson 1976
	difficulties of treatment of prostatitis	Arvis 1976
Radiotherapy	prognosis in radiotherapeutic management	Lipsett et al. 1976
	radiation therapy	Perez 1976, McGowan 1977, Taylor 1977
	megavoltage radiation	Neglia et al. 1977
	definitive radiotherapy	Birkhead 1978
	latent residual tumor following external radiotherapy	Nachtsheim et al. 1978
	use of a caliper to determine dimensions of the volume to be implanted with 125 iodine	Wheeler et al. 1978
	extended-field radiotherapy	Bagshaw et al. 1977
	interstitial radiation therapy using iridium 192 wires	Court et al. 1977
	needle biopsy after irradiation for stage C	Cox et al. 1977
Prevention and control	preoperative antibiotic therapy on bacterial prostatitis after transurethral prostatectomy	Landes et al. 1976

Table 6. Summary of some experimental models used to study prostatic carcinoma.

Species	Parameters	Studies, concepts and techniques	Authors
General	Experimental models	cell kinetics	Weisman et al. 1977
		carbon-11-labeled methylated polyamine analogs	Welch et al. 1977
		Dunning R3327H prostatic adenocarcinoma	Smolev et al. 1977
		Animal model for prostatic carcinoma	Fingerhut et al. 1977
		Animal models for human disease	Pollard 1977
Rat	Ultrastructure cytology	Ultrastructure cytology	Celesk et al. 1977
	Enzymology	Enzyme activity and distribution	Muntzing et al. 1978
	Chemotherapy	Transplantable adenocarcinoma (R-3327) of the Copenhagen rat	Block et al. 1977
	Pathology	Response to chemically induced prostatic tumors to stilbestrol and orchiectomy	Butz et al. 1976

Table 6. (continued)

Species	Parameters	Studies, concepts and techniques	Authors
	Immunology	Experimental studies R3327 adenocarcinoma of Copenhagen rats	Pollard et al. 1977 Claflin et al. 1977 Lubaroff et al. 1977 Lopez et al. 1977
	Metabolism	Lipoprotein-associated cytoxicity C-19 steroid Steroid hormone receptors	Chan et al. 1978 Shain et al. 1977 Markland et al. 1978
	Chemically induced	Sex hormones in producing experimental tumor Latent carcinoma receiving cyclophosphamide and azathioprine Steroids as a cause of adenocarcinoma of the dorsal prostate	Higuchi 1977 Elliot et al. 1977 Noble 1977
Mouse	Drug therapy	Reversal of methylcholanthrene-induced changes in vitro by retinoic acid and its analogues	Lasintzki 1976
	Prevention and control	Prevention and control beta-Retinoic acid	Chopra et al. 1977
Dog	Metabolism	Androgen receptor	Shain et al. 1978

REFERENCES

Ablin RJ: Serum antibody in patients with prostatic cancer. Br J Urol 48: 355, 1976.

Ablin RJ et al.: Evaluation of cellular immunologic responsiveness in the clinical management of patients with prostatic cancer. I. Thymic-dependent lymphocytic blastogenesis. Urol Int 31: 374, 1976.

Ablin RJ, et al.: Evaluation of cellular immunologic responsiveness in the clinical management of patients with prostatic cancer. III. Inhibition of leucocyte migration. Urol Int 31: 444, 1976.

Ablin RJ, et al.: Evaluation of cellular immunologic responsiveness in the clinical management of patients with prostatic cancer. IV. Leucocyte adherence inhibition. Urol Int 31: 459, 1976.

Ablin RJ, et al.: Immunostaging of patients with prostatic cancer: correlation of immunostage and clinical stage. An interim report. Curr Ther Res 20: 674, 1976.

Ablin RJ, et al.: Serum proteins in prostatic cancer. V. Alterations in immunoglobublins and clinical responsiveness following cryoprostatectomy. Urol Int 32: 56, 1977.

Ablin RJ, et al.: Serum proteins in prostatic cancer. VI. Reduction of the suppressive (blocking) properties of serum on in vitro parameters of cell-mediated immunologic responsiveness following cryosurgery. Urol Int 32: 65, 1977.

Ablin RJ, et al.: Leukocyte adherence inhibition and immunoreactivity in prostatic cancer. I. Identification of antitumour cell-mediated immunity and 'blocking' factor. Eur J Cancer 13: 699, 1977.

Ablin RJ, et al.: Inhibition of leukocyte migration by extracts of malignant prostatic tissue and correlation of degree of in vitro sensitization to clinical responsiveness in prostatic cancer patients. Urology 11: 289, 1978.

Abrams PH: A double-blind trial of the effects of candicidin on patients with benign prostatic hypertrophy. Br J Urol 49: 67, 1977.

Abrams PH: Prostatism and prostatectomy: the value of urine flow rate measurement in the preoperative assessment for operation. J Urol 117: 70, 1977.

Ackerman R, et al.: Retrospective analysis of 645 simultaneous perineal punch biopsies and transrectal aspiration biopsies for diagnosis of prostatic carcinoma. Eur Urol 3: 29, 1977.

Addonizio JC, et al.: Perineal seeding of prostatic carcinoma after needle biopsy. Urology 8: 513, 1976.

Adolphs HD, et al.: Correlation between tumor stage, tumor grade, and immunocompetence in patients with carcinoma of the bladder and prostate. Eur Urol 3: 23, 1977.

Agarwal RA, et al.: Prostatic carcinoma: castration alters the metabolism of catecholamine and 5-hydroxytrayptamine. Gen Pharmacol 8: 197, 1977.

Airhart RA, et al.: Flutamide therapy for carcinoma of the prostate. South Med J 71: 798, 1978.

Alsheik HI, et al.: The effect of transurethral resection of the prostate on lymphocyte response in patients with prostatic cancer. J Urol 118: 1022, 1977.

Altwein JE: Radiotherapy, hormone therapy and palliative therapy of prostatic carcinomas. Med Welt 29: 1210, 1978.

Anderson JT, et al.: Detrusor and urethral dysfunction of prostatic hypertrophy. Br J Urol 48: 493, 1976.

Andersen JT, et al.: Combined cystometric, sphincter electromyographic and uroflowmetric studies before and after transurethral resection of the prostate. J Urol 116: 786, 1976.

Anderson RU, et al.: Physical and chemical determinations of prostatic secretion in benign hyperplasia, prostatitis, and adenocarcinoma. Invest Urol 14: 137, 1976.

Andersson L, et al.: Estramustine phosphate therapy in carcinoma of the prostate. Recent Results Cancer Res 60: 73, 1977.

Anikwe RM: Correlations between clinical findings and urinary flow rate in benign prostatic hypertrophy. Int Surg 61: 392, 1976.

Anikwe RM: The effect of a 6FG urethral catheter on urinary flow in benign prostatic hypertrophy. Int Surg 61: 417, 1976.

Anikwe RM: Patterns of urinary flow in benign prostatic

184

hypertrophy. Int Surg 61: 433, 1976.

Anikwe RM: Bladder wall tension in benign prostatic hypertrophy. Invest Urol 14: 452, 1977.

Anikwe RM: Effect of estrogen therapy on metastatic carcinoma of the prostate. Int Surg 62: 532, 1977.

Anikwe RM: Urodynamics in benign prostatic hypertrophy. Br J Urol 50: 20, 1978.

Arvis G: Difficulties of treatment in the chronic prostatitis. Prog Clin Biol Res 6: 417, 1976.

Arya SK, et al.: RNA tumor virus-like activities in human prostate; possible novel pharmacologic approaches. Cancer Treat Rep 61: 113, 1977.

Attah EB, et al.: Atypical stromal hyperplasia of the prostate gland. Am J Clin Pathol 67: 324, 1977.

Baba S, et al.: Antiandrogenic effects of spironolactone: hormonal and ultrastructural studies in dogs and men. J Urol 119: 375, 1978.

Bagshaw MA, et al.: Evaluation of extended-field radiotherapy for prostatic neoplasm: 1976 progress report. Cancer Treat Rep 61: 297, 1977.

Bandhauer K, et al.: Evaluation of prostatic cytology in primary diagnosis and clinical course of prostatic carcinoma. Prog Glin Biol Res 6: 329, 1976.

Baranowska B, et al.: Rose of hormonal factors in the pathogenesis of prostatic hypertrophy. Pol Tyg Lek 32: 251, 1977.

Bard DR, et al.: The influence of oestradiol on the metabolism of androgens by human prostatic tissue. J Endocrinol 74: 1, 1977.

Bartsch G, et al.: Possibilities of the quantitative structural analysis of prostate biopsies. Bull Schweiz Akad Med Wiss 33: 99 1977.

Bartsch W, et al.: Sex hormone binding globulin binding capacity, testosterone, 5-alpha-dihydrotestosterone, oestradiol and prolactin in plasma of patients with prostatic carcinoma under various types of hormonal treatment. Acta Endocrinol (Kbh) 85: 650, 1977.

Bartsch W, et al.: Hormone blood levels in patients with prostatic carcinoma and their relation to the type of carcinoma growth differentiation. Eur Urol 3: 47, 1977.

Bartsch G: Stereology, a new quantitative morphological approach to study prostatic function and disease. Eur Urol 3: 85, 1977.

Barzell W, et al.: Prostatic adenocarcinoma: relationship of grade and local extent to the pattern of metastases. J Urol 118: 278, 1977.

Bashirelahi N, et al.: Specific binding protein for 17 beta-estradiol in prostate with adenocarcinoma. Urology 8: 552, 1976.

Baumueller A, et al.: Rosamicin – a new drug for the treatment of bacterial prostatitis. Antimicrob Agents Chemother 12: 240, 1977.

Beck PH, et al.: Plasma testosterone in patients receiving diethylstilbestrol. Urology 11: 157, 1978.

Belville WD, et al.: Bone marrow acid phosphatase by radio-immunoassay. Cancer 41: 2286, 1978.

Benson RC Jr.: Treatment of prostatic carcinoma with estramustine phosphate (Estracyt). Wis Med J 75: 89, 1976.

Benson RC Jr., et al.: Primary yolc-sac (endodermal sinus) tumor of the prostate. Cancer 41: 1395, 1978.

Bhatti RA, et al.: Responsiveness of lymphocytes to soluble extracts of prostatic tumors and abrogation by serum-blocking factor(s). Urology 9: 314, 1977.

Bioorneklett A, et al.: Bone marrow metastases from prostatic cancer-marked cytolytic effect after only a few days of treatment with diethylstilbestrol. Scand J Haematol 17: 227,

1976.

Birkhead BM: Definitive radiotherapy of prostatic cancer: a progress report. J Ky Med Assoc 76: 118, 1978.

Bishop D, et al.: A study of transrectal aspiration biopsies of the prostate with particular regard to prognostic evaluation. J Urol 117: 313, 1977.

Bishop MC, et al.: Urine hydroxyproline excretion – a marker of bone metastases in prostatic carcinoma. Br J Urol 49: 711, 1977.

Bissada NK: Accuracy of transurethral resection of the prostate versus transrectal needle biopsy in the diagnosis of prostatic carcinoma. J Urol 18: 61, 1977.

Bissada NK, et al.: Prostatic mycosis: nonsurgical diagnosis and management. Urology 9: 327, 1977.

Bissada NK, et al.: Factors affecting accuracy and morbidity in transrectal biopsy of the prostate. Surg Gynecol Obstet 145: 869, 1977.

Block NL, et al.: Chemotherapy of the transplantable adenocarcinoma (R-3327) of the Copenhagen rat. Oncology 34: 110, 1977.

Blomback M, et al.: Blood coagulation studies in patients with advanced carcinoma of the prostate treated with 2,6-cis-diphenylhexamethylcyclotetrasiloxane or estramustine-17-phosphate. Urol Res 6: 95, 1978.

Blomgren H, et al.: Reductions of responder and stimulator capacities of peripheral lymphoid cells in the mixed lymphocyte culture following external radiotherapy. Int J Radiat Oncol Biol Phys 2: 297, 1977.

Boehme WM, et al.: Lack of usefulness of bone marrow enzymes and calcium in staging patients with prostatic cancer. Cancer 41: 1433, 1978.

Boileau M, et al.: The effect of human serum on 3H-thymidine incorporation in human prostate tumors in tissue culture. J Urol 119: 779, 1978.

Bonard M, et al.: Placebo-controlled double-blind study in human benign obstructive prostatic hypertrophy with flutamide. Eur Urol 2: 24, 1976.

Boxer RJ: Adenocarcinoma of the prostate gland. Urol Surv 27: 75, 1977.

Brannen GE, et al.: Tumor specific immunity in patients with prostatic adenocarcinoma or benign prostatic hyperplasia. Cancer Treat Rep 61: 211, 1977.

Brecher ML, et al.: Nonsurgical treatment of pelvic rhabdomyosarcoma: a case report. J Surg Oncol 9: 601, 1977.

Breslow N, et al.: Latent carcinoma of prostate of autopsy in seven areas. Int J Cancer 20: 680, 1977.

Broder LE, et al.: Placental proteins and their subunits as tumor markers prostatic carcinoma. Cancer 40: 211, 1977.

Bruce AW, et al.: Carcinoma of the prostate: a critical look at staging. J Urol 117: 319, 1977.

Bruckman JE, et al.: Re: radical prostatectomy for carcinoma of the prostate: 1951-1976. A review of 329 patients. J Urol 118: 692, 1977.

Buck AC, et al.: Follow-up of prostate carcinoma with serial bone scanning using cyclotron-produced 18-flourine. Recent Results Cancer Res 60: 91, 1977.

Buell GV, et al.: Chemotherapy trial with comp-F regimen in advanced adenocarcinoma of prostate. Urology 11: 247, 1978.

Burke WR, et al.: Seven year survival of child with rhabdomyosarcoma of prostate. Urology 8: 357, 1976.

Butz GW, et al.: Response to chemically induced prostatic tumors in rats to stilbestrol and orchiectomy. Surg Forum 27: 590, 1976.

Cadman E, et al.: Chemotherapy of skeletal metastases. Int J Radiat Oncol Biol Phys 1: 1211, 1976.

Caine M, et al.: The treatment of benign prostatic hypertrophy with flutamide (SCH:13521): a placebo-controlled study. J Urol 114: 564, 1975.

Caine M, et al.: The use of alpha-adrenergic blockers in benign prostatic obstruction. Br J Urol 48: 255, 1976.

Catalona WJ, et al.: Surgical considerations in treatment of intraductal carcinoma of the prostate. J Urol 120: 259, 1978.

Catalona WJ, et al.: Carcinoma of the prostate: a review. J Urol 119: 1, 1978.

Catane R, et al.: Oral estramustine phosphate. Prolonged therapy for advanced carcinoma of prostate. NY State J Med 76: 1978, 1976.

Catane R, et al.: Disappearance of osteoblastic metastases in prostatic carcinoma following estramustine therapy. JAMA 237: 2471, 1977.

Catane R, et al.: Combined therapy of advance prostatic carcinoma with estramustine and prednimustine. J Urol 117: 332, 1977.

Catane R, et al.: Indium choride bone-marrow scanning in advanced prostatic carcinoma. NY State J Med 77: 1413, 237: 2471, 1977.

Catane R, et al.: Combined therapy of advanced prostatic cancer. Br J Urol 50: 29, 1978.

Cauda F, et al.: Retrograde urethrography with double contrast medium in the differential diagnosis of prostatic adenoma and carcinoma. Minerva Urol 29: 53, 1977.

Celesk RA, et al.: Ultrastructural cytology of prostate carcinoma cells from Wistar rats. Invest Urol 14: 95, 1977.

Chan SY, et al.: In vitro effects of lipoprotein-associated cytotoxic factor on rat prostate adenocarcinoma cells. Cancer Res 38: 2956, 1978.

Chica G, et al.: Mucinous adenocarcinoma of the prostate. J Urol 118: 124, 1977

Chisholm GD, et al.: The treatment of oestrogen-escaped carcinoma of the prostate with estramustine phosphate. Br J Urol 49: 717, 1977.

Chopra DP, et al.: Prevention and Control beta-Retinoic acid inhibits and reverses testosterone-induced hyperplasia in mouse prostate organ cultures. Nature 265: 339, 1977.

Christoffersen JC, et al.: Prostatic desiccation used in poor-risk patients with benign and malignant prostatic obstruction. Eur Urol 2: 229, 1976.

Chu TM: Serum acid phosphohydrolase (phosphatase) and ribonuclease in diagnosis of prostatic cancer. Antibiot Chemother 22: 98, 1978.

Chu TM, et al.: Immunochemical detection of serum prostatic acid phosphatase. Methodology and clinical evaluation. Invest Urol 15: 319, 1978.

Chung LS, et al.: Androgen glucuronide. II. Differences in its formation by human normal and benign hyperplastic prostates. Invest Urol 15: 385, 1978.

Claflin AJ, et al.: The Dunning 0327 prostate adenocarcinoma in the Fisher-Copenhagen F1 rat: a useful model for immunological studies. Oncology 34: 105, 1977.

Claflin AJ, et al.: Inhibition of growth and guanylate cyclase activity of an undifferentiated prostate adenocarcinoma by an extract of the balsam pear. Natl Acad Sci USA 75: 989, 1978.

Clark P, et al.: Subcapsular orchidectomy for carcinoma of the prostate. Br J Urol 49: 419, 1977.

Collier D, et al.: Doxorubicin hydrochloride, cyclophosphamide, and 5-fluorouracil combination in advanced prostate and transitional cell carcinoma. Urology 8: 459, 1976.

Court B, et al.: Interstitial radiation therapy of cancer of the prostate using iridium 192 wires. Cancer Treat Rep 61: 329, 1977.

Cox JE, et al.: The significance of needle biopsy after irradiation for stage C adenocarcinoma of the prostate. Cancer 40: 156, 1977.

Crisp J: Random bone marrow biopsy in the staging of carcinoma of the prostate. Br J Urol 48: 165, 1976.

Dajani YF, et al.: Leukemic infiltration of the prostate: a case study and clinicopathological review. Cancer 38: 2442, 1976.

Denis L, et al.: Radical prostatectomy: choice or chance. Eur Urol 4: 18, 1978.

Denis L, et al.: Progestogens in prostatic cancer. Eur Urol 4: 162, 1978.

Dennis M, et al.: Plasma sex hormone-binding globulin binding capacity in benign prostatic hypertrophy and prostatic carcinoma: comparison with an age dependent rise in normal human males. Endocrinol (Kbh) 84: 207, 1977.

Dermer GB: Basal cell proliferation in benign prostatic hyperplasia. Cancer 41: 1857, 1978.

Deutsch E: Disseminated intravascular coagulation in prostatic disease. Prog Clin Biol Res 6: 313, 1976.

DeWys WD, et al.: Comparative trial of adriamycin and 5-fluorouracil in advanced prostatic cancer: progress report Cancer Treat Rep 61: 325, 1977.

Dhom G: Pathology and classification of prostatic carcinoma. J Prog Clin Biol Res 6: 111, 1976.

Dhom G: Classification and grading of prostatic carcinoma. Recent Results Cancer Res 60: 14, 1977.

Dias R, et al.: Survival of patients with unsuspected prostatic carcinoma after open prostatectomy. Urology 11: 599, 1978.

Dilley WG, et al.: Hormone response of benign hyperplastic prostate tissue in organ culture. Invest Urol 15: 83, 1977.

Dmochowski L, et al.: Search for oncogenic viruses in human prostate cancer. Cancer Treat Rep 61: 119, 1977.

Donohue RE, et al.: Pelvic lymphadenectomy in stage A prostatic cancer. Urology 9: 273, 1977.

Dounis A.: Extremely high serum acid phosphatase level in carcinoma of prostate. J Urol 118: 500, 1977.

Drach GW: Sexuality and prostatitis: a hypothesis. J Am Vener Dis Assoc 3: 87, 1976.

Dunzendorfer U, et al.: Septicemic states and infections after transurethral resection and adenomectomy of the prostate. J Urol Nephrol 82 Suppl 2: 119, 1976.

Dunzendorfer U. et al.: Altered polyamine profiles in prostatic hyperplasia and in kidney tumors. Cancer Res 38: 2321, 1978.

Eagan RT, et al.: Adriamycin (NSC-123127) versus 5-fluorouracil (NSC-19893) and cyclophosphamide (NSC-26271) in the treatment of metastatic prostate cancer. Cancer Treat Rep 60: 115, 1976.

Earnster VL, et al.: Race, socioeconomic status, and prostatic cancer. Cancer Treat Rep 61: 187, 1977.

Elhilali MM, et al.: Urodynamic evaluation of prostatic obstructions. Union Med Can 106: 000, 1977.

Elliott GB, et al.: Latent carcinoma of the prostate in a 24 year old man receiving cyclophosphamide and azathioprine. Can Med Assoc J 116: 651, 1977.

Epstein NA: Prostatic biopsy. A morphologic correlation of aspiration cytology with needle biopsy histology. Cancer 28: 2078, 1976.

Epstein NA: Prostatic carcinoma. Correlation of histologic features of prognostic value with cytomorphology. Cancer 38: 2071, 1976.

Epstein NA: Primary papillary carcinoma of the prostate: report of a histopathologic, cytologic and electron microscopic study on one case. Acta Cytol 21: 543, 1977.

Ernster VL, et al.: Prostatic cancer: mortality and incidence rates by race and social class. Am J Epidemiol 107: 311, 1978.

186

Ernster VL, et al.: Cohort mortality for prostatic cancer among United States nonwhites. Science 200: 1165, 1978.

Evans CM, et al.: Immunological tests in carcinoma of the prostate. Proc R Soc Med 70: 417, 1977.

Fair WR, et al.: The prostatic antibacterial factor: identity and significance. Prog Clin Biol Res 6: 383, 1976.

Farnsworth WE, et al.: Prolactin and prostate cancer. Urology 10: 33, 1977.

Feld RD, et al.: Presence of creatine kinase BB isoenzyme in some patients with prostatic carcinoma. Clin Chem 23: 1930, 1977.

Fingerhut B, et al.: An animal model for the study of prostatic adenocarcinoma. Invest Urol 15: 42, 1977.

Firusian N, et al.: Results of 89 strontium therapy in patients with carcinoma of the prostate and incurable pain from bone metastases: a preliminary report. J Urol 116: 764, 1976.

Forman WB, et al.: Transurethral resection in a patient with a dysfibrinogen: fibrinogen cleveland I. J Urol 118: 885, 1977.

Forshell GP, et al.: The absorption metabolism, and excretion of Estracyt in patients with prostatic cancer. Invest Urol 14: 128, 1976.

Fossa SD, et al.: Hormone changes in patients with prostatic carcinoma during treatment with estramustine phosphate. J Urol 118: 1013, 1977.

Foti AG, et al.: Isozymes of acid phosphatase in normal and cancerous human prostatic tissue. Cancer Res. 37: 4120, 1977.

Foti AG, et al.: Detection of prostatic cancer by solid-phase radio-immunoassay of serum prostatic acid phosphatase. N Engl J Med 297: 1357, 1977.

Foti AG, et al.: Counterimmunoelectrophoresis in determination of prostatic acid phosphatase in human serum. Clin Chem 24: 140, 1978.

Franks LM: The natural history of prostatic cancer. Prog Clin Biol Res 6: 203 1976.

Frick J: Surgical and hormonal therapy of prostatic carcinoma. J Wien Med Wochenschr 127: 480, 1977.

Frick J, et al.: Hormonal status in prostatic disease. Prog Clin Biol Res 6: 143, 1976.

Frick J, et al.: Prostatitis: congestion, T-mycoplasma infection. Prog Clin Biol Res 6: 405, 1976.

Frost P, et al.: An isotope release cytotoxicity assay applicable to human tumors: the use of illindium. Oncology 34: 102, 1977.

Gaeta JF et al.; Scanning electron microscopic study of prostatic cancer. Cancer Treat Rep 61: 277, 1977.

Geder L et al.: Cytomegalovirus and cancer of the prostate: in vitro transformation of human cells. Cancer Treat Rep 61: 139, 1977.

Geller J et al.: Using antiandrogen therapy in benign prostatic hypertrophy. Geriatrics 32: 63, 1977.

Gerard GF et al.: Detection in human ovary and prostate tumors of DNA polymerase activity that copies poly(2'-o-methylcytidylate) oligodeoxyguanylate. Cancer Res 28: 1008, 1978.

Ghanadian R et al.: The use of methyltrienolone in the measurement of the free and bound cytoplasmic receptors for dihydrotestosterone in benign hypertrophied human prostate. J Steroid Biochem 9: 325, 1978.

Gibbons RP et al.: Prostatic carcinoma. Relationship between primary tumor, histologic grade, and response to chemotherapy. Urology 8: 222, 1976.

Goerttler K et al.: Monodispersal and deoxyribonucleic acid analysis of prostatic cell nuclei. J Histochem Cytochem 25: 560, 1977.

Goerttler U: Prostatic gland arteriography. Vascular supply, diagnosis and differential diagnosis of adenoma and carcinoma of the prostate. Radiologe 17: 256, 1977.

Grayhack JT et al.: Lactate dehydrogenase isoenzymes in human prostatic fluid: an aid in recognition of malignancy? J Urol 118: 204, 1977.

Greene LF et al.: Primary transitional cell carcinoma of the prostate. J Urol 116: 761, 1976.

Greene LF; Selection patients for transurethral prostatic resection. Geriatrics 33: 55, 1978.

Gregoir W: Haemostatic prostatic adenomectomy. Eur Urol 4: 1, 1978.

Gustafson A et al.: Treatment of oral estramustine phosphate (Estracyt) in prostatic carcinoma: influences on lipid and carbohydrate metabolism. Invest Urol 15: 220, 1977.

Gustafsson JA et al.: Demonstration of a progestin receptor in human benign prostatic hyperplasia and prostatic carcinoma. Invest Urol 15: 361, 1978.

Habib FE et al.: Metal-androgen interrelationships in carcinoma and hyperplasia of the human prostate. J Endocrinol 71: 133, 1976.

Habib FK et al.: Androgen levels in the plasma and prostatic tissues of patients with benign hypertrophy and carcinoma of the prostate. J Endocrinol 71: 99, 1976.

Hallemans E et al.: Transrectal ultrasono-tomography. Eur Urol 3: 37, 1977.

Hammond GL: Endogenous steroid levels in the human prostate from birth to old age: a comparison of normal and diseased tissues. J Endocrinol 78: 7, 1978.

Hampel N et al.: Primary lymphosarcoma of prostate. Urology 9: 461, 1977.

Handelsman H: The limitations of model systems in prostatic cancer. H Oncology 34: 96, 1977.

Hara S et al.: Prostatic caruncle: a urethral papillary tumor derived from prolapse of the prostatic duct. J Urol 117: 303, 1977.

Harada M et al.: Preliminary studies of histologic prognosis in cancer of the prostate. Cancer Treat Rep 61: 223, 1977.

Haschek H: Cryosurgery of prostate adenoma: evaluation of the method. Prog Clin Biol Res 6: 80, 1976.

Hawkins EF et al.: Steroid receptors in the human prostate. Detection of tissue-specific androgen binding in prostate cancer. Clin Chem Acta 75: 303, 1977.

Heaney JA et al.: Prognosis of clinically undiagnosed prostatic carcinoma and the influence of endocrine therapy. J Urol 118: 283, 1977.

Hellman L et al.: The effect of flutamide on testosterone metabolism and the plasma levels of androgens and gonadotropins. J Clin Endocrinol Metab 45: 1224, 1977.

Hensle TW et al.; Minocycline diffusion into benign prostatic hyperplasia. J Urol 118: 609, 1977.

Herbert JT et al.: Herpes simplex virus type 2 and cancer of the prostate. J Urol 116: 611, 1976.

Herr HW: Immunologic reactivity of lymph nodes regional to prostatic cancer: preliminary observations. J Surg Oncol 9: 509, 1977.

Herr HW: Immune reactivity of lymph nodes regional to prostatic cancer. J Surg Res 24: 409, 1978.

Herr HW et al.: Rectal invasion by benign prostatic hyperplasia. J Urol 118: 497, 1977.

Higuchi M: On the significance of sex hormones in producing experimental prostate tumor in the rat. Recent Results Cancer Res 60; 27, 1977.

Hoag G et al.: The production of creatine kinase isozyme BB in sera of a patient with prostatic carcinoma and in tumor homogenates. Clin Biochem 11: 38, 1978.

Hodgson NB: Long term survival from Müllerian duct carcinoma. Trans Am Assoc Genitour Surg 67: 94, 1975.

Hofstetter A: Tumor classification according to the TNM system in the region of the urogenital tract. 3. Prostatic neoplasma. A Fortschr Med 96: 1066, 1978.

Hohenfeller R: Prostatic carcinoma. Therapeutic concept. Med Welt 29: 1189, 1978.

Hollenberg GM: Extraosseous multiple myeloma simulating prostatic neoplasm. J Urol 119: 292, 1978.

Holmes EJ: Crystalloids of prostatic carcinoma: relationship to Bence-Jones crystals. 39: 2073, 1977.

Holmes FF et al.: Cancer data service. Prostate carcinoma distantly metastatic at diagnosis, 1945-1974. J Kans Med Soc 78: 423, 1977.

Houghton AL et al.: Melphalan in advanced prostatic cancer: a pilot study. Cancer Treat Rep 61: 923, 1977.

Houghton AL et al.: Sex hormone binding globulin in carcinoma of the prostate. Br J Urol 49: 227, 1977.

Houghton AL et al.: Advanced carcinoma of the prostate. Does the pretreatment Leydig cell function determine the response to orchidectomy? Postgrad Med J 54: 261, 1978.

Ishibe T: Liver function in prostatic carcinoma patients. Int Urol Nephrol 8: 135, 1976.

Ishibe T: Prognostic usefulness of serum lactic dehydrogenase and its fifth isoenzyme levels in carcinoma of the prostate. Int Urol Nephrol 8: 221, 1976.

Ishibe T: Alterations of serum lactic dehydrogenase and its isoenzyme V fraction levels following hyperglycemic condition in patients with genitourinary neoplasms. Urol Int 32: 393, 1977.

Ishimaru T et al.: Altered metabolism of androgens in elderly men with benign prostatic hyperplasia. J Clin Endocrinol Metab 45: 695, 1977.

Ito TY et al.: Adenocarcinoma of the prostate in paraplegics. Paraplegia 14: 101, 1976.

Jacobi GH et al.: Bromocriptine and prostatic carcinoma: plasma kinetics, production and tissue uptake of 3H-testosterone in vivo. J Urol 119: 240, 1978.

Jacobo E et al.: Comparison of flutamide (SCH-13521) and diethylstilbestrol in untreated advanced prostatic cancer. Urology 8: 231, 1976.

Jacobs SC et al.: Effects of immunosuppression on the rejection of methylcholanthrene tumor isografts. J Surg Oncol 9: 353, 1977.

Jakubik J et al.: Application of silicone implants in plastic surgery in Czechoslovakia.

Jameson RM: Regression of penile mestastases of prostatic carcinoma with cyproterone acetate therapy. Br J Urol 48: 268, 1976.

Javadpour N et al.: Common antigens found on fetal cells and viral transformed adult prostatic tissue. J Surg Oncol 10: 245, 1978.

Jobsis AC et al.: Demonstration of the prostatic origin of metastases: an immunohistochemical method for formalin-fixed embedded tissue. Cancer 41: 1788, 1978.

Johansson H: Chemical sympathectomy with phenol for chronic prostatic pain. Eur Urol 2: 98, 1976.

Johnson DE et al.: National randomized study of chemotherapeutic agents in advanced prostatic carcinoma: a progress report. Cancer Treat Rep 61: 317, 1977.

Johnson DE et al.: Phosphorus-32 for intractable pain in carcinoma of prostate. Analysis of androgen priming, parathormone rebound and combination therapy. Urology 9: 137, 1977.

Jonsson G et al.: Treatment of advanced prostatic carcinoma with estramustine phosphate. Scand J Urol Nephrol 11: 231, 1977.

Jordan WP Jr et al.: Reconsideration of orchiectomy in the treatment of advanced prostatic carcinoma. South Med J 70: 1411, 1977.

Kadohama N et al.: 5alpha-Reductase as a target enzyme for antiprostatic drugs in organ culture. Oncology 34: 123, 1977.

Kadohama N et al.: Estramustine phosphate: metabolic aspects related to its action in prostatic cancer. J Urol 119: 234, 1978.

Kambal A; Prostatic obstruction in Sudan. Br J Urol 49: 139, 1977.

Kane RD et al.: Serial carcinoembryonic antigen assays in patients with metastatic carcinoma of prostate being treated with chemotherapy. Urology 8: 559, 1976.

Kane RD et al.: Multiple drug chemotherapy regimen for patients with hormonally-unresponsive carcinoma of the prostate: a preliminary report. J Urol 117: 401, 1977.

Kane RD et al.: Radioisotope bone scanning characteristics of metastatic skeletal deposits of prostatic adenocarcinoma. J Urol 117: 618, 1977.

Khan R et al.: Bone marrow acid phosphatase: another look. J Urol 117: 79, 1977.

King DG et al.: Embryonal rhabdomyosarcoma of the prostate. J Urol 117: 88, 1977.

Kirchheim D: A critical review of histochemical and electromicroscopical studies of total prostatectomy specimens. Prog Clin Biol Res 6: 357, 1976.

Kjeldsberg CR et al.: A qualitative and quantitative study of monocytes in patients with malignant solid tumors. Cancer 41: 2236, 1978.

Kline TS et al.: Prostatic carcinoma and needle aspiration biopsy. Am J Clin Pathol 67: 131, 1977.

Kodama T et al.: Androphilic proteins in cytosols of human benign prostatic hypertrophy. Endocrinol Jpn 24: 565, 1977.

Kongtawng T et al.: Radiographic evaluation of treatment of advanced carcinoma of the prostate. South Med J 71: 247, 1978.

Kopper B et al.: Therapy of prostatic carcinoma. Dtsch Med Wochenschr 102: 1423, 1977.

Krarup T et al.: Prostatic carcinoma treated with 2,6-cis-diphenylhexamethylcyclotetrasiloxane (Cisobitan). Scand J Urol Nephrol 12: 11, 1978.

Krieg M et al.: Quantification of androgen binding, androgen tissue levels, and sex hormone-binding globulin in prostate, muscle and plasma of patients with benign prostatic hypertrophy. Acta Endocrinol (Kbh) 86: 300, 1977.

Krieg M et al.: Human prostatic carcinoma: significant differences in its androgen binding and metabolism compared to the human benign prostatic hypertrophy. Acta Endocrinol (Kbh) 88: 397, 1978.

Kuss R et al.: The effect of transurethral resection of the prostate on lymphocyte response in patients with prostatic cancer. J Urol 120: 388, 1978.

Kvols LK et al.: Evaluation of melphalan, ICRF-159, and hydroxyurea in metastatic prostate cancer: a preliminary report. Cancer Treat Rep 61: 311, 1977.

Kwart AM et al.: Blood vascular invasion: a poor prognostic factor in adenocarcinoma of the prostate. J Urol 119: 138, 1978.

Landes RR et al.: Effect of preoperative antibiotic therapy on bacterial prostatitis after transurethral prostatectomy. Urology 8: 352, 1976.

Landgarten S et al.: Hypercalcemia corrected by orchiectomy in a patient with carcinoma of the prostate. J Okla State Med Assoc 71: 288, 1978.

Lapides J: Prostatitis. Prog Clin Biol Res 6: 363, 1976.

Lasintzki I: Reversal of methylcholanthrene-induced changes in

188

mouse prostates in vitro by retinoic acid and its analogues. Br J Cancer 34: 239, 1976.

Lee CI et al.: A solid-phase fluorescent immunoassay for human prostatic acid phosphatase. Cancer Res 28: 2871, 1978.

Lee LW et al.: Granulomatous prostatitis. Association with isolation of Mycobacterium kansasii and Mycobacterium fortuitum. JAMA 237: 2408, 1977.

Leisering W: Therapeutic and prognostic aspects of cancer of the prostate detected incidentally in the course of adenoma enucleation. W Int Urol Nephrol 10: 23, 1978.

Lerner HJ et al.: Hydroxyurea in stage D Carcinoma of prostate. Urology 10: 35, 1977.

Levin AB et al.: Chemical hypophysectomy for relief of bone pain in carcinoma of the prostate. J Urol 119: 517, 1978.

Lin JI et al.: Basal cell adenoma of prostate. Urology 11: 409, 1978.

Lipsett JA et al.: Factors influencing prognosis in the radio-therapeutic management of carcinoma of the prostate. Int J Radiat Oncol Biol Phys 1: 1049, 1976.

Little C et al.: Bone marrow acid phosphatase concentrations in individuals with prostatic carcinoma or other disorders. Can Med Assoc J 119: 259, 1978.

Lo MC et al.: Metastatic prostatic adenocarcinoma of male breast. Urology 11: 641, 1978.

Loening SA et al.: A comparison between lymphangiography and pelvic node dissection in the staging of prostatic cancer. J Urol 117: 752, 1977.

Lopez DM et al.: Adenocarcinoma R-3327 of the Copenhagen rat as a suitable model for immunological studies of prostate cancer. Cancer Res 37: 2057, 1977.

Louis JF et al.: Contribution of osseous scintigraphy in the determination of metastases of cancer of the prostate. J Urol Nephrol 82 Suppl 2: 459, 1976.

Lubaroff DM et al.: R3327 adenocarcinoma of the Copenhagen rat as a model for the study of the immunologic aspects of prostate cancer. J Natl Cancer Inst 58: 1677, 1977.

Madduri SD et al.: Biologic and pathophysiologic prognosti-cating indices in prostatic cancer. Am Surg 44: 290, 1978.

Mainwarin WI: The relevance of studies on androgen action to prostatic cancer. Curr Top Mol Endocrinol 4: 152, 1976.

Markland FS et al.: Characterization of steroid hormone recep-tors in the Dunning R-3327 rat prostatic adenocarcinoma. Cancer Res 38: 2818, 1978.

Mathes GL et al.: An alternative to radical surgery for cancer of the prostate. Geriatrics 33: 53, 1978.

Mawhinney MG et al.: Androgens and estrogens in prostatic neoplasia. Adv Sex Horm Res 2: 141, 1976.

McCombs RM: Role of oncornaviruses in carcinoma of the prostate. Cancer Treat Rep 61: 131, 1977.

McDuffie RW Jr et al.: Radical retropubic prostatectomy: 59 cases. J Urol 119: 514, 1978.

McGowan DG: Radiation therapy in the management of lo-calized carcinoma of the prostate: a preliminary report. Cancer 39: 98, 1977.

McMillen SM et al.: The role of repeat transurethral biopsy in stage A carcinoma of the prostate. J Urol 116: 759, 1976.

McNeal JE: Origin and evolution of benign prostatic enlarge-ment. Invest Urol 15: 340, 1978.

McRoberts JW et al.: Carcinoma of the prostate. J Ky Med Assoc 76: 127, 1978.

Merino MJ et al.: Penile Paget's disease and prostatic carcinoma. J Urol 120: 121, 1978.

Merrin C: Treatment of advanced carcinoma of the prostate (stage D) with infusion of cis-diammin-edichloroplatinum (II NSC-119875): a pilot study. J Urol 119: 522, 1978.

Merrin C et al.: The clinical value of lymphangiography: are the

nodes surrounding the obturator nerve visualized? J Urol 117: 762, 1977.

Michigan S et al.: Ureteral obstruction from prostatic carci-noma: response to endocrine and radiation therapy. J Urol 118: 733, 1977.

Mickey DD et al.: Morphologic and immunologic studies of human prostatic carcinoma. Cancer Treat Rep 61: 133, 1977.

Migdalska B et al.: Serum levels and urine excretion of corticoids in patients with prostatic hypertrophy. Endokrynol Pol 28: 53, 1977.

Mittelman A et al.: New steroidal alkylating agents in advanced stage D carcinoma of the prostate. Cancer Treat Rep 61: 307, 1977.

Mobbs BG et al.: Androgen receptor assay in human benign and malignant prostatic tumor cytosol using protamine sulphate precipitation. J Steroid Biochem 9: 289, 1978.

Moller JT: Transrectal cytological aspiration biopsy in prostatic disease. Int Urol Nephrol 9: 235, 1977.

Morfin RF et al.: Correlative study of the morphology and C19-steroid metabolism of benign and cancerous human prostatic tissue. Cancer 29: 1517, 1977.

Morfin RF et al.: Precursors for 6beta- and 7 alpha-hydroxyl-ations of 5alpha-androstane-3beta, 17beta-diol by human normal and hyperplastic prostates. Biochimie 59: 637, 1977.

Morfin RF et al.: Comparison of testosterone, 5alpha-dihydro-testosterone and 5alpha-adrostane-3beta, 17beta-diol metab-olisms in human normal and hyperplastic prostates. J Steroid Biochem 3: 345, 1978.

Morganstern S et al.: Large prostatic hematomas associated with carcinoma of the prostate. J Urol 117: 622, 1977.

Morin ME et al.: Lymphocele: a complication surgical staging of carcinoma of the prostate. AJR 129: 333, 1977.

Muntzing J et al.: Enzyme activity and distribution in rat prostatic adenocarcinoma. Urology 11: 278, 1978.

Murphy GP: Chemotherapy of advanced prostatic cancer. Rev Surg 34: 75, 1977.

Murphy GP et al.: Prostatic cancer; evolution of treatment at a comprehensive center (1970-1974). Urology 8: 357, 1976.

Murphy GP et al.: Chemotherapy of advanced prostatic cancer today. Prog Clin Biol Res 6: 285, 1976.

Murphy GP et al.: A comparison of estramustine phosphate and streptozotocin in patients with advanced prostatic carcinoma who have had extensive irradiation. J Urol 118: 288, 1977.

Nachtsheim DA Jr et al.: Latent residual tumor following external radiotherapy for prostate adenocarcinoma. J Urol 120: 312, 1978.

Nagel R: Therapeutic concept in prostatic adenoma. Med Welt 29: 1194, 1978.

Nagel R et al.: Treatment of advanced carcinoma of the prostate with Estracyt. Prog Clin Biol Res 6: 267, 1976.

Nagel R et al.: Treatment of advanced carcinoma of the prostate with estramustine phosphate. Br J Urol 49: 73, 1977.

Naik KG: Patterns of tumors of the male genitalia in Zambia. Int Surg 62: 356, 1977.

Narayana AS et al.: Sarcoma of the bladder and prostate. J Urol 119: 72, 1978.

Neglia WJ et al.: Megavoltage radiation therapy for carcinoma of the prostate. Int J Radiat Oncol Biol Phys 2: 873, 1977.

Neumann R et al.: Antiandrogens and prostatic tumors (experi-mental base and clinical use). Prog Clin Biol Res 6: 169, 1976.

Nicholson TC et al.: Pelvic lymphadenectomy for stage Bl adenocarcinoma or the prostate: justified or not? J Urol 117: 199, 1977.

Nicolescu D et al.: Improved suprapubic vesical drainage in transvesical prostatectomy. Eur Urol 4: 230, 1978.

Nienhaus H: Aspiration biopsy cytology of prostate carcinoma.

H Recent Result Cancer Res 60: 53, 1977.

Nishimura T et al.: Immunoglobulin A in split ejaculates of patients with prostatitis. Urology 9: 186, 1977.

Nissen HM et al.: The prognosis in carcinoma of the prostate, judged on the basis of clinical classification into stages and histological grading. Int Urol Nephrol 9: 17, 1977.

Noble RL: The development of prostatic adenocarcinoma in Nb rats following prolonged sex hormone administration. Cancer Res 37: 1929, 1977.

Noble RL: Sex steroids as a cause of adenocarcinoma of the dorsal prostate in Nb rats, and their influence on the growth of transplants. Oncology 34: 138, 1977.

Nolten WE et al.: The effects of diethylstilbestrol and medroxy-progesterone acetate on kinetics and production of testosterone and dihydrotestosterone in patients with prostatic carcinoma. J Clin Endocrinol Metab 43: 1226, 1976.

O'Donoghue EP et al.: Lymphography and pelvic lymphadenectomy in carcinoma of the prostate. Br J Urol 48: 689, 1976.

O'Donoghue EP et al.: Early diagnosis of prostatic carcinoma: the role of transurethral resection. Br J Urol 49: 705, 1977.

Ohtsuki Y et al.: Virus-like particles in a case of human prostate carcinoma. J Natl Cancer Inst 58: 611, 1976.

Ohtsuki Y et al.: Particle-lamella complexes in a case of human benign prostate hyperplasia: brief communication. J Natl Cancer Inst 60: 299, 1978.

Oka M et al.: Endocrine therapy and serum urinary testosterone levels, as a monitoring, in patients with carcinoma of the prostate. Nippon Gan Chiryo Gakkai Shi 12: 336, 1977.

Olsson AM et al.: Advanced cancer of the prostate combined with hypercalcaemia. Scand J Urol Nephrol 11: 293, 1977.

Owen WL et al.: Health services delivery to prostatic cancer patients. J Okla State Med Assoc 70: 436, 1977.

Palanca E et al.: Conservative treatment of benign prostatic hyperplasia. Curr Med Res Opin 4: 513, 1977.

Pasqualucci V et al.: Result of hypophyseal neuroadenolysis in a 1st group of cancer patients. Minerva Anestes 44: 263, 1978.

Paul BD et al.: New agents for prostatic cancer activated specifically by prostatic acid phosphatase. Cancer Treat Rep 61: 259, 1977.

Peison B et al.: Acute urinary obstruction secondary to pseudolymphoma of prostate. Urology 10: 478, 1977.

Perez CA: Radiation therapy in the management of carcinoma of the prostate. Curr Probl Cancer 1: 30, 1976.

Perlstein GB: Case profile: ectopic bone formation in prostatic carcinoma. Urology 11: 651, 1978.

Pervaiz N et al.: Cutaneous metastases from prostatic carcinoma. Urology 11: 403, 1978.

Petersen DS et al.: Biopsy and clinical course after cryosurgery for prostatic cancer. J Urol 120: 308, 1978.

Pfau A et al.: Chronic bacterial prostatitis: new therapeutic aspects. J Urol 48: 245, 1976.

Pietila J et al.: Weight, stroma to gland ratio, and mitotic activity of the human hyperplastic prostate. Inves Urol 15: 90, 1977.

Pollard M: Animal model of human disease: metastic adenocarcinoma of the prostate. Am J Pathol 86: 277, 1977.

Pollard M et al.: Investigations on prostatic adenocarcinomas in rats. Oncology 34: 129, 1977.

Pond HS et al.: Defense of the radical perineal prostatectomy. South Med J 71: 541, 1978.

Pontes JE et al.: Indirect immunofluorescence for identification of prostatic epithelial cells. J Urol 117: 459, 1977.

Potsaid MS et al.: (32P) diphosphonatase determination in patients with bone metastases from prostatic carcinoma. J Nucl Med 19: 98, 1978.

Pretlow TG et al.: Separation and characterization of epithelial cells from prostates and prostatic carcinomas: a review. Cancer Treat Rep 61: 153, 1977.

Prout GR Jr et al.: In vitro uptake of 3H-testosterone and its conversion to dihydrotestosterone by prostatic carcinoma and other tissues. J Urol 116: 603, 1976.

Pytel IuA et al.: Use of supravital staining of the epithelial cells of the urine of prostatic cancer. Lab Delo 2: 80, 1978.

Quinnan GV Jr et al.: Prostatic carcinoma presenting as pericardial tamponade. Cancer Treat Rep 61: 1607, 1977.

Rader ES: Hematologic screening tests in patients with operative prostatic disease. Urology 11: 243, 1978.

Ramzy I et al.: Prostatic duct carcinoma: exfoliative cytology. Acta Cytol 21: 417, 1977.

Rao MS et al.: Multiple urethral metastases from prostatic carcinoma causing urinary retention. Urology 10: 566, 1977.

Ravich A: Point of view-misleading reports on Japanese incidence of prostatic cancer. Urology 11: 542, 1978.

Ray GR: Adenocarcinoma of the prostate: the need for standardized, controlled, prospective trials and less empiricism. Int J Radiat Oncol Biol Phys 2: 1041, 1977.

Reddy AN et al.: Intermittent cholestatic jaundice and non-metastatic prostatic carcinoma. Arch Intern Med 137: 1616, 1977.

Resnic ME et al.: Recent progress in ultrasonography of the bladder and prostate. J Urol 117: 444, 1977.

Resnick MI et al.: Recent progress in ultrasonography of the bladder and prostate. Trans Am Assoc Genitourin Surg 68: 8, 1976.

Rhodes RH et al.: Malacoplakia of the prostate following chronic urinary tract infection. J Urol 117: 808, 1977.

Robin PE: Major endocrine ablation for carcinoma of the breast and prostate. Clin Otolaryngol 3: 213, 1978.

Robinson MR et al.: Experimental cellular allergic reactions in normal canine and malignant human prostate. Clin Exp Immunol 26: 137, 1976.

Robinson MR et al.: Adjuvant immunotherapy with B.C.G. in carcinoma of the prostate. Br J Urol 49: 221, 1977.

Rotkin ID: Studies in the epidemiology of prostatic cancer; expanded sampling. Cancer Treat Rep 61: 173, 1977.

Rummelhardt S: Prostatic cancer as an incidental finding on prostatectomy. Prog Clin Biol Res 6: 95, 1976.

Sadlowski RW: Early stage prostatic cancer investigated by pelvic lymph node biopsy and bone marrow acid phosphatase. J Urol 119: 89, 1978.

Sandberg AA et al.: Some new approaches to potential test systems for drugs against prostatic cancer. Cancer Treat 61: 289, 1977.

Sande van, M et al.: On the presence of cysteinesulfinic acid and 2-aminoethanesulfinic acid in human adenomatous prostate. Eur Urol 4: 204, 1978.

Sanford EJ et al.: In vitro culture of human prostatic tissue. Urol Res 5: 207, 1977.

Sanford EJ et al.: Evidence for the association of cytomegalovirus with carcinoma of the prostate. J Urol 118: 789, 1977.

Sanford EJ et al.: Humoral and cellular immune response of prostatic cancer patients to cytomegalovirus-related antigens. J Surg Res 24: 404, 1978.

Sanford EJ et al.: The effects of castration on adrenal testosterone secretion in men with prostatic carcinoma. J Urol 118: 1019, 1977.

Scerbakov AP: Objective interpretation of the pneumocystograms on prostata-adenoma. Radiol Diagn 19: 87, 1978.

Schaffer DL et al.: Comparison of enzyme, clinical, radiographic, and radionuclide methods of detecting bone metastases from carcinoma of the prostate. Radiology 121: 431, 1976.

Schirmer HK et al.: Irradiation therapy of stage B and C

prostatic cancer mode of action, rationale and clinical results. Prog Clin Biol Res 6: 347, 1976.

Schnorr D et al.: Endocrine effects of oestrogen treatment in patients with prostatic cancer. Eur Urol 2: 85, 1976.

Schroder FH et al.: Prostatic adenoma and carcinoma in cell culture and heterotransplantation. Prog Clin Biol Res 6: 301, 1976.

Schwarz H: Prostatitis. Prog Clin Biol Res 6: 365, 1976.

Scott MB et al.: Papillary adenocarcinoma of prostate. Urology 8: 227, 1976.

Scott WW et al.: The continued evaluation of the effects of chemotherapy in patients with advanced carcinoma of the prostate. Trans Am Assoc Genitourin Surg 68: 24, 1976.

Shain SA et al.: C19-steroid metabolism by spontaneous adenocarcinoma of the AXC rat ventral prostate. J Natl Cancer Inst 58: 747, 1977.

Shain SA et al.: Androgen receptor content of the normal and hyperplastic canine prostate. J Clin Invest 61: 654, 1978.

Shain SA et al.: Characterization of unoccupied (R) and occupied (RA) androgen binding components of the hyperplastic human prostate. Steroids 31: 541, 1978.

Shiraiwa Y et al.: Freezing index in cryosurgery on the prostate gland. Tohoku J Exp Med 123: 49, 1977.

Silverton NP: Testicular metastasis from prostatic carcinoma. Br J Urol 48: 498, 1976.

Sinha AA et al.: Freeze-fracture observations on the membranes and junctions in human prostatic carcinoma and benign prostatic hypertrophy. Cancer 40: 1182, 1977.

Sinha AA et al.: A critical analysis of tumor morphology and hormone treatments in the untreated and estrogen-treated responsive and refractory human prostatic carcinoma. Cancer 40: 2836, 1977.

Sinowatz F et al.: A histochemical study of glycosidases in benign prostatic hyperplasia and in prostatic carcinoma in the human. Urol Res 6: 103, 1978.

Sirett DA et al.: Androgen binding in cytosol and nucleus of cells from human benign hyperplastic prostate. J Endocrinol 75: 25P, 1977.

Sirett DA et al.: Androgen binding in cytosols and nuclei of human benign hyperplastic prostatic tissue. J Endocrinol 77: 101, 1978.

Smolev JK et al.: Characterization of the Dunning R 3327H prostatic adenocarcinoma: an appropriate animal model for prostatic cancer. Cancer Treat Rep 61: 273, 1977.

Smolev JK et al.: Experimental models for the study of prostatic adenocarcinoma. J Urol 118: 216, 1977.

Smyth PP et al.: Effect of stilboestrol therapy on thyrotrophin-releasing hormon (TRH) responsiveness in males. Clin Endocrinol 1: 139, 1977.

Snochowski M et al.: Characterization and measurement of the androgen receptor in human benign prostatic hyperplasia and prostatic hyperplasia and prostatic carcinoma. J Clin Endocrinol Metab 45: 920, 1977.

Sonnenschein R: The effectiveness of transrectal aspiration cytology in the diagnosis of prostatic cancer. Eur Urol 1: 189, 1975.

Spaulding JT et al.: Extended total excision of prostatic adenocarcinoma. J Urol 120: 188, 1978.

Sprenger E et al.: The significance of DNA flow-through fluorescence cytophotometry for the diagnosis of prostate carcinoma. Beitr Pathol 159: 292, 1976.

Stallwood G et al.: Leiomyosarcoma of the rectum and prostate. Can J Surg 20: 446, 1977.

Staquet M: The randomized clinical trial: a prerequisite for rational therapy. Eur Urol 2: 265, 1976.

Steg A et al.: Recurrent benign prostatic hypertrophy. Prog Clin Biol Res 6: 81, 1976.

Stone KR et al.: Isolation of a human prostate carcinoma cell line (DU 145). Int J Cancer 21: 274, 1978.

Stone MP et al.: Scanning and transmission electron microscopy of human prostatic acinar cells. Urol Res 5: 185, 1977.

Sweitzer S et al.: Carcinoma of the prostate diagnosed initially as carcinoma of the rectum. Am Surg 43: 751, 1977.

Szymanoski J et al.: Study of the interdependence between prostatic hypertrophy and disorders in hormone levels. 1. Study of blood testosterone. J Urol Nephrol 82: 827, 1976.

Taylor EW et al.: Granulomatous prostatitis: confusion clinically with carcinoma of the prostate. J Urol 117: 316, 1977.

Taylor WK: Radiation oncology: cancer of the prostate. Cancer 39: 856, 1977.

Tejada F et al.: 5-fluorouracil versus CCNU in the treatment of metastatic prostatic cancer. Cancer Treat Rep 61: 1589, 1977.

Tulinius H: Epidemiology of prostate carcinoma. Recent Results Cancer Res 60: 3, 1977.

Van Hoff DD et al.: Estramustine phosphate: a specific chemotherapeutic agent. J Urol 117: 464, 1977.

Vassilakis GB: Pure leiomyoma of prostate. Urology 11: 93, 1978.

Veenema RJ et al.: Bone marrow acid phosphatase: prognostic value in patients undergoing radical prostatectomy. J Urol 117: 81, 1977.

Ventura M et al.: Transrectal prostatic biopsy using Franzen's needle in the cytologic diagnosis of prostatic cancer. J Urol Nephrol 83: 858, 1977.

Vincente J: Approach of transurethral adenomectomy: diagnosis and therapy. J Eur Urol 3: 310, 1977.

Wajsman A et al.: Blood group distribution in prostatic cancer patients. J Surg Oncol 9: 289, 1977.

Wajsman Z et al.: Clinical significance of serum alkaline phosphatase isoenzyme levels in advanced prostatic carcinoma. J Urol 119: 244, 1978.

Ward AM et al.: Acute phase reactant proteins in prostatic cancer. Gr J Urol 49: 411, 1977.

Weismann RM et al.: Cell kinetic studies of prostatic cancer: adjuvant therapy in animal models. Oncology 34: 133, 1977.

Welch MJ et al.: Carbon-11-labeled methylated polyamine analogs: uptake in prostate and tumor in animal models. J Nucl Med 18: 74, 1977.

Wenk RE et al.: Ectopic ACTH, prostatic cell carcinoma and marked hypernatremia. Cancer 40: 773, 1977.

Wheeler RR et al.: Use of a caliper to determine dimensions of the volume to be implanted with 125 iodine in the treatment of prostatic carcinoma. J Urol 120: 306, 1978.

Williams RD et al.: Production of carcinomaembryonic antigen by human prostate epithelial cells in vitro. J Natl Cancer Inst 58: 115, 1977.

Wilson CS et al.: Pelvic lymphadenectomy for the staging of apparently localized prostatic cancer. J Urol 117: 197, 1977.

Witherington R: Transvesical prostatic adenomectomy: a modification of Lower, Harris and Hryntschak techniques. Am Surg 43: 330, 1977.

Workman P: Inhibition of human prostatic tumour acid phosphatase by N,N-p-di-2-chloroethylaminophenol, N,N-p-di-2-chloroethylaminophenyl phosphate and other dysfunctional nitrogen mustards. Chem Biol Interact 20: 103, 1978.

Yamamoto KR and BM Alberts: Steroid receptors: Elements for modulation of eukaryotic transcription. Annu Rev Biochem 45: 721, 1976.

Yunda IF et al.: Testosterone excretion in chronic prostatitis. Andrologia 9: 89, 1977.

Zimel H et al.: Scanning of the prostate with Stilbostat-131I. Endocrinologie 15: 127, 1977.

INDEX*

A

Accessory sex organs 150
Acid phosphatase 9, 17-19, 29, 31, 45-47, 52, 79, 98-107, 125, 127, 131
  plasma levels 9
  prostatic 131
  secretion 50f, 102, 106
  serum levels 9, 29, 79, 131
Acini 6, 23, 116-118f, 148
  irregular secretory 7
  isolated 156
  prostatic 46, 54
Acute inflammatory changes 14
Acute prostatitis 20t
Adenocarcinomas 19, 62, 116-117, 145
  grading of 116-117
  of prostate grade 54f
  prostatic 116-117
  prostatoductal 25
Adenosine triphosphate 84
A_2 diffuse microcarcinoma 44
Adrenal androgens 17
Adrenal cortex 61
Age of tumor 63
Age-related changes 21
Albarran's subcervical glands 6f
Alcian blue staining technique 55
Aldolase syntheses 101
Alkaline 127
Alkaline phosphatase (ALP) 51, 83
Aliphatic polyamines 17
Alveoli 14, 167-170
Aminopeptidases 47, 50-53
Amylase 9, 83
Anaplasis (anaplastic) 168
  alterations 166
  cancer 44
Androgens (androgenic) 10, 15, 17, 23, 32, 59, 61, 90, 98, 107
  action
    biochemical markers for 99, 100
    mechanism of 98
  binding of 162
  binding protein
    molecular weight 163
  in circulating blood 160
  control
    of the prostate 102
    of the ventral prostate 98-107

  deprivation 15, 62
  estrogen ratio 26
  levels 91
  metabolism 99f, 162
  nuclear 26
    in the prostate 163
  pool estrogen 26
  in prostatic tissues 160
    uptake of 162
  receptors 10, 61, 88-91, 164
  regulation
    in the prostate of Rhesus monkey 160-164
  serum 161
  stimulation 163
  synthetic 163
Andrology 11
Androstenediols 23
5α-androstane 3α, 17β-diol 99
3α-androstanediol 102
3β-androstanediol 105, 107
Androstenedione 15, 161, 163
Aneuploid cell lines
  treatment of 170
Animal models 33
Anti-androgens 10
  agents 166
  atrophy 10
  therapy 64
Antibody requirements 133
Antigen 31
  requirements 133
Antimicrobials 113
Apex 13
Apical plasmalemma 7
Arterial blood supply 6
Ascending urethral infection 23
Aspiration biopsy 109

B

Basal cells 7, 9
Basal lamina 9
Benign 115
  hypertrophy 6
  nodular hyperplasia 7, 20
Benign proliferative lesions 19
  prostatic hypertrophy (BPH) 23, 30, 72
Benzo treatment 170
Beta-glucuronidase 51
Beta-glycerophosphate 125
Binding proteins 90-93

* f = figure; t = table

192

Biochemical techniques 29
Biopsy (of the prostate) 110
 perineal 109, 110
 retropubic (open) 110
Biosynthesis (polyamine) 101
Bladder 6
Blood groups 86
Blood markers 79
Bodansky method 125
Bone alkaline phosphatase isoenzyme value 83
Bone marrow 124-125
 acid phosphatase 31, 124-129
 markers in 88
Bone metastases 65
Bone scanning 125
Bound estradiol 92
2-bromo-α-ergocryptine 102
Bulbous urethra 15

C
Calcium 127
Cancer of the prostate
 see prostatic carcinoma
Carcinoembryonic antigen (CEA) 85
Carcinogenesis 154
 mechanism of 145-146
Carcinogens 146, 166-173
 effect of 166-173
 environmental 146
 induced 170
 potential of chemicals 166
 on prostatic explants 166-173
 treatment 170
Carcinoma 6, 38
 metastatic 9, 47
 occult 30
 prostaglandular 20t
Carcinomatous lesions 27
Carcinomatous prostates 10
Carcinosarcoma 62
Cardiovascular complications 60
Castration 10, 15, 18, 23
 of animals 62
 of rodents 11
Caudal lobes 162
Caudal prostate 162
Cell
 culture systems 166
 kinetic studies 62
 models (malignant) 157
 multiplication 154
 proliferation (stimulation) 168
 renewal 10
Central zones 6
Chemical agents 166
Chemical carcinogens
 application of 62
Chemotherapeutic agents 166
Chemotherapy 33, 158
 summary of 180
Chromatin
 nuclear 32
Chromatography 162
Chronic debilitating disease 21
Chronic granulomatous prostatitis 20t

Chronic inflammatory changes 14
Chronic nongranulomatous prostatitis 20t
Citrate 101, 106
 acid 9
Clinical carcinoma 30
 detection 27f
 examination 27
 markers 79-93
 response 62
 staging 28
Cloaca 5
Coagulase 18
Colcemid metaphase arrest technique 168
Collagen
 physiological breakdown 147
Collagenase 147, 148
Colon
 cancer of 86
Congenital cysts of the prostate 14, 15
Connective tissue
 capsule 9
 invaded by cancer cells 53
 stroma 53
Corpora amylacea 9-11, 14, 16f, 23
Corpora calculi 14, 16f
Corticosteroids
 treatment with 85
Counterimmunoelectrophoresis (CIEP) 80, 81, 128, 132
Cowper's gland
 duct of 15f
Cranial prostate 162
Creatine kinase 84
Creatine phosphokinase 84
Cribriform prostatic carcinoma 54
Cyproterone acetate
 administration of 85
Cytochemical localization of prostatic acid 155
Cytology (cytologic)
 diagnosis of prostatic secretions 40
 examination 109
 grading 110
 regressions 41
 studies 38
Cytopathology 29
Cytoplasm 167
 androgen receptor 26
 changes 38
 supranuclear 7, 168
Cytosol 61
Cytosolic androgen receptors 98

D
DaFano's silver impregnation method 52
Debilitating disease 19
Dehydroepiandrosterone 161
Dehydrogenase 127
Development of the prostate 5
Diagnostic procedures 26-27
Diethylstilbestrol 92
Differentiation of prostate carcinoma 19
Diffuse atrophy 19
Dihydrotestosterone 161-162
5α-dihydrotestosterone (5α DHT) 32, 98-102, 105, 155-156, 162
 effects of 154
Dilated prostatic ducts 16f

Diseased prostatic tissues 90
DNA content 10
  degradation in spermatozoa 9
  synthesis 98
Dog
  approaches to drug therapy 33
Drug therapy
  approaches 32-34
Duct of Cowper's gland 15f
Ducts 7
Ductus deferens 5-6

E
Ejaculate 9
Ejaculatory ducts 5, 6f, 13, 15f
Embryology 5
  embryological lobes 5
  embryologic origins 5f
Endocrine aspects 59-65
  imbalance 23
  parameters 15-17
  profile 32
  summary of 176
  therapy 59-65, 92
Endogenous steroids 89
Endoplasmic reticulum (RER) 7, 168
Environmental carcinogens 146
Enzymes
  markers 79
  oxidative 51
  profile 44
  proteolytic 9, 51
  respiratory 15
Enzymology
  summary of 176
Eosinophilic large nucleoli 29
Epidermal growth factor 156
Epithelium 5, 7, 11, 116-118, 170
  atrophic 118f
  atrophy 23
  of carcinogen-treated explants 168
  cells 14, 146, 148, 166
    growth 148
  cuboidal 116
  cylindrical 116
    isolation of 147
  lesions (malignant) 166
  prostatic (human) 147, 149, 151, 153-154
    post-pubertal 148
  pseudostratified 7
Esterases 51
Estradiol 62
Estrogens 10, 59, 60, 102, 119-120
  administration of 63
  binding component 164
  receptors 92
  stimulation 63
  therapy 32, 166
  treatment 33, 60, 64, 85, 119-120
Excretory ducts 7
Experimental animals 62

F
Fibrinolysin 18
Fibroadenoma 62

Fibroblasts 153, 166
Field experiment 73
  Franzen-needle 38
FSH 33
Functional Anatomy
  of the prostate 5-11, 13-34
Functional biochemistry 17

G
Geographical differences 13
Gestonorone 60
Giant nuclei 41
Glandular prostate 23
  -glucuronidase 89
Gland weight 10
Glycolytic activity 15
Glycosaminoglycans (muco-polysaccharide) 55
Glycosidases 51
Golgi apparatus 52
Golgi complex 153
Golgi cysternae 45
Golgi region associated enzymes 52
Gonadotropin
  inhibition of 102
Granulomatous prostatitis
  chronic 20t
Gross anatomy 6-7

H
Hematogenous infection 23
Heparan sulfate (HS) 56
Histochemistry 44-56
  methodology 50
  of prostatic acid phosphatase 45
Histology (histological) 7-9
  carcinoma 146
  changes 115
  classification 20
Histopathology 29
Histophysiology 9-11
Hormone
  levels
    seasonal rhythm of 160
  manipulation 61, 63
  markers 84
  receptors 17, 31
  steroid-peptid 19
  therapy 32, 38, 155
    clinical 65
  treatment 63
17α-hydroxyprogesterone 15
  serum levels 32
Hypercholesteroluria 87
Hyperchromatism (nuclear) 29, 40f
Hyperplasia 10, 63, 168, 170
  alterations 166
  changes 168
  lesions 170
  lobular 30
  postsclerotic 31
Hyperproliferation 168, 170
Hyperprolactinemia 17
Hypertrophy 10
  benign 6, 23, 30, 72
  prostatic gland 119f

Hypervitaminosis 153
Hypogastric plexus
  inferior 7

I
Immuno-histochemistry 51
Immunodiffusion 128
Immunology
  summary of 176
Incidental ages of prostatic cancer 72
Incidental carcinoma 30
Inferior hypogastric plexus 7
Infertility (male) 14
Inflammatory cells
  mononuclear 23
Inflammatory changes
  acute 14
Innervation 7, 9
Insulin 152, 153, 156
  effects of 150
Interstitial cells 61
Interstitial stroma 63
In vitro models 145-158
Isoenzymes 45
  lysosomal 102
Isolated acini 156
Isolation of normal prostatic epithelium 147

K
Keratinization 153

L
Lactic dehydrogenase 127
Leydig cells 26
LH 33
Lobation pattern 6
Lobular hyperplasia 30
Lumen 10, 45
Lymph 6, 126
Lymphadenectomy (pelvic) 126
Lysosomal isoenzyme 102
Lysozyme 9

M
Male infertility 14
Malignant 115
  cell models 155, 157
  epithelial lesions 166
  prostate 19
Marital status 13
Marrow 124-125
Mass screening
  experiments 74t
  programs 73
    for prostatic diseases 72
  system 71
Mesenchyme 5
Mesonephric ducts 5
Metaplasia 5
Metaplastic squamous epithelium 42f
Metastatic carcinoma 9
Metastatic prostatic cancers 47
3-methylcholanthrene 168
Methyltrienolone 163
Mitochondria 167

Mitotic
  activity 10, 154
  inhibition 10
  stimulatory (effect of) 168
Model experiment 72
Monkey 33
Mononuclear inflammatory cells 23
Mortality rate 13, 21, 60
  summary of 176
Mucopolysaccharides 14
Mucopolysaccharides of connective tissue 55
Müllerian ducts 5, 20
Müllerian inhibiting factor 5

N
Needle biopsy 109, 111
Neoplastic prostatic cells 11
Nervous innervation 7, 9
Neuraminic acid 86
Nodes 126
Nodular prostatic hyperplasia (NPH) 20-22, 30
Non-carcinogens
  effects of 168
Non-hormonal treatment 65
Nonmyelinated nerve fibers 9
Normal cell models 145, 156
  mechanism of transformation 145
Normal prostatic acinus 46, 54
Normal prostatic epithelium 147, 149, 151, 153-154
Nuclear androgen receptor 26
Nuclear chromatin 32
Nuclear hyperchromatism 29
Nucleoli
  wasting of 41
Nucleoside-diphosphatases 52

O
Objective regression (partial) 65
Occult carcinoma 30
Open biopsy of the prostate 110
Open perineal biopsy 110
Open retropubic biopsy 110
Orchiectomy 59, 63, 64, 85, 166
Organ culture models 166
Ornithine decarboxylase 101
Oxidative enzymes 51

P
Paraprostate 13
Parenchyma 14
Pathological prostates 91
  summary of 179
Partial objective regression 65
Pelvic lymphadenectomy 126
Perineal aspiration biopsy of the prostate 109, 110
Perineal biopsy (open) 110
Perineal prostatectomy 110
Perineural invasion 29
Peripheral zone 6, 7
Periurethral gland mass 13
Phosphatase 124-125
Physiomorphology (regional) 13-34
Physiopathology
  of human prostate 13-34
  mechanisms 23

of prostatic diseases 19
  quantitative 13-34
  summary of 179
Pituitary 61
Placental proteins 86
Plasma level
  seasonal rhythm 161
  testosterone 161
Plasminogen activator 9
Polyamines 86, 87, 101
Postsclerotic hyperplasia 31
Premalignant epithelial lesions 166
Preneoplasia 168
Preneoplastic hyperplasia 154
Primitive urethra 5f
Principal cells 7
Production Rate
  in man 161
  in monkey 161
Progesterone 15, 60
  receptors 93
Progestin
  cytosolic receptors 91
  receptors 91
Prolactin 11, 15, 17, 33, 85, 98, 102
Prophylactics 166
  effects of 170
Prostaglandins 17, 18
Prostaglandular carcinoma 20t
Prostate (prostatic)
  acid phosphatase 29, 65, 88, 131-138, 156
    cytochemical localization of 155
    immunoassay values 136
    immunological assay 132
    isoenzymes 82
    in non-prostatic disorders 139
  acini 29, 46, 54, 147, 148f
  adenocarcinoma 33, 54
  in baboon 163-164
  biochemical markers (hormonal control) 98-107
  biopsy 109-113, 115-122
  calculi (exogenous) 14
  carcinoma 137, 176
    clinical detection of 27f
    cribriform 54
    cytologic grades 41
    differentiation of 19
    estrogen (treatment) 121f
    etiology of 145
    follow-up of 38-43
    grading of 116-117
    incidence of 145
    incidental age of 146
    staging of 45
    summary of (classification, complications, diagnosis,
      grading, etiology, immunology, enzymology, metabolism,
      mortality, occurrence, pathology, structure) 178-179
    therapy of 166
    treatment of 92, 155
    ultrasonotomogram 76, 77f
  cells 90
    neoplastic 11
  concretions 14
  cysts 14
  cytology 38-43

development of 5
diseases 71, 115-122
  mass screening of 71-78
  physiopathology of 19
ducts 23
  dilated 16f
epithelium 18, 146-147, 151, 153, 154, 168
  cells 10f, 50, 149
  characterization 155
  growth of 151
  hyperplasia 19
  isolation of 147
  post-pubertal 148
explants 168-170
  morphology of 167
  system 168
  treatment of 166
fluid 9, 18, 19, 88
  markers in 87
gland 10, 45, 51-53, 60, 61, 98, 166
  changes of 42f
  epithelium 138
  hypertrophied 116, 119f
  mass 13f
  preoperative 116
  of the rhesus monkey 160
growth 61
histology 116-117
hormonal control 98-107
hormone treated 38
hyperplasia 26
hypertrophy (benign) 115
lobe zones 15
malignant 19
massage 28, 79
mouse 167
needle biopsies 92
neoplasm (summary of) 179
open biopsy of 110
organ culture 167-168
pathologically normal 91
physiopathology of 13-34
proper 7
secretions 9, 10, 17, 19
  cytologic diagnosis of 40
squamous metaplasia 20
stroma 93
tissue 90
  diseased 90
  markers in 88
utricle 5
weight 100
Prostatectomies 148
perineal 110
Prostatitis 20, 23, 72
acute 20t
Prostatoductal
  adenocarcinoma 25
  adenomatoid hyperplasia 30
  carcinoma 20t
  fibroadenoid hyperplasia 30
  hyperplasia 30
  papillary hyperplasia 30
  planophytic hyperplasia 30
  regenerative atypia 30

Prostatoglandular carcinoma   13, 23, 24, 28
   staging of   28
Protein hormone action   17
Proteolytic enzymes   9, 51
Pseudostratified epithelium   7
Puberty   6
Puboprostatic ligaments   6

Q
Quantitative physiopathology   13-34

R
Racial differences   13
Radial immunodiffusion   128
Radiation therapy   41, 166
Radioactivity   162
Radioimmunoassay (RIA)   80, 128, 131-138
Radiotherapy   38, 120-122
   following biopsy   121-122
   summary of   180
Rat   34
   prostate   98
      steroid mechanism of   99f
Rectal examination   6, 2f
Rectal palpation (of the prostate)   75
Rectovesical septum   6
5α-reductase   88, 89, 162
Refractory cells   170
Regan isoenzyme   82
Regional physiomorphology   13-34
Regressive stage   40f
Remission   65
Respiratory enzymes   15
Resting fluid   19
Retinoids   166f, 170
   acid   171
   comparative activity of   171
   effects of   166
   on prostatic explants   166
   toxic effects of   171
Ribosomes   167
Roentgenologic examinations   27
Roy method   129

S
Scanning (bone)   125
Sclerotic atrophy   19
Secondary male sex traits   17
Secondary (postatrophic hyperplasia)   30
Secretions (secretory)
   acid phosphatase   102, 106
   cells   45, 167
   epithelial cells   153
   isoenzymes   102
   of the prostate   6, 9, 10, 17
   prostatic acinus   53
Seminal
   coagulum   9
   fluid   19
   plasma (prostatic contribution)   19
   seminin   9
   vesicles   5, 6f, 15, 17
Serial biopsies
   in follow-up   120-121
   variations and significance   120-121

Serial prostatic biopsies   120-121
   significance of changes in   121-122
Sertoli cells   26
Serum
   acid phosphatase   29, 79
   amylase   83
   androgens   161
   glycoproteins   86
   prolactin   85
   ribonuclease activity (RNase)   83
   selection of   149
   steroids   84
   testosterone level   161
Sex hormone   84
Sodium   129
Solid phase immunofluorescence (SPIF)   80
Spermatozoa   19, 52
Spermidine   101
Spermine   17, 19, 101
Sperm metabolism   19
Sperm motility   14
Squamous metaplasia   153, 168
   benign   41
Steroid contents   90
   hormone receptors data   90
   metabolism   99f
   metabolizing enzymes   100
   oxido-reductase enzymes in prostatic tissue   88
Steroid-peptide hormone (lactogen)   19
Steroid receptors   59-65, 92
Stroma   7, 9, 11
   invasion   44-56
Supranuclear cytoplasm   7
Synthetic analogs   166

T
Tartrate   80, 103, 105, 106f
Testicles   52
Testicular steroidogenesis   59
Testis   23, 61
Testosterone   10, 11, 17, 33, 60, 61, 98, 102, 150, 154, 163
   administration   101
   binding globulin   84
   biosynthesis   102
   conversion of   162
   injections   106
   plasma   160
   production   160
Therapy   63
   effects   170
   radiation   41, 166
   summary of   180
Thymolphthalein   126
Toxic side effects   166
Tracheal organ cultures   170
Transducer tube   73f
Transitional zone   7
Transperineal needle biopsy   112
Transrectal aspiration biopsy   38, 41, 109
Transrectal needle biopsy   112
   accuracy of   112
   complications of   113
Transrectal ultra sonotomography   71
   chair type scanner   72
Transurethral biopsy   111

Transurethral prostatectomy 111
Travenol disposable biopsy
    needle 111f
Travenol needle 112
Treatment of prostatic cancer 92, 155
True prostate 7
Tubuloacinar gland 7
Tumor
    age of 63
    cells 154
    growth 33
    mass 65

U
Ultrasonotomography
    transrectal 71, 72
Ultrastructure 7-9
    differentiation 20
    summary of 176
Urethra 6, 7
    infection (ascending) 23
    primitive 5f
Urine (urinary)
    cholesterol levels 87
    hydroxyproline 87
    markers in 87
Urogenital diaphragm 6, 15

Urogenital sinus 5
Urorectal septum 5
Utricle 6

V
Vacuoles
    large empty 39
    melting of 39
Venous plexus 6
Vertebral plexus 6
Vesical orifice 13f
Vesical plexus 7
Vitamin A 154, 156, 166
    deficiency 171
    effects of 153

W
Wolffian ducts 5

Z
Zinc 9, 11, 17, 18, 31, 52, 53, 101, 102, 106
    albumin 19
    binders 93
    in the epithelium 101
    ions 19
    levels 91